SECOND EDITION

Physical Education for Lifelong Fitness

The Physical Best Teacher's Guide

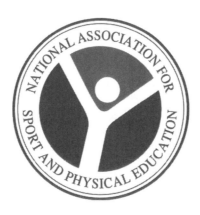

NATIONAL ASSOCIATION FOR SPORT AND PHYSICAL EDUCATION

HUMAN KINETICS

Library of Congress Cataloging-in-Publication Data

Physical Best (Program)
  Physical education for lifelong fitness : the Physical Best teacher's guide / National Association for Sport and Physical Education, an association of the American Alliance for Health, Physical Education, Recreation and Dance.-- 2nd ed.
    p. ; cm.
  Includes bibliographical references and index.
  ISBN 0-7360-4807-3 (soft cover)
  1. Physical education and training--Study and teaching--United States. 2. Physical fitness--Study and teaching--United States. I. Title: Physical Best teacher's guide. II. National Association for Sport and Physical Education. III. Title.
  GV365.P4992 2004

613.7--dc22   2004006081

ISBN-10: 0-7360-4807-3
ISBN-13: 978-0-7360-4807-1

Acquisitions Editor: Bonnie Pettifor; **Developmental Editor:** Jennifer Sekosky; **Assistant Editor:** Ragen E. Sanner; **Copyeditor:** Patrick W. Connolly; **Proofreader:** Kathy Bennett; **Indexer:** Bobbi Swanson; **Permission Manager:** Dalene Reeder; **Graphic Designer:** Robert Reuther; **Graphic Artist:** Angela K. Snyder; **Photo Manager:** Kareema McLendon; **Cover Designer:** Robert Reuther; **Photographer (cover):** Kelly J. Huff; **Photographer (interior):** Kelly J. Huff, unless otherwise noted; **Art Manager:** Kelly Hendren; **Illustrator:** Argosy; **Printer:** United Graphics

We would like to thank Stephen Decatur Middle School in Decatur, Illinois, for assistance in providing the location for the photo shoot for this book. We would also like to thank the faculty of Johns Hill Magnet School and Douglas MacArthur High School in Decatur, Illinois, for assistance in providing the models.

Printed in the United States of America   10   9   8

Human Kinetics
Web site: www.HumanKinetics.com

United States: Human Kinetics
P.O. Box 5076
Champaign, IL 61825-5076
800-747-4457
e-mail: humank@hkusa.com

Canada: Human Kinetics
475 Devonshire Road, Unit 100
Windsor, ON N8Y 2L5
800-465-7301 (in Canada only)
e-mail: info@hkcanada.com

Europe: Human Kinetics
107 Bradford Road
Stanningley
Leeds LS28 6AT, United Kingdom
+44 (0)113 255 5665
e-mail: hk@hkeurope.com

Australia: Human Kinetics
57A Price Avenue
Lower Mitcham, South Australia 5062
08 8372 0999
e-mail: info@hkaustralia.com

New Zealand: Human Kinetics
Division of Sports Distributors NZ Ltd.
P.O. Box 300 226 Albany
North Shore City, Auckland
0064 9 448 1207
e-mail: info@humankinetics.co.nz

CONTENTS

PREFACE

As a physical educator, you have an awesome opportunity to have a powerful and positive impact on hundreds of young people each year. By teaching them the skills and knowledge they need to live physically active lives, and by giving them the appreciation and confidence to do so, you are preparing them to avoid many major diseases and to live healthier, less stressful, and more productive lives than those who live sedentary lives.

And what greater preparation can a teacher give students than readiness for a healthy life? In 300 B.C., Herophiles (considered the "father of anatomy") stated, "When health is absent, wisdom cannot reveal itself, art cannot become manifest, strength cannot be exerted, wealth is useless, and reason is powerless." For all the technological advances that have taken place since 300 B.C., this one constant remains—without one's health, all else is useless.

The role physical education plays in preparing students for lifelong health is clear—there is a direct link between participation in regular physical activity and good health. Physical education in the schools affords the best opportunity to reach the majority of the population. However, for a physical education program to successfully prepare students for healthy lives, it must be far more than the "roll-out-the-ball" programs that are stereotyped in the media, remembered by some adults from their experiences with physical education, and sadly, still seen in a few schools today.

This book was written to provide a comprehensive guide to successfully incorporating health-related fitness and lifetime physical activity into physical education programs. It provides a conceptual framework based on recent research and includes a wealth of examples from experienced physical educators. It provides specific advice on integrating all aspects of a quality health-related fitness education program. For example, it will show how to teach fitness concepts through enjoyable physical activities and how to use fitness testing as an educational and motivational tool.

For veteran teachers, this book outlines strategies for placing a greater emphasis on health-related fitness while still maintaining all the excellent components of an existing program. For new teachers, this book details all aspects of creating an excellent fitness education program, illustrating these details with specific examples from master teachers.

In part I, we provide an introduction to health-related fitness, including an in-depth look at physical activity behavior and motivation. We also examine the basic training principles for fitness. Because nutrition is an essential component of body composition, part I concludes with an overview of nutrition that includes the foundations of a healthy diet, categories of nutrients, and dietary tools.

An overview of health-related physical fitness concepts is provided in part II. Specifically, we address aerobic fitness, muscular strength and endurance, flexibility, and body composition as they relate to the teaching of kindergarten through 12th-grade students. Because knowledge of fitness has been rapidly evolving and some disagreement still exists (even among exercise physiologists) about appropriate exercise protocols, we provide discussions of controversial topics along with recommendations for addressing these issues in your program.

In part III, we outline strategies for developing a health-related fitness education curriculum that will serve your needs whatever your unique situation. We also examine effective teaching methods that allow for the inclusion of all students, whether in the gymnasium, on the field, or in the classroom.

Assessment is an important component of effective teaching, and in part IV, we provide a detailed look at assessing health-related fitness. This includes using fitness testing appropriately, assessing knowledge of fitness concepts, assessing participation in physical activity, and assessing evidence of growth in the affective domain.

The book concludes with a glossary, appendixes that provide ready-to-use worksheets and masters, and a reference list that can be used as a reading resource guide.

How This Edition Was Developed

Good teaching is both an art and a science. We developed the first edition by combining extensive research on the science of physical activity for children and young adults with the vast knowledge and experience of master physical education teachers from across the country. This second edition builds on that information by focusing on updated research and current guidelines for youth physical activity and fitness. This edition provides enhanced practical tools and information throughout. Chapter reorganization was another focus for this edition. Information was therefore updated and streamlined while maintaining the high-quality publication and practical focus that made the first edition such a valuable resource for physical educators, teacher educators, and preservice students. Please see page vii for a listing of physical educators who were involved in the editing of this edition. The Physical Best Activity Guides, described further in chapter 1, have also been updated with many new activities and chapters at both levels.

Your Physical Best

As a physical educator, you have a very important job, one that can literally shape the future health of the nation. It is our hope that you will find this book both informative and inspirational in being the best physical educator you can be.

Scott Wikgren
Director
Health, Physical Education,
Recreation and Dance Division
Human Kinetics

Gayle Claman, MS
Professional Services Manager
NASPE/AAHPERD

ACKNOWLEDGMENTS

Many physical educators contributed their time and expertise to this project. That started with reviews of the first edition by many of the Physical Best Steering Committee members and Physical Best Instructors from around the country. We would like to thank Jennie Gilbert, who wrote the report for this book, synthesizing feedback from multiple sources and detailing a comprehensive list of recommendations for the second edition.

In addition to the overall guidance of the Physical Best Steering Committee, many researchers and educators generously shared their ideas and experiences, which are referenced throughout the book. Gayle Claman, Professional Services Manager for NASPE, who played a significant role in coordinating the revision, and the following individuals dedicated countless hours and content expertise as chapter editors for this edition:

Debra Ballinger
Rhode Island
Chapters 2, 12, 13, 14

Jennie Gilbert
Illinois
Chapters 3, 5, 6, 7

Melody Kyzer
North Carolina
Chapters 4, 8

Joan Morrison and Ginny Popiolek
Maryland
Chapter 11

Diane Tunnell
Washington
Chapters 1, 9, 10

The Physical Best program has been reviewed by the American Heart Association and is consistent with their science and recommendations for physical activity.

American Heart Association®

Learn and Live SM

Foundations of Health-Related Fitness and Physical Activity

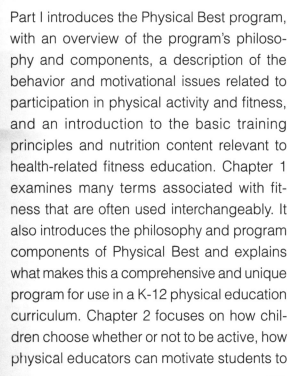

Part I introduces the Physical Best program, with an overview of the program's philosophy and components, a description of the behavior and motivational issues related to participation in physical activity and fitness, and an introduction to the basic training principles and nutrition content relevant to health-related fitness education. Chapter 1 examines many terms associated with fitness that are often used interchangeably. It also introduces the philosophy and program components of Physical Best and explains what makes this a comprehensive and unique program for use in a K-12 physical education curriculum. Chapter 2 focuses on how children choose whether or not to be active, how physical educators can motivate students to ☞

be active in an age-appropriate manner, and how that information connects to the Physical Best program. Information about putting the philosophical and behavioral concepts of the program to work is presented in chapters 3 and 4. This includes an overview of the basic training principles to follow when implement-

ing the aerobic fitness, muscular strength and endurance, and flexibility components of health-related fitness. It also includes the basics of nutrition that are important to know when implementing the body composition component of health-related fitness.

1

Introduction to Physical Best

The scientific and empirical evidence is indisputable—lifelong participation in physical activity has a significant positive impact on people's health and well-being. In turn, improved health and well-being have significant positive consequences for both individuals and society as a whole. Health-minded organizations such as the American Academy of Pediatrics, the American Medical Association, the American Heart Association, the Centers for Disease Control and Prevention, the President's Council on Physical Fitness and Sports, and the U.S. Department of Health and Human Services, as well as the allied health community, emphasize the importance of lifelong physical activity to good health. This is true for all people, including those with physical and mental challenges, the sedentary population, and even elite athletes, who need to understand the health benefits of lifelong physical activity so they do not become sedentary after completing their athletic careers.

Benefits of Lifelong Participation in Physical Activity

According to the CDC report, *Promoting Lifelong Physical Activity* (USDHHS 2000c), "the percentage of young people who are overweight has almost doubled in the past 20 years," "inactivity and poor diet cause at least 300,000 deaths a year in the United States," and "adults who are less active are at a greater risk of dying of heart disease and developing diabetes, colon cancer, and high blood pressure." While students must know the risks of a sedentary lifestyle, it is also crucial—and more meaningful—for them to know about the many benefits of getting enough physical activity and remaining active for life. It is especially important to emphasize the benefits they will see today. Regular physical activity can (adapted from USDHHS 1996)

- increase muscular strength and endurance,
- increase aerobic fitness,
- increase flexibility,
- help control weight,
- decrease stress, and
- increase feelings of well-being and self-esteem.

Beyond the many positive benefits associated with adequate physical activity, students need to know what diseases can be prevented by being active for life. According to the U.S. Department of Health and Human Services (2000b), regular physical activity can reduce or prevent health problems such as:

- premature death in general,
- death caused by heart disease,
- diabetes,
- high blood pressure,
- some types of cancer, and
- high cholesterol levels.

Not only does physical activity provide tremendous individual health benefits, a physically active population also benefits society as a whole by enabling people to be more productive. Physically active people have healthier attitudes, which allows the larger problems associated with work or home to be handled in a more positive, reflective manner. A happy, healthy person is a productive person.

In recent years, society as a whole has shown an unprecedented interest in health. Newspaper articles discussing health issues appear on a daily basis; more and more "healthy living" classes are being offered through community resources and are being advertised in the daily newspapers; television stations are devoting segments of time on their newscasts to promoting health issues in addition to airing "fitness classes" in their weekly lineup; technology has allowed quick access to the latest health reports or Internet sites to answer your questions on health; government documents such as *Promoting Better Health for Young People Through Physical Activity and Sports: A Report to the President* (USDHHS, USDOE 2000) are being published and disseminated on a regular basis; and professional organizations such as the American Alliance for Health, Physical Education, Recreation and Dance (AAHPERD) and the Centers for Disease Control and Prevention (CDC) are actively researching and publishing data on the importance of physical activity. The time seems right for physical education to significantly affect the physical activity and health of children and adolescents. This concept is not new; there is plenty of documentation from 20 to 25 years ago calling for physical education reform. The best opportunity to prepare the majority of children and adolescents to live physically active and healthy lives is through physical education in the schools. Schools have at least three advantages in the targeting of physical activity:

- Schools work with people at ages where change is most likely to occur.
- Schoolwide strategies should enable virtually all members of an age group to be targeted.
- A delivery structure is already in place, mainly through physical education, but also available through other curriculum areas and school practices (Vanden Auweele et al. 1999).

Physical educators should help community members understand these advantages so that physical education doesn't get the "short end of the stick" when it comes to financial decisions. They should garner support from others who understand this concept, such as physicians and allied community health practitioners, and let their community know that physical activity can help save society money and help prevent drug abuse, violence, and depression. In fact, if people think of a school as a child's "workplace," a health-related physical fitness education program that teaches children about a wide range of healthy habits is similar to a business instituting a workplace health promotion program. Children in school deserve the same assistance in being healthy as adults receive in the workplace, and school is a good time to reach them in order to prevent the development of bad habits.

What Is Physical Best?

In the early 1980s, AAHPERD recognized a need to create a program that would assist physical educators in helping youth understand the importance of a lifetime of activity. It wanted a program that would focus on educating *all* students, regardless of their abilities, from a health-related viewpoint. Thus, in 1987, AAHPERD developed Physical Best.

Physical Best is a comprehensive health-related fitness education program. It provides a series of activities and conceptual information that is critical for a quality physical education program. From a curriculum standpoint, Physical Best helps teach-

Practical

Health related

Youth fitness education

Standards based

Inclusive

Comprehensive

Age appropriate

Lifestyle emphasis

Behavioral approach

Enjoyable!

Self responsibility

Teaching energy balance

ers assist students in meeting the National Association for Sport and Physical Education (NASPE) national standards for physical education pertaining to health-related fitness. The goal of the program is to assist students in achieving their individual physical best.

To fully understand the mission of the Physical Best program, you must first be able to recognize the difference between a few frequently used terms. Though you often encounter the words *fitness*, *physical activity*, and *exercise*, many reports, particularly in the popular media, fail to distinguish among these terms.

- **Health-related fitness** is a measure of a person's ability to perform physical activities that require endurance, strength, or flexibility. It is achieved through a combination of regular exercise and inherent ability. The components of health-related physical fitness are aerobic fitness (cardiorespiratory endurance), muscular strength, muscular endurance, flexibility, and body composition as they relate specifically to health enhancement.

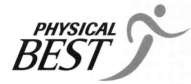

Physical Best's Mission

The mission of the Physical Best program is to foster healthier youth by providing quality resources and professional development for educators. The mission incorporates partnerships with like-minded programs and organizations. The program emphasizes teaching health-related fitness concepts and attitudes through activity, in a manner that is inclusive of all children, is enjoyable, and promotes a physically active lifestyle.

■ **Skill-related fitness** is often confused with "health-related" fitness components. Skill-related components often go hand in hand with certain physical activities and are necessary for one to accomplish or enhance a skill or task. The skill-related components include agility, coordination, reaction time, balance, speed, and power. An individual can still achieve and maintain a healthy lifestyle and lifelong participation in physical activity without possessing a high degree of skill-related components. Health-related and skill-related components are not mutually exclusive, but the Physical Best program primarily focuses on the health-related components of fitness (see figure 1.1).

Further, the USDHHS (1996) offers technical definitions of these terms:

■ **Physical activity** is strictly defined as any bodily movement produced by skeletal muscles that results in an expenditure of energy. It includes a broad range of occupational, leisure time, and routine daily activities—from manual labor to gardening, walking, or household chores. These activities can require light, moderate, or vigorous effort and can lead to improved health if they are practiced regularly.

■ **Exercise** is physical activity that is planned, structured, and repetitive bodily movement done to improve or maintain one or more of the components of health-related fitness.

Michael Pratt summarizes these terms succinctly: "In a nutshell, physical activity is something you do. Physical fitness is something you acquire—a characteristic or an attribute one can achieve by being physically active. Exercise is structured and tends to have fitness as its goal" (USDHHS 1999).

Definitions aside, since research shows that participants, in general, may view the word *exercise* in a negative light (CDC 1995), the Physical Best program has been developed to counter this view. The program focuses on the positive benefits of physical activity (not just exercising), offers a variety of enjoyable activities, and teaches the skills needed to be confident and reasonably successful in a wide range of movement forms.

Current Issues Within Physical Education

There are many excellent physical educators who have been using the Physical Best approach for years—in fact, these experts helped create the Physical Best resources and program. Unfortunately, however, many more physical educators in the United States have been doing more harm than good, because they have turned children off to physical activity as a lifestyle choice. In some districts, the physical education programs have not significantly changed from when the teachers and administrators were children. Physical education has been associated with fitness testing, comparing one person to another, touting the "no pain, no gain" philosophy, and using fitness activities for punishment and embarrassment. Many programs have not made a change from when the goal was preparing for war—when fitness status was critical to our military strength, and programs were focused on physical "training" rather than the "education" necessary to maintain personal health in a new and high-tech age.

Components of health-related fitness

Aerobic fitness
Muscular strength and endurance
Flexibility
Body composition

Components of skill-related fitness

Agility
Coordination
Reaction time
Balance
Speed
Power

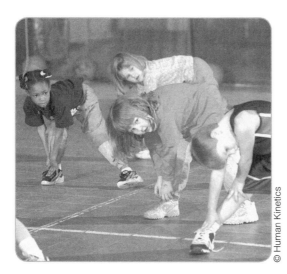
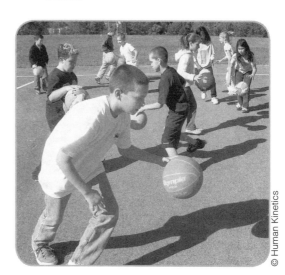

Figure 1.1 Elements of health-related fitness and skill-related fitness.

Because of this, physical education in the nation's schools has been getting shortchanged at a time when an increasing number of American adults view exercise as important to their health. It should come as no surprise, then, that the availability of physical education and the rate of physical activity among young people are declining:

- Almost half of young people ages 12 to 21 do not participate in vigorous physical activity on a regular basis (CDC 2000).

- Approximately one-fourth of high school students participate in moderate physical activity on four or more days a week (CDC 2000).

- Approximately 44 percent of high school students are not even enrolled in a physical education class; enrollment declines from 79 percent in the 9th grade to 37 percent in the 12th grade (Secretary of Health and Human Services and Secretary of Education 2000).

- In schools requiring physical education, approximately 30 to 40 percent of the teachers teaching it are not physical education teachers, with the largest percentage of non–physical education teachers at the high school level (CDC 2000).

- At the very best, physical education classes account for less than 1.75 hours of physical activity per week (ILSI 1997).

- In many states, requirements for physical education are gradually being reduced (NASPE 1993).

Thus, not surprisingly, children carry more body fat than ever and are more likely to display one or more risk factors for developing heart disease in the future. According to the 2001 *Youth Risk Behavior Surveillance Report of the Centers for Disease Control and Prevention*, only about one-third of students nationwide attend physical education class daily (see figure 1.2, a-d).

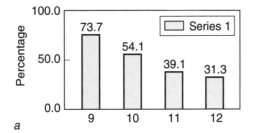

Percentage of students enrolled in a physical education class (by grade)

a

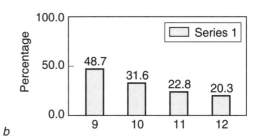

Percentage of students who attended a physical education class daily (by grade)

b

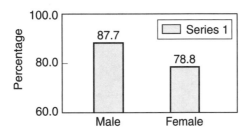

Percentage of students who exercise for 20 minutes or more (by gender)

c

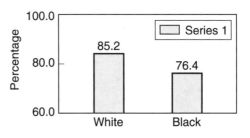

Percentage of students who exercise for 20 minutes or more (by race)

d

■ **Figure 1.2**   According to this research, (a) enrollment in physical education class declines significantly from 9th grade to 12th grade, as well as (b) percentage of students who attended daily. Exercise is also more common (c) for males than for females and (d) for white students than black students.

Centers for Disease Control and Prevention. Surveillance Summaries, June 28, 2002. MMWR 2002:51 (No. SS-4).

The key issue is, How should we be preparing children and adolescents for daily physical activity? According to the U.S. Department of Health and Human Services (USDHHS 1999), young people *must be taught* the skills, knowledge, attitudes, and behaviors that lead to regular participation in physical activity. As a physical educator, you know the value of physical education; you've seen it with your own eyes. Unfortunately, fitness is temporary, and being fit as a child does not guarantee fitness as an adult unless the person remains active. Teaching students *how to remain fit* is the essential component of physical education and a major focus of the Physical Best program.

What Makes Physical Best Unique?

The comprehensiveness of the Physical Best program is what makes it truly unique—combining the latest scientific research with practical experience and activities of physical educators from around the country. The following list highlights the program's many features that make it a valuable tool for physical educators and for students.

■ *Comprehensive conceptual framework*—Physical Best provides a framework for educators to teach conceptual information about physical fitness and nutrition within the activity setting. It provides students with information to help them understand and value the concepts of physical fitness and its relationship to a healthy lifestyle. It also provides information on assessment, goal setting, and motivational strategies. In addition, the Physical Best program offers ideas and suggestions for integrated curricula (across subject areas, in the three learning domains: cognitive, affective, and psychomotor) as well as parental and community involvement.

■ *Active participation*—The activities are designed so all students are involved and remain active a majority of the time. Teams are limited in size (two to four students per team) so each student has numerous practice opportunities. Multiple stations are set up so students do not have to wait long for a turn.

■ *Individualized activities*—Activities are designed so students can work at their own fitness or activity level. The program also provides avenues for students to excel by moving beyond the minimum. The activities may provide various levels to achieve, different practice times, variety in the number of trials, choices of task difficulty, and so forth. Individuals have the opportunity and freedom to choose activities that are interesting to them. They can also modify an activity to suit their needs, goals, and abilities without losing the health-related benefits of the activity. In short, Physical Best emphasizes enjoyment in participation and encourages students to strive for personal success in a positive learning atmosphere.

■ *Tools for lifelong activity*—Students will gain the knowledge, skills, and self-motivation to regularly engage in one or more physical activities as an ongoing lifestyle choice.

■ *Health-related physical activity* (fitness and skill development)—Students are provided with safe and sequential activities that will help maintain or improve the components of health-related physical fitness (aerobic fitness, muscular strength and endurance, flexibility, and body composition). Activities focus on personal improvement rather than attaining unrealistic standards. The program incorporates the latest fitness testing (*FITNESSGRAM*) and combines assessment and activities into a plan for individual improvement.

■ *Adherence to standards*—Physical Best was developed to help teachers meet national standards for physical education, health education, and dance education (see chapter 9). It also supports the "Healthy People 2010" objectives as well as the 1996 *Surgeon General's Report on Physical Activity and Health.*

In the past, some physical educators have said, "I teach football, basketball, volleyball, and softball." Physical Best teachers say, "I teach children and young adults the *how* and *why* of a physically active, healthy lifestyle." The "how" and "why" components are combined into a comprehensive K-12 health-related fitness education program, with resources and professional development training, to make the Physical Best program truly unique—and truly valuable for student and teacher success!

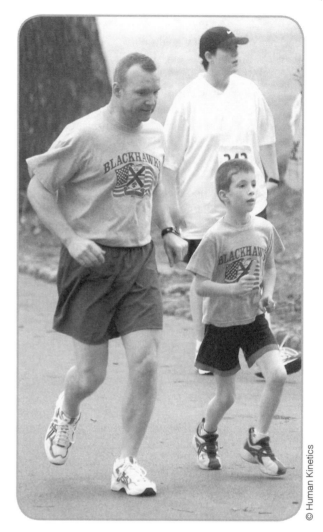

© Human Kinetics

Students must be taught the skills, knowledge, and attitudes that set the groundwork for daily physical activity.

Physical Best Companion Resources

With the foundation of knowledge in health-related fitness that this book provides, you will be ready to move on and motivate students with the *Physical Best Activity Guides* and to assess and self-assess with *FITNESSGRAM/ACTIVITYGRAM*. These are companion resources to the Physical Best Teacher's Guide and are described in the following section.

Physical Best Activity Guide: Elementary Level

This guide contains the information you need to help kindergarten through 5th-grade students gain the knowledge, skills, appreciation, and confidence to lead physically active, healthy lives. The easy-to-use instructional activities have been developed and used successfully by physical educators across the United States. You will find competitive and noncompetitive activities, demanding and less demanding activities, and activities that allow for maximum time on task. Above all, the activities are designed to be educational and fun! Packaged with the book is a CD-ROM containing reproducible charts, posters, and handouts that accompany the activities. New features for the second edition include many new activities in each chapter, a sample newsletter for each component of fitness, as well as the addition of a new chapter, titled "Special Events," containing activities that coincide with national holidays and health observances throughout the school year.

Physical Best Activity Guide: Middle and High School Levels

This guide is similar in scope to the elementary guide but is geared toward 6th- through 12th-grade students. The information is more in-depth and allows for a deeper and richer understanding of the importance of daily physical activity. The middle school and high school level guide contains an additional section focused on personal health and fitness planning. This provides students with an introduction to the skills needed to be physically active for life after they graduate from high school. Other features for the second edition include the addition of a CD-ROM containing printable materials that supplement the activities, many new activities in each chapter, and the addition of a new activity chapter, titled "Combined Component," that incorporates multiple health-related fitness components.

Related Resources

During a typical school year, many educators will use more than one program and a variety of teaching resources, overlapping different approaches on a day-to-day basis. With this in mind, it may be reassuring to know that although Physical Best is designed to be used independently for teaching health-related fitness, the following resources can also be used in conjunction with the Physical Best program. *FITNESSGRAM/ACTIVITYGRAM*, *Fitness for Life*, and the NASPE products listed below are suggested resources to complement Physical Best.

FITNESSGRAM/ACTIVITYGRAM

FITNESSGRAM/ACTIVITYGRAM (developed by the Cooper Institute) is a comprehensive health-related fitness and activity assessment as well as a computerized reporting system. All elements within *FITNESSGRAM/ACTIVITYGRAM* are designed to assist teachers in accomplishing the primary objective of youth fitness programs, which is to help students establish physical activity as a part of their daily lives.

FITNESSGRAM/ACTIVITYGRAM is based on a belief that extremely high levels of physical fitness, while admirable, are not necessary to accomplish objectives associated with good health and improved function. It is important for all children to have adequate levels of activity and fitness. *FITNESSGRAM/ACTIVITYGRAM* is designed to help all children and youth achieve a level of activity and fitness associated with good health, growth, and function.

FITNESSGRAM/ACTIVITYGRAM resources are published and available through Human Kinetics, as are the materials for the Brockport Physical Fitness Test, which is a health-related fitness assessment for students with disabilities.

Fitness For Life

Fitness for Life is a complete set of resources for teaching a lifetime fitness and wellness course at the secondary level. It is compatible with the Physical Best program in philosophy, with the goal of lifelong physical activity habits, and *Fitness for Life* is a program that has been shown by research to be effective in promoting physically active behavior after students finish school.

Fitness for Life and Physical Best complement one another effectively, because the *Physical Best Activity Guide: Middle and High School Levels* can be used both before and after a *Fitness for Life* course, as well as during the course to provide supplemental activities. Both programs are based on the HELP philosophy, which promotes health for everyone with a focus on lifetime activity of a personal nature. In fact, the two programs are so compatible that the Physical Best program offers teacher training for Fitness for Life course instructors.

NASPE Resources

NASPE publishes many useful resources that are available by calling 800-321-0789 or through the online AAHPERD store at www.aahperd.org. These resources include the following:

- *Moving Into the Future: Standards for Physical Education,* 2nd edition.
- *Beyond Activities: Learning Experiences to Support the National Physical Education Standards*
- *Appropriate Practices Documents (Elementary, Middle School, and High School)*
- Assessment series (titles relating to fitness and heart rate)
- *Physical Activity for Children: A Statement of Guidelines for Children Ages 5-12.*

Physical Best Certification

Physical Best provides accurate, up-to-date information and training to help today's physical educators create a conceptual and integrated format for health-related fitness education within their programs. NASPE/AAHPERD offers a certification program that allows physical education teachers to become Physical Best Health-Fitness Specialists. The Physical Best certification has been created specifically for the purpose of updating physical educators on the most effective strategies for helping their students gain the knowledge, skills, appreciation, and confidence needed to lead physically active, healthy lives. It focuses on application—how to teach fitness concepts through developmentally and age-appropriate activities and the *FITNESSGRAM* assessments.

To earn certification through NASPE/AAHPERD as a Physical Best Health-Fitness Specialist, you will need to do the following:

- Attend the one-day Physical Best Health Fitness Specialist Workshop.
- Read this book, *Physical Education for Lifelong Fitness: The Physical Best Teacher's Guide, FITNESSGRAM/ACTIVITYGRAM Test Administration Manual,* and one of the *Physical Best Activity Guides.*
- Using the required resources just mentioned, complete a take-home examination and submit it to NASPE/AAHPERD. Successful and timely completion and submission of the examination will result in certification.

For more information on certification as a health-fitness specialist, or to learn about becoming a Physical Best Health-Fitness Instructor (to train other teachers), call Physical Best at 800-213-7193.

Summary

Physical Best complements and supports existing physical education programs by teaching and applying health-related physical fitness concepts to promote lifelong physical activity. Physical Best excels at providing this component of a well-rounded physical education curriculum by

- basing its philosophy and materials on current research and expert, field-tested input,
- teaching the benefits of lifelong physical activity,
- offering national certification (the Physical Best Health-Fitness Specialist),
- focusing on the positive (such as student strengths and enjoyable activities), and
- individualizing instruction so that all students may benefit and succeed.

The Physical Best approach enhances the likelihood that students will pursue healthy, physically active lifestyles after they leave your program and into adulthood.

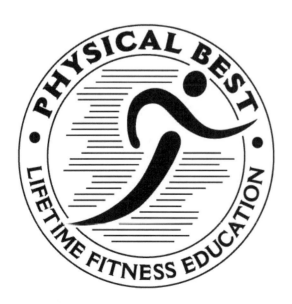

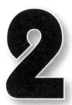

CHAPTER

2

Physical Activity Behavior and Motivation

❝ Even though most kids are oriented to the present, learning to choose and stay with activities that meet both long- and short-term interests and needs in some balance is one of the hallmarks of mature self-direction. ❞

—Don Hellison (2003, 32)

Adults have various reasons for being physically active or inactive, and, of course, children do too. In this chapter, we look at motivational factors affecting physical activity levels. Some of these factors are common to both children and adults, but others are not. Using the acronym MOTIVATIONAL PE, we offer strategies for helping students learn to set goals, and we show how this important tool can help teachers influence children and adolescents to increase and maintain a health-enhancing level of physical activity.

Why Children Choose to Be Active

Children seem to be the most active age group in our society; even so, physical activity declines in early adolescence—especially during the ages of 11 to 13 years (CDC 2001b; USDHHS 1999). Why are some children more physically active than others? Why do some children stay more physically active than their peers during adolescence? Is activity level always a choice? Or do factors outside of the child's control have more influence on activity levels? The answers to these questions lie within the habitual patterns of behavior of children and adolescents. The behaviors of individuals are influenced by both internally and externally controlled factors. If teachers are to become effective facilitators of behavioral change, they must first understand the factors that are influential in the formation of physical activity habits.

"A healthy lifestyle is achieved by eliminating unhealthy behaviors; this requires behavior modification" (Powers and Dodd 1997, 157). This sounds like a simple solution, but modifying behaviors, especially those behaviors that have become habitual, is one of the most difficult challenges people face. Research has found that physical activity levels in children can be influenced by both **internal** or "personal" (i.e., biological and psychological) and **external** or "environmental" (i.e., social and physical) **factors.** Understanding personal and environmental influences on children's behaviors can help teachers encourage students to develop more physically active lifestyles. Teachers must not only understand how these differences affect student activity behaviors, but, more important, they must be able to teach students about how these individual differences will affect their efforts toward becoming their physical best.

Internal Factors Influencing Physical Activity Behavior

Internal factors, sometimes called personal factors, can be grouped into biological and psychological categories.

Biological Factors

As shown in table 2.1, gender, age, and race have been studied as possible biological influences on physical activity behavior. Studies investigating gender and age factors have shown fairly clear-cut trends: Boys are generally more active than girls (CDC 2001b; CDC 2003), and a substantial decline in physical activity levels occurs between the ages of 6 and 18. Recent survey results report a steady decline throughout the high school years (CDC 2001b; CDC 2003; Grunbaum et al. 2002). A biological explanation would point out that this change parallels the onset of puberty and therefore may be caused by the changes in biological factors (hormonal, growth) as well as social and lifestyle factors. The International Life Sciences Institute (ILSI 1997) has also confirmed these trends.

Once individuals enter the workforce, rates of physical activity drop off further: In 1999, 64.7 percent of teens reportedly engaged in vigorous physical activity, but by age 21, these rates drop off to 40 percent for men and 30 percent for women (Jackson et al. 2004). Further variance is seen when examining differences in obesity levels among adolescents by race. Little research has focused on differences related to race or ethnicity, although recent studies cited by the CDC in *Profiles of the Nation's Health* (2001a) report that black females are more likely to be overweight (16.3 percent) than white females (9.0 percent) between the ages of 12 and 19. This trend reverses, however, in adolescent males, with white males 12 to 19 years old being more likely to be overweight (12 percent) than black males (10.4 percent). Although evidence shows a relationship between obesity and physical activity levels in adolescents and teens, not enough longitudinal study has been done to understand whether obese youth were always prone to inactivity or if they became inactive only after they became obese. What is known is that obese children prefer low-intensity activities and obese children with obese parents view endurance activities more negatively than do lean children with lean parents (Epstein et al. 1989). More research on the play habits of children with obese parents might help determine whether the obese child is inhibited from being active by the environment or parental interests, or if the child is truly predisposed to obesity from birth. We do know that genetics plays a role as well. In answer to the question, "Are physical activity habits inherited?" Jackson et al. (2004) wrote, "Only about 20 percent of the variation in a person's physical activity is explainable by genetic inheritance. . . . " Yet, children with obese parents are likely to become obese adults at a much higher rate than those with leaner parents.

Youth and Physical Activity Statistics

Although youth are a more active population, two particular factors make it less likely for adolescents to continue an active lifestyle into adulthood. First, physical activity levels in both males and females decline steadily during high school. Second, American high school students do not engage in regular physical activities that maintain or improve their aerobic fitness, strength, and flexibility (CDC 2003).

These trends are shown in the results of the 2001 national school-based Youth Risk Behavior Surveillance (YRBS) system:

- 9.5 percent of the students had no vigorous or moderate activity during the previous seven days (previous to the survey date).

- Only 32.2 percent of the high school students had daily physical education.

- 13.6 percent of the students were "at risk" for becoming overweight due to dietary and exercise behaviors, while 10.5 percent were already overweight.

- And in a possibly related area, male students (41.8 percent) were more likely than female students (35 percent) to have watched television for more than three hours per day. This gender difference was identified for white students and students in ninth grade.

CDC 2003: Summary of 2001 Youth Risk Behavior Survey Results. http://www.cdc.gov/nccdphp/dash/yrbs/2001/youth01online.htm

Research has also shown differences in strengthening exercise behavior among students (Grunbaum et al. 2002).

- 53.4 percent of students had done strengthening exercises (e.g., push-ups, sit-ups, and weightlifting) on more than three of the seven days preceding the survey.

- Male students (62.8 percent) were significantly more likely than female students (44.5 percent) to have participated in strengthening activities. This gender difference was identified for all the racial/ethnic and grade subpopulations.

- White students (54.8 percent) were significantly more likely than black students (47.9 percent) to have participated in strengthening activities.

- Students in grade 9 (58.7 percent) were more likely than students in grades 10, 11, and 12 (53.9 percent, 51.1 percent, and 48 percent, respectively) to have participated in strengthening activities.

Grunbaum, J., Kann, L., Kinchen, S., Williams, B., Ross, J., Lowry, R., & Kolbe, L. (2002) Youth Risk Behavior Surveillance—United States, 2001. June 28, 2002/51 (SS04); 1-64 (retrieved Nov. 30, 2003:http://www.cdc.gov/mmwr/preview/mmwrhtml/ss5104a1.htm.

TABLE 2.1 Biological Factors and Children's Physical Activity

	Percentage of students who did not participate*	Interpretation
Gender	Males – 24.3	Females are less active than males.
	Females – 37.9	
Race	White – 29.3	Nonwhite high school students are less active than white high school students.
	Black – 36.4	
	Hispanic – 35.4	
	Other – 33.3	
Age	9th graders – 24.3	Activity level declines with age and grade throughout high school.
	10th graders – 29.6	
	11th graders – 34.4	
	12th graders – 38.9	
Overall	31.2	Altogether too many students are not participating in the minimum recommended amount of physical activity.

*Percentage of students that did not participate in at least 20 minutes of vigorous physical activity on three or more of the past seven days and did not do at least 30 minutes of moderate physical activity on five or more of the past seven days.

Center for Disease Control (2003) Summary of 2001 Youth Risk Behavior Survey Results, www.cdc.gov/nccdphp/dash/yrbs/2001/summary_results/usa.htm (August 4, 2003) retrieved November 30, 2003.

Psychological Factors

Psychological factors also affect physical activity behaviors. Researchers have studied the relationship of many cognitive and psychological variables to physical activity participation in children and adolescents. For adults, knowledge about the benefits of physical activity has been recognized as a powerful influence on exercise behaviors. But, knowing that it's healthy to be physically active does not always influence the physical activity levels of adults, and for children, this knowledge is even less of an influence. Children place more importance on the value of an activity and on whether or not they feel competent and satisfied during the activity. Table 2.2 summarizes some of the research in this area.

Teachers are usually adept at teaching about the benefits of activity and about the skills used in many activities. But to actually influence changes in children, teachers need to know how to motivate students to put forth effort in all of their activities, and how to help students achieve satisfaction or feel successful following that effort. Recent research on children in sport and exercise psychology provides the physical education teacher with a much better understanding

of how children and adolescents are motivated. This understanding can help teachers develop classroom strategies that may help to reverse the trend toward physical inactivity in adolescents.

For students to persist in physical activities as they grow, the research clearly demonstrates that children and adolescents must feel generally competent in physical activities and must feel confident in their ability to achieve a specific goal (self-efficacy). They need to feel that they have a chance to succeed and that they have some control over the outcomes of their efforts (Harter 1999).

To feel competent, younger children must be guided through skill acquisition and provided with many opportunities to practice at their own level, without emphasis on competition. Young children have a tendency to believe that effort controls outcome. Teachers can use this information by rewarding the efforts or attempts in younger children. However, as children learn and develop, they understand that effort does not always lead to success, and the reward system must be changed to award outcomes or achievement of goals. This developmental change is the reason that

TABLE 2.2   Psychological Factors and Children's Physical Activity

Variable	Relationship to motivation for physical activity
Self-efficacy	Belief that they can succeed will lead to attempts to participate in specific activities.
Self-control (internal control)	Belief that they have control over the outcome leads to persistence in activity.
Intrinsic motivation	Individuals differ on levels of curiosity and preference for challenge or mastery of goals.
Value of activity	Students who perceive an activity to be important are more motivated to pursue it.
Global self-esteem and global self-worth	Related to motivation, but only in trying new activities—persistence depends on success or achievement and value of activity.
Satisfaction	Satisfaction is an outcome of success experiences in valued activities.

older children need to be given more choices of activities—so that they can find activities in which they can succeed. Persistence will stop as children learn that effort doesn't always lead to success.

To develop "physical activity self-efficacy," children must be provided with a variety of activities from which they can choose. This will enhance the chances of finding activities matched to personal factors such as strength, height, endurance, or other biological factors. Self-control is also enhanced when teachers provide students with choices of activities, including individual or team activities, and various levels of competitive or noncompetitive activities. Teachers should create a psychologically safe classroom where children and adolescents can be successful, are given regular helpful feedback to increase their performance of physical skills, and have choices of activities used to accomplish fitness goals. This will create the psychological climate for students to persist in activities both in the physical education classroom and during after-school hours.

External Factors Influencing Physical Activity Behavior

Naturally, the world a child lives in influences his or her physical activity level and choices. Social and physical surroundings (environmental factors) must therefore also be taken into consideration.

Social Factors

Parents and siblings greatly influence a child's choices in life, but an adolescent is more likely to seek peer approval and support. "Families can also transmit a home culture that promotes or hinders physical activity" (Jackson et al. 2004). Parents must serve as role models—the ILSI survey revealed that very physically active parents have very physically active children. Two-thirds of parents who reported that they felt their children were not active enough blamed lack of interest and competition from TV, video games, and computers (ILSI 1997). Other adults, including teachers, coaches, and physicians, also influence a child's choices. All of these influences affect physical activity behavior.

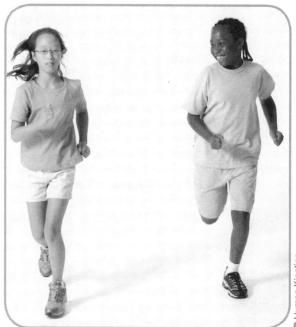

© Human Kinetics

Social interaction can be motivating to students. You should help students learn that fitness can be social as well as good for their physical health.

The various people in a child's life can influence physical activity behavior in many ways:

- Peers—Naturally, if a child's friends are out biking or in-line skating, the child is more likely to be doing the same. By the same token, if a child's friends are more interested in television or video games, these will probably be the child's interests too. The older the child, the more likely it is that peers will significantly influence physical activity behavior.

- Parents and siblings—As with peers, if a child's family is out hiking or playing basketball regularly, the child is more likely to feel competent in these areas. The child is more likely to be physically active if the family is active and the child is exposed early to activity. Conversely, if the child's family is sedentary and avoids physical activity, the child is less likely to be motivated to be physically active. Parents also influence a child's physical activity level by being able or unable to finance community-based physical activities. As any parent knows, chauffeuring for these activities alone can require a tremendous commitment of time and energy.

- Teachers—Most people can think of at least one teacher who greatly influenced life choices they have made in one area or another. In relation to physical activity behavior, Sallis (1994) writes, "It is likely that physical educators who are active and enthusiastic about teaching will be more successful in stimulating their students' enjoyment of physical activity." Coaches usually have the same degree of influence.

- Physicians—Although knowledge of the need for physical activity is definitely not a motivator, apparently even adolescents have great respect for the authority of their physicians and will follow their doctor's advice regarding physical activity (Sallis 1994). Doctors have even written prescriptions for physical activity, and this seems to be a powerful motivator for most kids. In addition, physicians, like physical educators, should be physically active and fit themselves, serving as role models in the community.

Environmental Factors

Many different environmental factors may promote or discourage physical activity. This is an especially important area to consider because most physical activity must take place outside of physical education class and school itself. (Table 2.3 summarizes the research into the influences in this area.) The neighborhood a child lives in can greatly influence physical activity behavior. For example, in many urban environments, parents are reluctant or unwilling to allow their children to play outdoors because of safety concerns. Indoor activities, such as watching television, reading, or playing computer games, keep children entertained and occupied but are sedentary in nature, rather than active. In a rural area, facilities and friends may be several miles away, so transportation can be a barrier to participating in physical activities that require more than one individual. In contrast, the child living in a suburban neighborhood is likely to have greater freedom as well as more attractive and conveniently located physical activity facilities, such as parks, gymnasiums, and swimming pools. Temperatures that are too hot in summer or too cold in winter can also influence activity levels in various parts of the country. Teachers who recognize the limitations associated with such environmental factors often alter their curricular offerings to provide knowledge and experience in a variety of activities that correspond with the resources of their students.

TABLE 2.3   Physical Environment Factors and Children's Physical Activity

Variable	Relation to physical activity
Day of week	Probably more active on weekends
Season	Most active in summer, least active in winter
Setting	More active outdoors
Organized programs	More active when involved in organized programs.
Television and video games	Probably less active when more time is spent watching television or playing video games

Reprinted, by permission, from R. Pate and R. Hohn, 1994, *Health and fitness through physical education* (Champaign, IL: Human Kinetics), 36.

Overcoming Barriers to Physical Activity for Children With Disabilities

"Easier said than done" could be the motto for many families who try to provide expanded opportunities to participate in physical activity to their children with disabilities. Although the Individuals with Disabilities Act (see chapter 11) mandates accessibility to public buildings and accessible transportation for all, it still takes a lot of resolve for families to facilitate getting these children into the arena of physical activity. Here are some examples:

- James, a teenager with cerebral palsy, wanted to prepare for a swim meet, and this required him to travel alone by bus to the pool. His mother felt comfortable with this because James is able to communicate clearly, but the bus driver refused to help James position his heavy wheelchair to use the lift. James' mother had to fight to get the bus company to change its "policy," forcing the bus driver to give James the assistance he needed.

- Sara's father wanted her to play soccer, but the city league was not receptive to including a child with a disability. Sara's father organized his own special team, which thrived for many years because of this parent's dedication.

Contributed by Aleita Hass-Holcombe, Corvallis (Oregon) School District.

Why Physical Activity Decreases With Age

Young children naturally want to move. What happens, then, to this natural inclination to be physically active as children grow into early adolescence?

Developmental changes occur over a life span. The decrease in physical activity seen from childhood to adolescence, and on into adulthood, is likely influenced by a combination of factors that may be developmental in nature. Cognitive, social, and psychological development leads to changes in interests and motivational factors. Physical development leads to changes in functions and abilities. Environmental factors are interspersed within each of these areas. Changing the downward trend in activity levels with age involves examining all factors influencing activity levels, and then tailoring the curriculum and environment to meet these changing needs. While this may seem like an impossible task, expert teachers and researchers have responded to the challenge and have identified strategies incorporated into Physical Best and *FITNESSGRAM/ACTIVITYGRAM* that can be useful in reversing trends.

When asked why they don't exercise more, the reasons teens give for low activity levels are much like those adults give: lack of time [or so they perceive] and interest (Sallis 1994). Teens also say, "I don't care for all the competition" and "It's (physical activity is) not fun anymore." Virgilio (1997) offers the following explanation:

As children reach about 10 years of age, they discover various interests and hobbies that may pull them away from physical activity. Moreover, they resist being labeled a 'child,' and so they may stop playing active childhood games. Too often, parents and teachers convey the message that physical activity must have a purpose, such as joining a team to compete or taking karate lessons to become a black belt. Children who are not very athletic may become inactive if they feel incompetent and unsupported. We must stop treating 10-year-olds as miniature adult athletes and start letting them develop as children who need to move freely and express their physical selves (3).

Teens may also have suffered through years of boring or developmentally inappropriate physical education programs, and once given the choice, they avoid physical activity as much as possible. Moreover, teens may lack the knowledge they need to be physically active in safe and interesting ways. In other words, they may not know how to set up a personal physical activity program that meets their individual needs, how to set goals, how to monitor their own progress, or how to reward themselves appropriately and effectively. In addition, teens may not have learned the basic physical skills that lead to physical activity success and confidence.

Students need to understand that although mastering physical skills obviously helps them achieve more success in activities and therefore helps them to be more confident, people do not need to be highly skilled to enjoy the benefits of physical activity. For example, the person finishing last in a 5K run is still gaining health benefits and enjoyment from participating. Likewise, players on the company basketball team might not be able to even touch the rim, but they still benefit from and enjoy the activity. Not everyone can or needs to perform at an elite level; when it comes to a person's health and well-being, it is better to have played and lost than not to have played at all. In addition, because self-confidence is so important to participation in physical activity, perceived competence may be even more important than actual competence. Moreover, all students can learn and improve. So encourage all students, regardless of their levels of natural ability, to participate in physical activities. This can be done by individualizing instruction (see chapter 11). Also keep in mind that students tend to gravitate toward partners of their own skill levels. In an appropriate setting in which they can succeed, students learn that enjoyment and reward lie in the participation itself.

Therefore, the question to ask when assessing the value of a physical education program is, "Does the particular program contribute to increased physical activity when a child reaches adulthood?" (Pate 1995). Pate goes on to assert that "The three primary self-management skills are self-monitoring of behavior, self-evaluation through goal setting, and self-reinforcement. . . . This type of training is especially critical for high school students who will soon leave structured physical education programs" (p. 131). In general, then, physical education programs must focus on teaching students to apply what they're learning to real-life community settings and activities available to adults, while helping students develop the basic skills they need for their activities of choice. Note that focusing on preparing students for the rest of their lives usually coincides with a school's overall mission, because learning self-responsibility is an invaluable life skill.

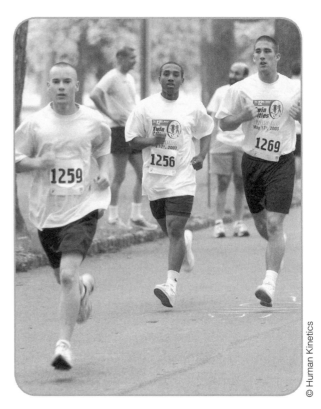

Involvement with peers in community events can be a powerful motivator for getting young people to be active.

Motivating Students to Be Active for Life

How can teachers prevent their students' levels of physical activity from decreasing as the students get older?

For more than 30 years, psychologists have examined extrinsic and intrinsic motivation as critical determinants influencing behavioral change. Extrinsic motivation, requiring the use of rewards, tokens, or social reinforcers, is effective. However, reliance on extrinsic motivation leads to dependence on others for behaviors to become habitual. Intrinsic motivation comes from within—from the child's own desire to succeed, to grow, and to be independent. Teachers have spent countless hours debating which type is best to effect learning and behavioral change. The question is best answered by recognizing that the job of teachers is to foster independence and to empower their students—and intrinsic motivation is increased as self-confidence and self-esteem are enhanced, and as students assume responsibility for their own behaviors (Hellison 2003).

Extrinsic Motivation

Extrinsic motivation occurs when a desired object or socially enhancing consequence is presented to increase the likelihood that a behavior will be repeated. Extrinsic motivational tools include the use of rewards or tokens and the use of public praise and recognition by teachers or others. Extrinsic motivators work well with younger children and initially can enhance the value of an activity to adolescents. Stickers (at the elementary level) and T-shirts (at the middle and high school levels) are often effective in rewarding effort or conveying the sense of belonging to the group. Although extrinsic rewards motivate children to achieve activity goals to some extent, they tend to lose their effectiveness over time. When extrinsic rewards are used too often, children come to view the rewards as the reason to participate in activities they might have chosen to do on their own anyway (Raffini 1993). When used appropriately, extrinsic rewards must be selected carefully—they must be valued by the recipient and directly related to the activity.

Active Lifestyle Program

For teachers who wish to incorporate extrinsic rewards as part of student motivation, AAHPERD has developed partnerships with national

---

Physical Best Summer Shape-Up Challenge

Each summer Nancy Raso-Eklund runs a Summer Shape-Up Challenge for her students in Green River, Wyoming. Examples from one summer's program are shared on pages 22 – 23. This program encourages students to take the initiative to participate in summer activities like basketball or swimming.

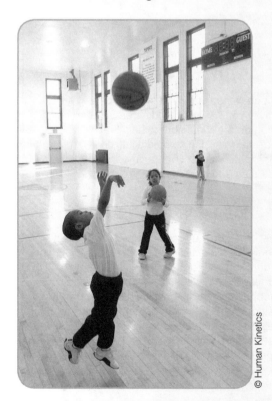

© Human Kinetics

Dear Students and Parents,

Welcome to the Physical Best Summer Shape-Up Challenge.

This program is designed as an incentive to keep your bodies in good physical condition during the summer. I hope you all accept the challenge to stay fit. Set your goals high! Be responsible for a healthy, active lifestyle. This is how it works:

Accept at least 3 of the 6 challenges. You can do more if you'd like. Each time you participate, jot the information down on the fitness log the best that you can. Return your Physical Best Summer Shape-Up Challenge contract and log sheet when school starts and you will receive your certificate.

Let's work together to establish a lifetime of fitness and health. Good luck, have fun, and be your physical best!

Healthfully yours,
Nancy Raso-Eklund
PE Specialist

Physical Best
Summer Shape-Up Challenge

In order to earn the Physical Best Summer Shape-Up Challenge certificate, I will complete at least 3 of the 6 Summer Shape-Up Challenges.

_____   _____
Student Signature   Parent Signature

Summer Shape-Up Challenge

1. The Vacation Run

Select a relative or friend you'd like to visit who lives in a nearby town. Determine the distance to their house. Draw a map to plot the course of your trip. As you run or walk this summer, log and chart your mileage until you've reached your destination.

2. Parents Like to Play, Too

To complete this challenge, you must participate with one or both parents or guardians at least 1 day per week for 10 weeks. Your activity session should be at least 20 minutes long.

3. Wheels in Motion

Using your bike, scooter, roller skates, in-line skates or skateboard, challenge yourself to log 20 miles between June 5 and August 24. Record the date and distance.

4. Try Something New

The challenge is for you to participate in an activity you have not tried before. Find a friend or family member to help teach you necessary skills to complete this challenge. Participate at least 5 more times and log the dates and time spent.

5. The Green River Float Trip

The challenge is to log two miles of the Green River by swimming laps in the pool. Each time you go swimming, do some lap swimming. One lap = 2 lengths; 30 laps or 60 lengths = 1 mile.

6. Keep the Log Rolling

Keep a log of your favorite activities. Challenge yourself to three activities a week at 20 minutes in duration. Record date and time spent. Suggested activities: ballet, basketball, baseball or teeball, bowling, golf, gymnastics, hiking, jogging, hula hoop, jump rope, karate, playing catch, soccer, tennis, dance class, waterskiing, wrestling.

Physical Best Summer Shape-Up Challenge

A quality physical fitness education program prepares students to take self-responsibility for engaging in healthful physical activities. It also encourages students to choose activities they enjoy. The Summer Shape-Up Challenge provides students the opportunity to take responsibility and make choices regarding their physical activity levels.

**Activity Log
for Summer Shape-Up Challenge**

Name _____

Date	Activity	Time/Distance	Challenge
6/1	Walk	30 min.	1
6/1	Bike ride	2 miles	3
6/3	Bike ride	3 miles	3
6/4	Jump rope	30 min.	2
6/5	Bike ride	3 miles	3
6/6	Basketball practice	1 hour	6
6/7	Bike ride	3 miles	3
6/8	Basketball game	3 hours	6
6/9	Bike ride	3 miles	3
6/12	Bike ride	3 miles	3
6/13	Walking	1 hour	2
6/15	Hoop jump	30 min.	4
6/16	Bike ride	3 miles	3

organizations to provide ways to recognize student achievement. One such program—the Active Lifestyle program—provides recognition for exhibiting an active lifestyle.

The Active Lifestyle program is part of the President's Challenge, which is a program of the President's Council on Physical Fitness and Sports (PCPFS). The Active Lifestyle program was created to recognize the importance of regular physical activity. This program offers the Presidential Active Lifestyle Award (PALA) to recognize youth and adults who participate regularly in physical activity.

Presidential Active Lifestyle Award (PALA) The **PALA** is an embroidered blue presidential emblem accompanied by a certificate signed by the president of the United States. Students who are active for 60 minutes per day, five days a week, for six weeks are eligible to receive this award. The award can also be earned by keeping track of steps per day using a pedometer. Boys who take at least 13,000 steps per day and girls who take at least 11,000 steps per day are also meeting the daily requirement. Once the certificate has been earned, students can continue the program, and they are recognized by earning a series of stickers to place on the certificate indicating the number of times they have won the award. Adults can also earn the PALA (on their own or with children) by participating in physical activity at least 30 minutes per day (or 10,000 steps) for five days a week, over a six-week period. By earning this award,

adults enhance their own health, serve as role models, and encourage children and youth to live actively.

Active Lifestyle Model School Based on the results of the Active Lifestyle program and the objectives of Healthy People 2010, the PCPFS also offers schools the opportunity to become an Active Lifestyle model school. A model school is one where 35 percent or more of its school enrollment has earned the Presidential Active Lifestyle Award (PALA) two or more times during a school year. More information can be found by accessing the President's Challenge Web site at www.presidentschallenge.org.

FITNESSGRAM/ACTIVITYGRAM

The *FITNESSGRAM/ACTIVITYGRAM* program gives teachers the tools and the opportunity to create individualized and personalized student awards by printing certificates from the reports section of the Teacher's Edition. Basing the award on student achievement of important goals reinforces the importance of persistence and effort toward goals. It also allows each child to be recognized for progress. This system is especially beneficial for teachers working with students with disabilities because the certificates can be made to recognize behavioral changes, fitness

Reprinted by permission of The President's Challenge.

achievement, progress toward personal goals, skill accomplishment, or important social objectives such as teamwork or respect for others.

Intrinsic Motivation

When children choose to participate on their own, and they experience feelings of competence, then unexpected extrinsic rewards may help reinforce those feelings. This in turn enhances their intrinsic motivation to participate in physical activity. **Intrinsic motivation** is an individual's internal desire to perform a particular task (Ormrod 1995). A primary example is participating in an activity simply because a person enjoys it. Unlike extrinsic rewards, intrinsic motivators encourage long-term behavior changes fairly effectively. Intrinsically motivated children tend to view physical activity as a process, and this continual process can lead to feelings of personal satisfaction and competence. Master teachers have learned to initially reward physical activity behavior extrinsically (e.g., with stickers, ribbons, gift certificates) and to gradually substitute social reinforcers until the students understand the importance of physical activity. As children mature toward adolescence, learning about the personal rewards of becoming physically fit and active can help the student become more intrinsically motivated. This transition is best accomplished when goals and awards are focused on the process, such as being rewarded for being active,

rather than the product, such as achieving a fast time in the mile run (see also chapter 13). Keep in mind, however, that it is actually choice plus physical skill that creates a physically active person, regardless of extrinsic rewards.

In a summary of current motivational research, experts on motivation argue that an understanding of human drive is much more complex than a two-dimensional (extrinsic versus intrinsic) model. For example, Vallerand's (2001) model not only includes a third construct to explain human motives, that of amotivation, but also argues that motivation is multidimensional and hierarchical in nature. His work points out that to understand exercise (or activity) motivation, you need to know about the motives of individuals in other life contexts, such as education, leisure, and interpersonal relationships, as well as their perceptions of competence, autonomy, and relatedness (Vallerand 2001, 309).

Prochaska, Norcross, and DiClemete (1994) and others (Cardinal 2000; Carron, Hausenblas, and Estabrooks 2003) have examined motivation to change as it relates to stages of readiness and awareness (figure 2.1a) and have demonstrated that understanding the **stages of change** (SOC) can help adults be more successful in changing behaviors, such as achieving their exercise goals (figure 2.1b). The SOC or transtheoretical model may be useful for middle and high school level teachers working with more mature students; however, more

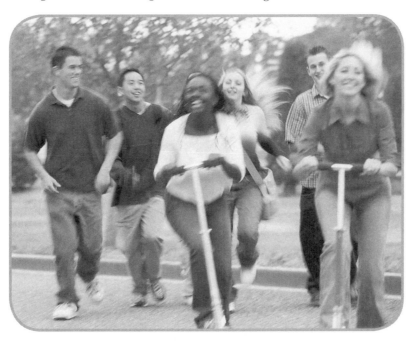

Having fun is the primary intrinsic reason students give for choosing to be physically active on their own.
DititalVision

Behaviors of Individuals at Each Stage of Change

Precontemplation

- Resist change
- Believe change is not needed
- Not really thinking about or intending to change behaviors

Contemplation

- Think about changing within six months; may be indecisive about change
- Gather information about pros and cons of change (benefits, barriers)

Preparation

- Have achieved desire to change, but don't know how
- Believe benefits outweigh cons
- Lack efficacy or confidence to maintain desired behaviors

Action

- Have a plan of action; have goals
- Are committed to new behavior
- Are at risk for relapse—easily discouraged
- Find confidence slowly increasing

Maintenance

- Have maintained behavior for six months
- Enjoy benefits of change—less likely to relapse
- Have increased confidence in new behavior
- Find temptations to relapse fewer and less enticing

a

What Teachers Can Do to Help Students Move Through the Stages

From precontemplation to contemplation

- Teach about benefits of healthy lifestyle
- Challenge unhealthy behaviors—show how they affect self and others
- Encourage students to self-assess behaviors and fitness (awareness enhances contemplation)
- Provide assessments

From contemplation to action

- Help students set goals
- Reward students for reaching goals

- Praise and recognize achievement of goals or change
- Encourage students when they are at risk for relapse
- Provide continued assessments

From action to maintenance

- Recognize sustained change
- Help to reassess; provide opportunities for assessment
- Provide options or choices of activities to enhance enjoyment

b

■ **Figure 2.1** The stages of change or transtheoretical model provides *(a)* typical behaviors of individuals at each stage and *(b)* recommendations for teachers helping students through the stages of change.

Adapted from J.O. Prochaska, J.C. Norcross, and C.C. DiClemente, 1994, *Changing for good: The revolutionary program that explains the six stages of change and teaches you how to free yourself from bad habits* (New York, NY: William Morrow.

research is needed on adolescent students to determine if the adult model applies to exercise behavior modification in teens.

Teachers must understand that **motivational factors** for children differ from those for adults. Harter (1999) and Harter, Waters, and Whitesell (1998) found that children's self-worth varied and was influenced greatly by their perceptions of the people near them (parents, teachers, students) and by their desire to please those people, or be accepted by them. Therefore, since the context or environment is always changing, the motivational climate will also change, depending on the time, place, or people around the child. As an example, a child might be motivated to participate in physical education class if she has a desire to please the teacher, but she may just as easily be amotivated to participate if her friends don't value physical activity. Simply put, teachers must know the needs of their students to be able to influence their behaviors, AND teachers must have a repertoire of motivational strategies to use with their students.

Creating Physical Education Programs That Motivate

The major intrinsic motivator for children is, of course, fun. Indeed, fun is the primary intrinsic reason students give for participating in physical activity. Enjoyable, intrinsically motivating activities have four characteristics: create challenge, provoke curiosity, provide control (chances for self-responsibility), and promote creativity (Raffini 1993). The activities you use should embody these characteristics. Another intrinsic motivator is the natural urge to learn. If the child learns from the class activity, he or she is more likely to be motivated to continue being physically active. Finally, don't forget skill teaching: It's not enjoyable to participate in an activity for which the student lacks the basic skills.

No matter your approach, however, students must perceive your physical education program in the right light to reach the goal of physical activity for life. Enhancing the intrinsic pleasures of physical activity is the strength of Physical Best.

Debating About Rewards and Awards

Whether or not to offer extrinsic rewards for physical activity participation or fitness test scores is a controversial topic. On the one hand, it is important to encourage students to do their best on tests and be more active overall. On the other hand, the research shows that intrinsic motivation is longer lasting. The following are some guidelines for using rewards and awards judiciously.

- Reward the performance, not the outcome.
- Reward the students more for their effort than for their actual success.
- Reward little things on the way toward reaching larger goals.
- Reward the learning and performance of emotional and social skills as well as health-related fitness endeavors.
- Reward frequently when youngsters are first learning to apply new concepts.
- Once physical activity and health-related fitness habits are well formed, you only need to reinforce them occasionally. In other words, you can use extrinsic rewards to change students' physical activity habits, then slowly "wean" them onto intrinsic appreciation of physical activity.
- Use rewards that have meaning to the recipients. Ask students what they might find reinforcing. Be age appropriate in your choices.
- Don't forget that rewards can be words of praise or chances to choose from a wider variety of activities, as well as more tangible items, such as stickers and T-shirts.

Reprinted, by permission, from R. Martens, 1997, *Successful coaching* (Champaign, IL: Human Kinetics) 36-38.

What Is "Fun"?

Throughout this book, we emphasize the importance of making physical activity "fun." You should note that fun is not a goal or objective of a quality physical education program. Rather, fun is a means to achieving the ultimate goal of having students adopt physically active, healthy lifestyles.

People are more likely to participate in activities they enjoy, and there is no reason why being physically active can't be enjoyable. Of course, what is fun for one person may not be fun for others. Some people like competition (e.g., playing team sports), some like cooperative social activities (e.g., participating in an aerobics class), while others prefer individual activities (e.g., running on a treadmill at home while watching television). The key is making physical education purposeful and enjoyable in order to achieve the goal of graduating students who will be physically active, healthy, and productive adults.

Dressed for Success

Remember the ugly old gym uniforms that used to be required? Talk about motivating students to skip physical education! Remember that students, especially at the middle school and high school levels, are very concerned about how they look. Consider allowing students to choose their own physical education clothes—within specific guidelines (e.g., appropriate for moving freely, purposeful, functional, appropriately fitting, safe, clean, and no offensive language or artwork)—or design a contemporary outfit that kids will like. Being able to dress in sharp workout clothes instead of really ugly uniforms can make a difference in the attitude of your students. You might work with a local sporting goods retailer to come up with a design that can be offered for a very reasonable price. Do keep in mind the attitude of students—at some schools, kids fight over trendy clothes. Work with your administrators and students to find solutions.

We cannot stress enough that too often in attempting to get children fit, physical educators turn them off to physical activity. Boring laps, the "no pain, no gain" philosophy, and comparisons to others have too often been deterrents to physical activity. The *Physical Best Activity Guides* help teachers explore enjoyable and interesting activities that promote a conceptual knowledge of fitness in a positive, fun, and developmentally appropriate manner. Through this type of experience, students will learn to make better decisions about their own health, and teachers will learn how to design and implement a health-related physical fitness education program that motivates students to be active for life.

Goal Setting

Goal setting is a mechanism that helps students understand their potential and feel satisfied with their accomplishments. Establishing goals is a good way to encourage changes in behavior that lead to improved health and fitness. Using goals created from personal assessments establishes ownership and fosters pride in the process. Written action plans help to establish a pathway to the destination that has been set. The types of behaviors (goals) students require for improving health-related fitness can be determined from a pretest. (See the Fitness Goals Contract and Activity Goals Contract in appendix A.) The goal-setting process is invaluable to physical education—as well as to other areas of life.

Goal setting, however, must be done carefully to successfully enhance motivation. It takes experience and practice for both students and educators. Many factors should be taken into consideration: gender differences, current fitness level, information about fitness improvement, and growth and maturation. The criteria-level (healthy fitness zone) charts provided in the *FITNESSGRAM* assessment (pages 61-62 in the third edition) reflect both gender and age differences. In general, the less fit a person is, the greater the gains may be. For the person who is more fit, smaller gains should be expected. Finally, remember to focus on personal improvement—and encourage students to do so as well—rather than on comparisons to others.

Goal-Setting Steps

1. Determine a baseline. The baseline is an accounting of the current fitness level or the behaviors needing change. Thus, in setting goals to enhance personal fitness, the first step is to assess the current level of fitness.

2. Clearly define the desired outcome. If in the initial assessment it is determined that improvement in flexibility in the right shoulder is needed, the student can use the *FITNESS-GRAM* healthy fitness zone charts as a guide in setting the desired outcome. The desired outcome would be that the student would be able to touch fingertips when reaching with the right hand over the shoulder.

3. List the activities to be performed or strategies needed to achieve the desired outcome. Using the FITT guidelines help the student ensure specificity in the setting of the activities: frequency (e.g., how many times per day or week a stretch will be performed); intensity (e.g., whether the stretch is to be performed by the person alone or with partner assistance); time (e.g., how long to hold the stretch); and type (e.g., the types of stretching that will enhance shoulder flexibility).

4. Identify a time line for reassessment and the accomplishment of the goal. Often, this is written at the beginning of the goal, as in the following: "At the end of six weeks, I will be able to touch fingertips when performing the right shoulder flexibility test."

5. Commit to the achievement of the goal. This is best accomplished by using goal partners (the teacher can also be the goal partner for younger students). The goal partner and the goal setter both sign the paper, and the paper is then posted in a place that reminds the individual to work toward the goal. Posting the paper on the inside of the student's locker door, the refrigerator at home (e.g., for a nutritional goal), or in a daily journal can serve as excellent reminders. Students should be told to check daily with their goal partner and to provide encouragement. This can be done via phone, in person, or using e-mail.

6. Reassess and reinforce. Reassessment should not occur only at the end of the time period, but should be made at least weekly. Reinforcement occurs daily from both the goal setter and the goal partner after each reassessment period. For students needing extrinsic motivation, the reinforcement might come in the form

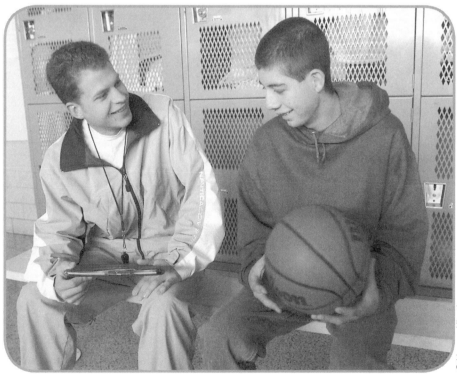

© Human Kinetics

Provide individualized motivation and support, but do so in a way that is perceived as helpful rather than stigmatizing.

of tokens (e.g., stickers) that can be exchanged at the end of the goal period for something of value—free time, choice of activities, points toward a grade, or even a day off.

MOTIVATIONAL PE

For goal setting to be effective, teachers must demonstrate that goals are important. The teacher must teach students the goal-setting process, and time must be provided in class for reassessment. Teach-

ers will need to help students identify areas of fitness that are priorities for the students and will need to help the students make decisions throughout the goal-setting process. Teachers who are new to using individualized goal setting might find the acronym MOTIVATIONAL PE helpful in teaching about setting good goals. It will also help them create a motivational climate that leads to successful achievement of student goals. The Goal-Setting Worksheet is an example of applying these concepts with students (see figure 2.2).

Goal-Setting Worksheet

Name:_____   Date:_____

M = Measure and monitor
In class, my *FITNESSGRAM* scores were as follows: _____

The scores below the healthy fitness zone were (list) _____ .

O = Outcomes defined that are optimally challenging
Based on my *FITNESSGRAM* scores, I wish to improve fitness in the following areas:
(Example: abdominal strength and endurance)

T = Time
I will accomplish my goal in _____ weeks.

I = Individualized
I will not compare my scores to my classmates' scores.
To reach the HFZ, I need to increase my score by _____ (the exercise).
(Example: 10 curl-ups)

V = Valuable
I have chosen a goal of _____ .
(Example: increasing abdominal strength)
This is important to me because . . .

A = Active
By completing this sheet, I am taking responsibility for increasing my health and fitness. _____
(initial)

☞

T = Type

The following activities will help me to reach my goal: (list several activities)
(Example: curl-ups, pelvic thrusts, oblique curls)

I = Incremental

I will add _____ (a number of exercises) to my score or add _____ minutes of _____ (activity) each week to achieve my goals.
(Example: 2 curl-ups each week or 5 minutes of jogging each week)

O = Overload

I will increase the weight or quantity of my activity each day by _____.
(Example: 10 curl-ups each day)

N = Necessary

The purpose of this activity is to help me . . .

A = Authentic assessment

Although I can perform the _____ test again to see my improvement, I can also know I am achieving my goal by
(Examples: measuring waist circumference, seeing my clothes fit better)

L = Lifestyle

Unhealthy behaviors that I would like to change in the future include the following:
(Examples: Inactive television viewing, snacking on unhealthy foods)

P = Posted but private

I will post this sheet or keep it _____, where I can see it each day.
My goal partner is_____ .

E = Enjoyable

I know that work on this activity may not always be easy or fun, but I will be happier when I am healthy.
My reward to myself when I achieve this goal is _____.
(Example: I will go see a movie with my best friend)

My signature:_____

Teacher signature*:_____

(*Teacher has reviewed goal and believes it to be achievable for student.)

■ **Figure 2.2** Students can use the Goal-Setting Worksheet to identify and track physical activity goals using the MOTIVATIONAL PE concepts. See appendix A for a reproducible version of this form.

Debra Ballinger, PhD., Associate Professor, University of Rhode Island

M = Measure and Monitor

As previously mentioned, the goal-setting process begins with measurement. Taking stock of student needs is the basis for effective goal setting and motivation. Once goals are set, they must be constantly monitored to determine if progress is being made toward their achievement. Goals must be written in measurable terms. The process must allow teachers time to monitor the progress of all students so the teacher can ensure that the students are having fun and are making progress toward goals. Too often teachers and students set goals but then do not revisit the goals, or set new ones, once the goals are met.

O = Outcomes Defined That Are Optimally Challenging

Use the *FITNESSGRAM* healthy fitness zone charts to identify achievable goals. Provide knowledge about why fitness is important and how it is achieved. Teachers must help students define the desired outcome. Teachers are accustomed to writing specific objectives that specify conditions and outcomes that are measurable, and this format is the basis for a good goal. To have fun and not be bored, students must be challenged with tasks or goals that are difficult but achievable (i.e., they must be optimally challenged). Goals that are too difficult will be discarded; those that are too easy will not have value.

T = Time

If a goal can't be reached within a specified time limit, then the goal is too difficult. Setting a time line for assessment is critical for appropriate monitoring of progress toward goal achievement. To remain motivated, students should have both short-term and long-range goals. The short-term goals should be achievable within one or two class periods, such as increasing the number of laps in the PACER test or increasing curl-ups by one per class session. Short-term goals are often process goals related to skill acquisition or form. Long-term goals should also have a time limit and should be achievable within a couple of weeks or a month. For students, focusing on a longer period of time may result in a loss of interest and enjoyment in the activity and the value of its outcome. The goals should specify the length of time needed to achieve the outcome, as well as a time line for reassessment.

I = Individualized

Teachers must remember that the student owns the goal, and it must be tailored to meet the needs of the individual. This means that goals should not be competitive and that goals will vary in level of difficulty, time, type of activity, and in the number of goals set. This individualization is especially valuable in helping students with special or diverse needs. Goals, like well-prepared classes, need to include variety to remain motivational. Allowing students to choose a variety of activities to meet their individual goals helps them avoid boredom and provides greater opportunities for success. Younger students may need more teacher guidance, but as students develop, they should have autonomy in setting goals for fitness and should have choices of the physical activities they will use to accomplish the goals.

V = Valuable

For a goal to have value, a student must first set the goal himself, and then must be able to determine the reward to be earned. For younger students, activities that are fun are valued, and providing rewards such as tokens that can be exchanged for "choice activity time" often increases the value of goal achievement. For adolescents, value is often enhanced when goals are linked with those of other students. Sharing goals and having goal partners validate success are great ways to enhance the social value of goal achievement.

A = Active

We would be remiss if we did not include "activity" as a component of the goal-setting process. Active refers to the process of goal setting as well as to the achievement of its outcome. Too often, teachers fail to trust students to determine their goals. They tell the students what the students should be able to do, what they must be able to learn, and even how they should feel. Students should select the aspect of fitness on which they wish to focus their efforts, record their own progress toward the goal, and have a say in the rewards received as a result of goal accomplishment.

T = *Type*

Providing choices (types) of activities that may be used to achieve the desired outcomes will enhance motivation to achieve the goal. Allowing choices can also help overcome barriers to success. Consider a goal leading toward enhanced aerobic fitness. A student might write that he will walk one mile each day, but then winter weather may prevent walking. Teaching the student different activities that are available to achieve the fitness goal would encourage him to substitute a different activity in this situation, such as riding an ergometer, walking 15 minutes on a treadmill, or doing 15 minutes of step-ups. Each activity will lead to the desired outcome, and providing choices will facilitate greater success than limiting activities to one type. In quality physical education, stations are used to provide choices for learning about and accomplishing skills. Similarly, students should be encouraged to use different types of activities to reach their fitness goals.

I = *Incremental*

Incremental refers to developmentally appropriate and safe progressions in levels of difficulty. When setting several goals, the easiest goal to accomplish should be the first goal. This will provide an initial success experience. For optimal success, goals should be written so that the difficulty increases incrementally.

O = *Overload*

Within each goal, steps should be included that outline the process to achieve the student's physical best. The principle of overload should be clearly stated in the wording of the conditions of the goal. The **overload principle** states that a body system (cardiorespiratory, muscular, or skeletal) must perform at a level beyond normal in order to adapt and improve physiological function and fitness. A sample goal is that the student will achieve a health-enhancing level of cardiorespiratory fitness (aerobic fitness) by adding one lap in the PACER per day (overload in time and distance).

N = *Necessary*

Adding to the concept of value is the point that the goal must be "necessary" or important to the student. By allowing the students to determine their own goals, the chances that the goals will be important to them are greatly enhanced. However, the teacher must also provide incentives through instruction about the importance of health-related fitness, in order for the student to have the capacity to understand which goals are important and necessary. Students should be challenged to respond to the question, "How will my life be different or better after I achieve my goal?" If the answer isn't obvious, then the necessity of the goal should be called into question.

A = *Authentic Assessment*

Assessment should be directly related to the goal and the outcome desired by the student, as well as provide a connection to the needs and interests of the student in life outside the physical education class. The creativity of the teacher will be challenged when helping students find real-life reasons and assessment strategies for their goals. Weight loss programs typically focus on reduction in inches rather than pounds because this is more "authentically" tied to what the client really wants to achieve—fitting into a certain dress or pant size (rather than reading a number on a scale). Authentic assessment is also closely tied to the "necessity" component of goal setting.

L = *Lifestyle*

Student goals must be tied to achieving a healthy lifestyle. You should teach students about why certain behaviors lead to healthy lifestyles and others lead to self-destructive behaviors. Using a journal to track behaviors and the feelings related to them should be a joint activity with goal setting. If goals don't include connections to behavioral change, they become less valuable. This is especially important when working with high school students. Help students see the connection between the goal and real changes affecting their futures. For younger students, linking goals with family activities and interests contributes to connections between school and home—and helps them better understand nutrition, exercise, and fitness from a global perspective.

P = Posted but Private

Commitment to the goal is critical. Commitment is best achieved by writing the goals and having them signed by the individual and a goal partner. The partner is a motivator in the process and a support system when progress isn't so obvious. Allow students to choose their goal partner, as well as the place for posting their goals. If lockers are truly private, posting the goals inside the locker door may work. Goal partners should be encouraged to check on progress daily (using e-mail or instant messaging can be an enjoyable tool for today's youth to communicate about goals). Goals should only be shared with the permission of the student, and privacy must be maintained throughout the process. Recognition in public is acceptable for some students when goals are accomplished; however, for others, public recognition can be embarrassing and counterproductive.

E = Enjoyable

Enjoyment comes not only from participating in chosen activities that are fun, but also from feelings of satisfaction in the accomplishment of challenging goals. Help students select activities that will ensure success as well as those that the students feel are fun. Pairing students with friends as goal partners also adds to enjoyment. Students don't even have to be in the same class to be paired. Enjoyment can also be enhanced for younger children by involving family members, parents, or other teachers in the process.

Promoting Physical Activity and Fitness Through Physical Best

Remember, children and adolescents are not mini-adults. Look for age-appropriate ways to tailor the general strategies described in the previous section to the realms of home, school, and community. Table 2.4 offers several specific suggestions that the Physical Best program endorses.

Finally, don't forget one of the most important keys: Emphasize enjoyment! If a child remembers only one thing from your class, it should be that being physically active is enjoyable and interesting. Teachers can find new and fun activities in the revised *Physical Best Activity Guides*, as well as through NASPE publications. Remember, enjoyment is an important key to a lifetime of fitness.

Fund-Raising Can Be Fun!

Fifty physical educators in Jacksonville, Florida, decided to jump on the advocacy bandwagon to promote physical education and make their programs more visible. One such effort involved selling bright yellow bumper stickers that read, "Physical Education . . . Knowledge to Last a Lifetime."

Their goal was to use the stickers to remind families and individuals of the value of exercising and making healthy choices. Purchasing a bumper sticker was an easy way for parents to get involved and show their support, especially after they realized that many physical education programs were in jeopardy following district budget cuts.

The bumper stickers were sold for one dollar each during school, community, statewide, and regional events. Organizers were also able to gain support from a large local amusement center, which gave them coupons for its entertainments to be included with each bumper sticker sold. The schools used the money raised to purchase much needed equipment. Most important, however, this fund-raiser generated a great deal of positive publicity for physical education within the community.

Reprinted, by permission, from J.S. Tipton and S.L. Tucker, 1998, *Journal of Teaching Elementary Physical Education* 9 (3): 14.

TABLE 2.4   Strategies for Promoting Physical Activity in Children

Setting	Objectives	Strategies
Home	Families will be active together	• Use PALA awards • Newsletters sent home • Set family activity goals • Homework: exercise with family • Journals to reflect on activity levels at home
	Parents will facilitate child's activity	• Arrange transportation and car pools • Set "family activity" time daily • Set limits on TV time per day • Teacher provides suggested weekly activities • School allows pedometer or heart rate monitor checkout for a 24-hour period
School	Students will maintain a health-enhancing level of physical activity each day on school days	• Use *ACTIVITYGRAM* • Use pedometers in school • Use heart rate monitors in school • Set class activity goals • Interclass competition for walking
Community	Access to safe and fun venues for all children	• Open school venues during nonschool days • Provide community programs • Link activity times for children with public transportation • Regularly inspect playground safety • Have police regularly patrol venues • Secure grants to fund inclusive programs for children with special needs
	Establish corporate partnerships	• Contact businesses to establish partnerships • Contact professional sport franchises to set up partnerships or special attendance nights

Reprinted, by permission, from R. Pate, 1995, Promoting activity and fitness. In *Child health, nutrition, and physical activity*, edited by L.W.Y. Cheung and J.B. Richmond (Champaign, IL: Human Kinetics), 143-144.

Leaving Behind America's Physical Activity Myths

For years Americans have heard the message that they should exercise vigorously for at least 20 minutes per day, three times per week. They believed that nothing less would do. Even though many people today might be able to recite the recommendation from memory, the vast majority of Americans have not successfully carried out the advice. And in the process, it is likely that a good many have given up trying.

Previous efforts by public and private organizations to promote physical activity have emphasized the importance of high-intensity physical activities. As a result, many people are convinced that they must engage in vigorous, continuous activity for at least 20 minutes three times a week to achieve any health benefits. Rather than do less than this, many people choose to do nothing at all. As people's perception of the effort required to perform an activity increases, their participation in physical activity seems to decrease (Dishman and Sallis 1994).

Therefore, if people with little confidence in their ability to be physically active were convinced that moderate-intensity activity counts and that "it's easier than you think" to fit activity into the course of a busy day, perhaps the number of people who are willing to adopt and continue a physically active lifestyle would increase. Perhaps if Americans felt more comfortable with their own ability to fit physical activity into their lives, they'd be more likely to spread the word and really get the ball rolling for a "fitness revolution." After all, studies show that people who have confidence in their ability to be physically active and who receive support from family members and friends are more likely to begin and continue exercise programs (Dishman and Sallis 1994).

Building a Fitness Program Around Student Goals

The Physical Best program is a model for establishing goals in physical fitness levels, activity participation, and the affective and cognitive domains. Teachers must teach students the goal-setting process and provide opportunities after assessments for students to set, revise, and evaluate goals. The Physical Best program recognizes the achievement of goals set by students as an important reinforcement for student motivation. Using goal-setting techniques and strategies helps students have positive experiences through

movement activities, feel good about themselves in physical activity, and carry positive fitness habits for a lifetime. Physical educators can support the students' use of goal setting to enhance their lives and fitness abilities.

Table 2.5 provides some examples for setting fitness goals. In the table, the level of fitness is based on the healthy fitness zone (HFZ):

- Low—initial level is far from reaching the HFZ
- Moderate—initial level is close to the low end of the HFZ
- High—initial level is within or above the HFZ

Teachers can aid students in focusing on appropriate fitness goals by ensuring that the healthy fitness zone wall charts (included with the *FITNESSGRAM* test kits) are posted on the wall where students can readily compare their scores to the healthy fitness zone for their age and gender

TABLE 2.5   Guidelines for Setting Reasonable Goals and Expectations

Fitness component	Pretest below HFZ*	Pretest close to or in lower end of HFZ*	Pretest in or above HFZ*
Aerobic fitness	Increase daily activity	Increase daily activity	Maintain activity levels
PACER	Increase laps by 2-4/wk	Increase laps by 2-4/wk	Continue behaviors
Flexibility	Stretch 2 or 3 × /day	Stretch 2 × /day	Maintain activity level
Back-saver sit-and-reach	Hold 8-10 sec	Hold 8-10 sec	Stretch all areas daily
Shoulder stretch— measure distance apart	Learn 2 yoga positions	Stretch w/partner 2 × /day	• Stretch daily • Continue daily activity
Muscular strength and endurance	• Perform strength activity on alternate days for low areas • Increase reps by 2-5/ set every other day	Increase weight 1 lb/day and increase reps by 2-5/set each day	• Maintain activities • Add 2 new exercises/wk • Encourage a classmate
Body composition	Increase activity time by 2 min/day until maintaining 30 min/day	• Increase activity by 5 min/wk • Add strength and flexibility or maintain if in HFZ	• Maintain activity level • Vary lifetime activities • Learn 1 new activity

* HFZ = The *FITNESSGRAM* healthy fitness zone

Sample Goals for Aerobic Fitness

- I will reduce my mile run by _____ seconds (outcome/product goal) by performing aerobic activity _____ times per week for at least _____ minutes each session (process component of goal).
- I will do push-ups four times a week, and each week I will increase the number of push-ups I do by at least one repetition, until I reach my healthy fitness zone (process goal).
- I will exercise aerobically _____ times a week, running the one-mile distance at least _____ times a week, timing and logging the results (process goal).
- I will perform aerobic activity _____ times a week, recording the amount of time, type of activity, and intensity of the activity (process).
- I will walk briskly _____ times a week for a total of _____ blocks (process and product). Each week I will increase the distance by _____ blocks (product).
- I will replace sedentary (inactive) habits with active habits at least three times per day (process).
- As I exercise, I will monitor my heart rate level to remain in my target zone (process).

The *FITNESSGRAM/ACTIVITYGRAM* software printouts offer more specific advice for students based on their age and their performance on the battery of tests. Use the *FITNESSGRAM* report to guide student goal setting. The *ACTIVITYGRAM* is useful for assessing school and nonschool daily activity levels and also for providing information about blocks of time that the students might be able to use for fitness development and maintenance. Both reports can form the basis for individual goal setting to help students achieve and maintain healthy lifestyles.

It's Okay to Excel

Throughout this book, we emphasize that lifelong physical activity is for all students, and that teachers especially need to work with students at low fitness levels who have long been ignored. We don't, however, want to forget about the highly motivated students who want to achieve a high level of fitness for a variety of reasons. Just as teachers want to provide opportunities for excellence to students interested in science or math, they should also provide the same types of opportunities to students who are interested in achieving excellence in fitness. For example, a teacher may create an individualized plan for a student who wants to compete at an elite level in tennis or track. Another example is having a student serve as a mentor to other students; this could help the

student decide if he or she would enjoy a career as a physical educator or personal trainer. The first key, of course, is that this is voluntary on the students' part. You should explore ways of individualizing programs for these students to help them safely achieve their goals. We provide examples in later chapters.

Finally, the unique circumstances of each student must be considered when establishing that student's goals. For example, two moderately fit students might establish goals for upper body strength that fall at the opposite extremes of the range. One student might have class only two times a week, not get much encouragement at home, and be somewhat overweight. The other student might have an hour-long class five times a week. You and your students will improve in the ability to set goals as you practice setting more goals and observing the outcomes.

Summary

Based on the research, the Physical Best program offers the following suggestions for motivating students to be physically active for life:

- Award the process of participation, rather than the product of fitness.
- Teach children and adolescents to set goals that are challenging yet attainable, enjoyable, and valuable.

- Develop students' basic skills by using developmentally appropriate progressions so that students become competent and feel confident when participating in physical activities that develop fitness for a healthy lifestyle.

- Use bulletin boards and visual aids to publicize items of interest in fitness. Recognize students for progress toward lifestyle changes and goals, rather than for competitive outcomes.

- Emphasize self-testing programs that teach children to assess and evaluate their own fitness levels.

- Provide multiple opportunities for success and monitoring of personal goals.

- Provide choices of activities to promote enjoyment and self-determination.

Throughout this book, we offer more specific suggestions for developing the desire within students to be physically active for life.

3

Basic Training Principles

Chapter Contents

As physical educators, we believe in the value of physical activity across the life span, although there is limited scientific evidence indicating physically active children become physically active adults. Whether or not activity patterns track into adulthood, a big part of producing physically active adults is to teach students the basic training principles, providing them with the tools they need to lead an active lifestyle throughout their lives. The FITT guidelines are the *hows* of physical activity that empower students to construct and tailor workouts that meet their individual health-related fitness needs. Many instructors are likely to be familiar with this information, but we have included this chapter as a quick reference to make the job of teaching the information easier. You may also want to share this concise summary when including colleagues, administrators, and parents in schoolwide physical activity events.

A growing body of literature indicates an increase in chronic disease in children, as well as an increasing number of overweight children. Also, there is evidence of declining physical activity across the life span and evidence that activity patterns developed early in childhood track into adulthood (Malina 1996; Malina 2001; Sallis 2000). Altering behavior appears to be a monumental task that takes time and involves changes in attitudes about physical activity, which is beyond the scope of this chapter. (See chapter 2 for more information on behavior and motivation.) However, teachers can encourage and educate children by providing them with the necessary tools to develop activity programs that grow and progress as they mature. The principles of training are important concepts (tools) that students will use across their life span.

Physical educators know how these training principles apply to adults; however, they must use caution when applying these same principles of training to children. It is important to use fun activities and strive for the development of positive attitudes toward physical activity instead of focusing on the "product"—fitness—since "aerobic and muscular strength improvements are relatively small, even after prolonged training regimens" (Rowland 1996, 100). Keep in mind that if a parent or coach decides that "training" is necessary to increase a child's athletic potential, then the program must follow the basic principles of training and must be designed using the child's stage of maturation rather than chronological age (Bompa 2000).

Understanding the Basic Training Principles

The principles of training (overload, progression, specificity, regularity, and individuality) govern how the body responds to the physical stress of physical activity across all five areas of health-related fitness (aerobic fitness, muscular strength, muscular endurance, flexibility, and body composition). The basic physiological changes that occur over the course of a training period are called **training adaptations**. Students must understand that to see changes in any area of health-related fitness, they must stimulate the specific physiological system involved (such as the cardiorespiratory, muscular, or skeletal system). Remember that these training principles apply to training and conditioning, and although they are the basis for health-related fitness activities, there are limitations to the magnitude of the physiological changes that will

occur in children, because they do not respond to training as adults do. Also, physical educators do not want children training in physical education classes at the high intensities (85 percent heart rate max) required to elicit these training changes (Rowland 1996). The principles of training are applied through manipulation of the frequency, intensity, duration, and mode of the activity performed. A key concept when applying these principles to your classroom activities is that they allow you (the instructor) to individualize the lesson to meet the needs of the athlete, the sedentary student, the disabled student, or the poorly motivated student. It is unrealistic to expect all students to be at the same fitness level or motivational level. Each student will respond to the activities in your lesson very differently, and application of the principles of training allows a very individualized approach to each lesson.

Overload The **overload principle** states that a body system (cardiorespiratory, muscular, or skeletal) must perform at a level beyond normal in order to adapt and improve physiological function and fitness. For example, to apply this principle to the cardiorespiratory system, a person must exercise at an intensity greater than the body is accustomed to; this in turn will develop a stronger and healthier heart capable of doing more work with less effort.

Progression **Progression** refers to how an individual should increase the overload (see figure 3.1, *a* and *b*). Proper progression involves a gradual increase in the level of exercise that is manipulated by increasing either frequency, intensity, or time, or a combination of all three components (see the next section). Emphasize that all progression must be gradual to be safe. If the overload is applied too soon, the body does not have time to adapt, and the benefits may be delayed or an injury may occur (both of which can discourage or prevent an individual from participating). Thus, for each component of health-related fitness, take the time to outline and model appropriate progressions. Emphasize that improving a person's fitness level is a continual, ongoing process. Keeping a training log provides an opportunity for students to see the gradual progression and track the dates a new overload was applied (see appendix A).

Specificity The **specificity principle** states that explicit activities that target a particular body system must be performed to bring about fitness changes in that area. For example, a person must perform exercises that stress the hamstring muscles in order to develop muscular strength or muscular endurance of the hamstrings.

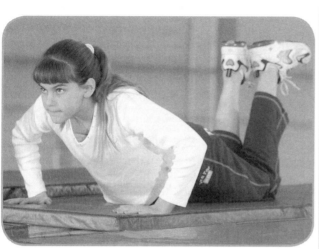

a

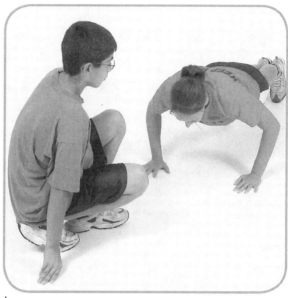

b

■ **Figure 3.1** A student demonstrates progression by increasing the intensity by moving from *(a)* a modified push-up to *(b)* a regular push-up.

Regularity The **regularity principle** is based on the old adage of "use it, or lose it" and states that physical activity must be performed on a regular basis to be effective. Any fitness gains attained through physical activity will be lost if the person does not continue to be active. The various body systems respond differently to discontinuation of training and physical inactivity, with the cardiovascular system and **stroke volume** (amount of blood ejected in one heart beat) being affected quickly (a return to baseline levels within one month) (Coyle et al. 1984; Coyle 1990; Mujika and Padilla 2001).

Individuality The **individuality principle** takes into account that each person begins at a different level of fitness, each person has different personal goals and objectives for physical activity and fitness, and each person has different genetic potential for change. Giving children plenty of opportunities to choose activities in your classroom is an important way to help children develop physical activity patterns that they may carry across the life span.

Applying the Training Principles

The American College of Sports Medicine (ACSM 2000) defines the **exercise prescription** as the process of designing a routine of physical activity in a systematic and individualized manner. You should keep in mind that children respond differently than adults, and that the traditional idea of an exercise prescription should not be stringently applied to children. To safely apply the principles of training to any area of health-related fitness, the FITT (frequency, intensity, time, and type) guidelines must be followed, and the emphasis should be on fun interactive activities that encourage high participation levels. By engaging in fun, high-participation activities, the training principles are applied and fitness will develop through the "process" of physical activity (not the "product" of forced, boring activities).

FITT Guidelines

The **FITT guidelines** describe how to safely apply the five principles of training: overload, progression, specificity, regularity, and individuality. Rowland (1996) states that altering physical activity patterns in children is—at least conceptually—simpler than altering physical fitness by engaging in a training program with variations in frequency, intensity, and time, as in the adult model. Keep in mind that the following guidelines (ACSM 2000) for the development of fitness (including frequency, intensity, and time) are based on an adult model and may not be applicable to younger children. These guidelines are included here because they are applicable to students at the middle and high school levels. Each of the health-related fitness component chapters (part II of this book) outlines the use of the FITT guidelines by age.

Frequency

Frequency describes *how often* a person performs the targeted health-related physical activity. For each component of health-related fitness, the beneficial and safe frequency is generally three to five days per week, with aerobic fitness activities being performed all or most days of the week. The exceptions are activities intended for increasing muscular strength and endurance. Most experts believe these activities should be limited to three nonconsecutive days per week, unless different muscle groups are exercised on alternating days (see chapter 6).

Intensity

Intensity describes *how hard* a person exercises during a physical activity period and depends on the age and fitness goals of the participant. Heart rate has traditionally been used as a measure of training intensity to develop aerobic fitness. But teachers must remember that the development of physical fitness in children should be a lifelong process of increased physical activity and the development of positive attitudes toward physical activity—not the product of "training." Therefore, teachers should reserve calculations and goals of meeting a specified target heart rate for high school level students (or at least late teen years). Also keep in mind that a child's heart rate max is age independent and is approximately 195 to 205 BPM regardless of age. Calculating a target heart rate based on 60 to 90 percent heart rate max will yield target heart rates, but these are not necessarily heart rates that improve fitness in children. More information on heart rates can be found in chapter 5.

You may, however, begin to teach concepts of intensity and heart rate monitoring—providing the student with opportunities to compare resting heart rate with exercise heart rate, to learn basic anatomy of the cardiovascular and respiratory systems, and to learn how increased physical activity helps children play longer without getting tired. Primary grade students can begin to monitor their intensity levels by placing a hand over the heart before, during, and after moderate to vigorous physical activity; they can note the general speed of the heartbeat using terms such as slow, medium, and fast or turtle and race car. Fourth- through sixth-grade students can begin to locate the carotid and radial arteries to count heart rate, but they should not use target heart rate zones. Most students seventh grade and up can be

expected to calculate target heart rate values, but you should still avoid the use of target heart rate zones (THRZ) as requirements for participation in physical activities. High school students can begin to use the THRZ to guide them in monitoring intensity of activity. Chapter 5 outlines specific guidelines for using heart rate as a measure of exercise intensity.

Intensity can be manipulated in different ways, depending on the health-related fitness component. For example, monitoring heart rate is one way to gauge intensity during aerobic activities at the middle and high school levels, but it gives no indication of intensity during flexibility activities. Appropriate intensity depends on the goals of the participant and the activity performed. Intensity and time work in opposition to each other. For example, higher intensity activities may be performed for shorter time periods, while lower intensity activities may be performed for longer time periods. The more intense the activity, the shorter the bout should be for younger or less-fit children (see the next section). Classroom concepts related to intensity should emphasize pacing and getting children to recognize that speed is not always necessary for success. Emphasizing high intensity or speed (trying too hard) may actually reduce the quality of performance and increase the likelihood of injury. Instead, teach students the appropriate range of intensity for each type of activity.

Time

Time describes *how long* the activity should be performed. As with other aspects of the FITT guidelines, time varies depending on the targeted health-related fitness component, and it is inversely related to intensity. Primary grade children will have difficulty understanding this concept comparable to older children. Not only will primary grade children have difficulty understanding time or **duration** of physical activity, but they are also less able than older children and adolescents to complete intense physical activities in one time period. Specific guidelines for each area of health-related fitness are discussed in chapters 5 through 8.

Type

Type refers to mode or *what kind* of activity a person chooses to perform for each area of health-related fitness (figure 3.2). For example, a person may choose walking to develop aerobic fitness or to work on body composition principles; station tasks may be used to develop muscular strength, endurance, or flexibility. Encourage students to select activities they enjoy and that specifically target their personal goals. Instructors of elementary and middle school students should provide a variety of activities that will facilitate future choices at the high school level. Most activity should be intermittent and come from levels 1 to 3 on the physical activity pyramid (figure 3.3 *a* and *b*). Continuous, vigorous activity is not recommended for most children (NASPE 2004).

FITT Age Differences

Most research examining the FITT guidelines is based on adult physiology. Overzealous adults often forget that children are still growing and are not miniature adults. "Anatomical, physiological, and psychological immaturity of children may place them at greater risk during athletic training and competition" (Rowland 1990, 253). Teachers and coaches of children should focus on age-appropriate activities (defined in chapter 5) that give

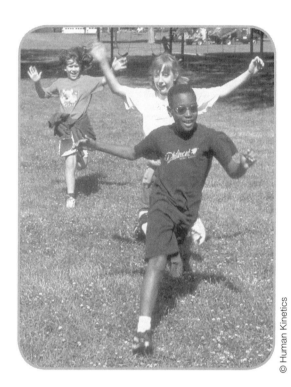

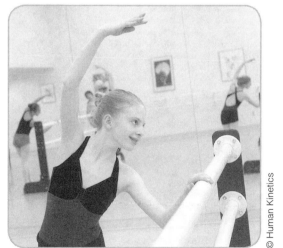

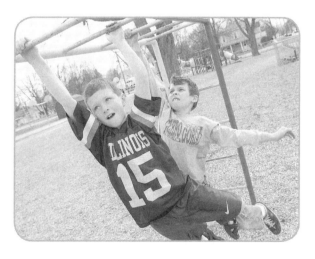

■ **Figure 3.2** Types of activity.

all participants an equal opportunity to play, make friends, and improve social skills, and at the same time improve their fitness. At the middle and high school levels, students are closer to adulthood and respond to training and conditioning much like the adult, so the FITT guidelines may be applied.

Self-Esteem

Adhering to the basic principles of training involves more than the physical aspects of training and conditioning or simply increasing physical activity; psycho-social components must also be considered. Generally, children do not choose to exercise or be physically active for the associated health benefits,

but they are more likely to be physically active if they perceive their physical abilities as high (NASPE 2004; Weiss and Horn 1990).

Although some research appears to indicate a positive relationship between physical activity and self-esteem, it has been difficult to establish a relationship that links increased physical fitness with improved self-esteem (Sonstroem 1984). Physical Best emphasizes development of lifetime physical activity and education calling attention to fitness as a lifelong process, rather than a product of isolated training and conditioning. Teachers must be especially careful to take self-esteem into consideration when working with children. Verbal encouragement must be provided and related specifically

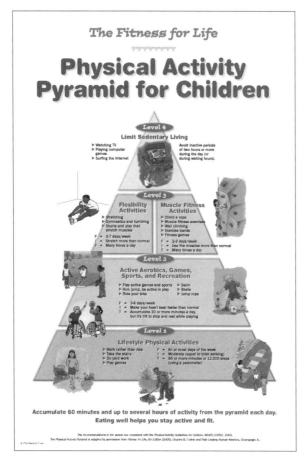

a

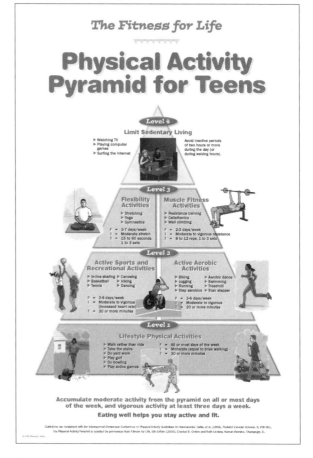

b

■ **Figure 3.3**   The physical activity pyramid, *(a)* for children and *(b)* for teenagers, is a tool that will help your students understand how to address each component of health-related fitness. The children's version is available for full-size printing on the *Physical Best Activity Guide: Elementary Level CD-ROM.* The teen's version is available for full-size printing on the *Physical Best Activity Guide: Middle and High School Levels CD-ROM.*

to performance; collective praise for the group or general praise for the individual is not effective. Verbal encouragement is especially important for younger children (under 10 years old) because they tend to evaluate their competence based on success in competition and parental praise, while older children (over 10 years old) rely on peer evaluation of performance (Horn and Hasbrook 1986, 1987; Weiss and Horn 1990).

Self-perceptions of competence decline as children get older. Jacobs and Eccles (2000) and Jacobs et al. (2002) indicate that as children become aware of other children's levels of competence, they begin to realize where they fall in relation to other students. Also, as the child gets older, there are fewer and fewer opportunities for success in sport and activity because the competition increases. The child becomes selective, participating in the few things considered opportunities to be successful. Physical Best activities provide ample opportunity for positive encouragement of individuals and provide success for each child, which fosters improved self-esteem and perceived competence. For more information on physical activity behavior and motivation, refer to chapter 2.

Components of a Physical Activity Session

Every physical activity session should incorporate a systematic approach not only to ensure safety but also to prepare the body for the rigors of physical activity. Properly warming up before and cooling down after the workout may also prevent injuries and aid in returning the body to a more rested state, respectively. The main physical activity must also be conducted appropriately for students to feel and understand, through participation, the importance of being physically active.

Warm-Up

A **warm-up** is a low-intensity activity done before a full-effort and may serve multiple purposes and should be organized to meet specific goals of the planned activity. A general warm-up—including activities such as walking, jogging, swimming, or cycling—may be used to prepare the cardiorespiratory and musculoskeletal systems for the stretching portion of the warm-up and the main physical activity that follows. The warm-up is also more effective

if the warm-up activities use the muscles that will be used in the main physical activity. The stretching portion of the warm-up should be preceded by 5 to 10 minutes of cardiorespiratory warm-up activity (ACSM 2000). A cardiorespiratory warm-up has the following benefits:

- Increases active muscle blood flow
- Increases blood flow to the heart
- Raises body temperature and may reduce the risk of muscular injury and muscle soreness
- Facilitates temperature regulation by causing earlier sweating

Physical Best activities can be used throughout the year as warm-up activities during other units besides fitness education. For example, if throwing is the main activity, a general warm-up such as Red Light, Green Light (page 23 in *Physical Best Activity Guide: Elementary Level*) could be used to explain to students, in age-appropriate ways, that warming up properly prepares the body for the main activity by gradually increasing heart rate and blood flow to the muscles and tissues of the body. A specific warm-up (figure 3.4) might include jumping jacks, jumping jills, and "angels in the snow" (Foster, Hartinger, and Smith 1992, 21) to specifically prepare the arms for throwing activities.

Although gentle stretching and walking or slow jogging for about five minutes are common and safe warm-up activities, you must vary the warm-up to prevent boredom and carelessness in the routine. For younger children (and to prevent discipline problems), plan and lead warm-ups that provide "instant activity" as the students arrive at the lesson site (Graham 1992). This might include challenge activities such as how many times students can jump back and forth across a line, how many successive turns of a jump rope the students can complete, a short circuit training course, or a dribbling activity. These "instant activities" may also work for older students by providing an opportunity for students to socialize while warming up. Also, for older students, post the warm-up in the locker rooms or at the lesson site and make the students responsible for carrying it out independently.

Main Physical Activity

The main physical activity is the core of the lesson or workout intended to improve or maintain one or more of the health-related fitness components. The type

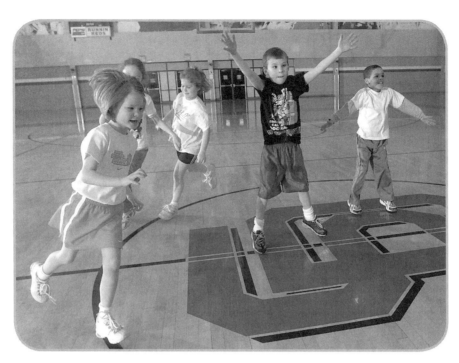

Figure 3.4   Jumping jacks, jumping jills, and angels in the snow.

of activity and the time and intensity of the workout depend on the goals of the lesson, the length of the class period, and the current fitness level of individual students. Whether teaching kindergarteners or high school seniors, you should explain the purpose of the lesson and how the day's activity will help students reach class goals or personalized goals.

Cool-Down

A proper **cool-down** includes a period of light activity following exercise that allows the body to slow down and return to near resting levels. Students must understand that the body needs this gradual recovery following exercise to reduce muscle stiffness and soreness, remove lactic acid, and prevent light-headedness, dizziness, or even fainting. Teach them to resist the urge to simply sit or lie down after physical activity; instead, they should gradually slow down their activity by walking or jogging for three to five minutes, or until the heart rate returns to near resting level. Continued light activity facilitates recovery by "milking" blood in the veins back toward the heart. An abrupt cessation of exercise facilitates pooling of blood in the extremities and decreases blood returning to the heart, and subsequently to the brain, leaving the individual susceptible to fainting. Stretching exercises should also be performed

during the cool-down because this is when the muscles are warmest and most pliable, therefore providing maximum benefit toward improving flexibility. Refer to chapter 7 in this book and to the *Physical Best Activity Guides* for examples of stretching exercises and activities. The cool-down is also an opportunity for the teacher to bring closure to the lesson by reviewing critical components and facilitating student self-evaluation of personalized goals for the workout.

In summary, for the prepubescent child, the emphasis should be placed on increasing physical activity, skill development, and access to a wide variety of sports and activities that may serve as a primer or foundation for conditioning programs during puberty and beyond. At the middle and high school levels, the emphasis may be placed on the FITT guidelines and the development of programs more in line with the adult model. Successive chapters of this book, isolating each area of health-related fitness, outline the minimum amount of physical activity that an individual should engage in to acquire health-related benefits as recommended by various organizations, including the Centers for Disease Control and Prevention (CDC), National Association for Sport and Physical Education (NASPE), and the American College of Sports Medicine (ACSM). And while it is crucial that students understand that these minimums are sufficient for a lifetime of health, wellness, and fitness, you will have certain students who are interested in achieving higher levels of health-related fitness. Some may want to further condition themselves in order to enjoy recreational sports, and some may be serious competitors who want to reach maximal levels of fitness. Note, however, that striving for higher fitness levels should be the personal choice of the individual, not that of a teacher, coach, or parent.

The best way to increase health-related fitness is to begin with increasing physical activity. At the elementary level, teachers should remove the stringent three-day-per-week training requirement, place less emphasis on minimum intensity levels, remove time limits frequently suggested as minimums for the development of fitness, and emphasize increased daily physical activity. This is not to say that the adult model FITT guidelines cannot be presented, but the emphasis should be on increasing physical activity. To prevent students from losing interest, or to keep them from losing the desire to become more physically fit, help each student explore a variety of recreational activities and different ways to vary workouts. Encourage students to become involved in school athletic programs and before- or after-school fitness or activity programs. Demonstrate active behavior and be a role model for your students. Take the stairs, park away from the building, or take your classes outside and walk the longest distance to the activity area. Explain to your students the importance of adding these activities to their lifestyle and how it directly relates to them. For example, explain how improved aerobic fitness will enable them to play longer without getting tired. Explain how improved muscular strength will help them perform their daily chores, such as taking out the trash, or how extra strength can help them play on the playground bars and equipment. In addition, act as a liaison between the student and the community, pointing out the various recreational programs available in your community away from the school setting (such as sport leagues, health clubs, and park district activities).

Balancing the Components of Health-Related Fitness

Children, like adults, will express and act on preferences among the many physical activities available.

We strongly encourage you to provide a wide variety of activities and to allow a wide range of personal choice in your program; however, you must ensure that your students understand the need to address each component of health-related fitness. In short, emphasize the importance of total fitness and the need to engage in an activity for each area of health-related fitness. The student who elects to swim laps instead of going cross-country skiing is addressing aerobic fitness appropriately, but this student still needs to work on flexibility, muscular strength and endurance (for muscle groups not addressed by the activity), and body composition. The physical activity pyramid (Corbin and Lindsey 2004) is an effective tool for teaching students how to weigh each component of health-related fitness as well as inactivity (see figure 3.3).

Safety Guidelines for Health-Related Fitness Activities

Students seeking any level of health-related fitness must be encouraged to listen to their body and slow down if feeling overtired, losing weight too rapidly (more than two pounds per week), or suffering soreness that is intense or lasts more than a day or so. Doing too much too fast, weakness, lack of flexibility, biomechanical problems, and improper footwear are common causes of injury. Teach students to use proper pacing—beginning gradually and at an easy intensity and then slowly progressing to activities that are more intense and are longer in duration. These concepts are difficult to get across, especially with younger children who still gauge success by "winners and losers" of competition. Beginners frequently ignore early warning signs of **overtraining** and fail to recognize that they are overdoing it until it is too late to prevent injury or avoid fatigue. Overtraining is the condition caused by training too much or too intensely and not providing sufficient recovery time. Symptoms include lack of energy, fatigue, depression, aching muscles, loss of appetite and proneness to injury.

In regard to flexibility and muscular strength and endurance, students must understand that concentrating on only a few muscle groups and neglecting others can make an individual more susceptible to injury. For example, only working on leg strength and leg flexibility can lead to shoulder or back injuries if the student plays a sport that involves the arms, such as basketball. What actually causes an imbalance in a particular individual depends on that individual's needs. So encourage students to take a whole-body approach to health-related fitness.

Summary

Remember, we are talking about health-related physical activity—not Olympic training. Students, regardless of age, should be presented with reasonable choices of how intense they will work during a given workout, based on their personal goals. Keep in mind that fitness is a journey, not a destination. All teachers want to see their students develop lifelong health-related physical activity habits. Moreover, it is vital that students understand the principles of training and the FITT guidelines so that, ultimately, they can choose to increase their performance and fitness levels as they desire—and know how to do so safely. The goal is to progress toward self-assessment and self-delivery of health-related fitness activities.

CHAPTER

4

Nutrition

The science of nutrition examines food, the level of nutrients and other chemicals in foods, and how these are used in the body. The substances in food affect growth as well as health. All people have the same general needs, but the amounts of specific nutrients needed may increase or decrease due to gender, age, growth, disease, or activity level. One of the factors that makes applying good nutrition principles more challenging is that food serves many purposes in our society other than nourishment. Americans eat to celebrate, to mourn, for entertainment, out of boredom, and for myriad other reasons. The key to good nutrition is for people to strive to meet their individual nutrient needs, while still remembering that food should be enjoyed.

Foundations of a Healthy Diet

Diet is the total intake of food and beverages consumed. No single food item or meal defines the diet. Throughout the average lifetime, a person spends 13 to 15 years of his waking hours eating (Wardlaw 1999). Food habits are learned early and will change throughout life. However, early in life, parents and family tend to shape food habits, and these habits may prove long lasting (see figure 4.1). These patterns are also affected by peers and marketing as children mature into adolescence. Eating habits and preferences established by adolescence tend to carry into adulthood.

The majority of foods have nutrient value and may fit into a healthful diet. In making sure a person takes in good nutrition, the primary goals are to

- provide a variety of different foods,
- supply all the nutrients in adequate amounts, and
- supply a level of calories that will maintain an ideal body weight.

The childhood years offer the best chance for parents and teachers to influence not only current but also future food choices, and thus to develop good eating behaviors. Food habits developed in childhood and adolescence often continue into adulthood. Parents are the gatekeepers; they control and influence the availability and choices of food in their children's environment. As a physical educator, you must actively help educate parents about nutrition and the concept of energy balance. It is critical that parents and teachers do what they can to help establish good eating and activity habits at the elementary school level and make students aware of the relationship among nutrition, activity, and health, both now and for the future. The concept of balance and moderation in eating combined with an active lifestyle are crucial to maintaining an appropriate body weight as well as maintaining optimal health.

An individual's total nutrient needs are greater during adolescence than at any other time of life, except perhaps pregnancy and lactation. According to the USDA guidelines, the majority of adolescent girls need approximately 2,200 calories a day, whereas boys require about 3,000 calories a day (Saltman, Gurin, and Mothner 1993). Nutrient needs rise throughout adolescence and then level off, or possibly even diminish slightly, as an adolescent becomes an adult (Institute of Medicine of the National Academies 2001).

Of course, adolescents make many more choices for themselves than young children do, both about their activity levels and what they eat. Social or peer pressures may push them to make both good and bad choices. Children and adolescents acquire information, and sometimes misinformation, on nutrition from personal, immediate experiences. They are concerned with how food choices can improve their lives and looks now, so they may engage in crash

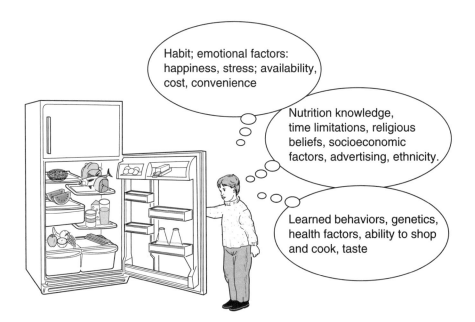

Habit; emotional factors: happiness, stress; availability, cost, convenience

Nutrition knowledge, time limitations, religious beliefs, socioeconomic factors, advertising, ethnicity.

Learned behaviors, genetics, health factors, ability to shop and cook, taste

Figure 4.1   Factors that may affect food choices.

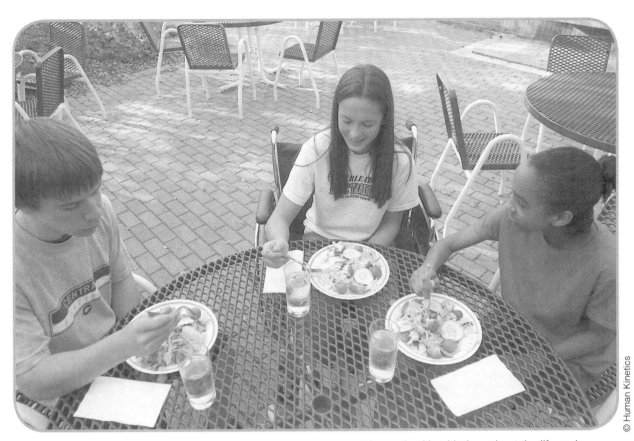

Nutrient requirements may vary by age, but good nutrition is essential to optimal health throughout the life cycle.

© Human Kinetics

dieting or the latest fad in weight gain or loss. Conversely, it is also common to see increased calorie consumption, especially of fats and carbohydrates, among adolescents.

A **kilocalorie** is actually a measure of heat energy. Technically, it's the amount of energy required to raise the temperature of one kilogram of water one degree Celsius. Popular sources often shorten the term *kilocalories* to simply *calories*. Different types of food have different energy values for equal weights.

Nutrient density refers to the amount of a given nutrient per calorie. A variety of foods with high nutrient densities should predominate in a diet. A sample listing of foods and nutritional information for each is included in table 4.1. As you can see, the reduced fat monterey cheese is more nutrient dense than the American cheese.

Categories of Nutrients

There are six categories of nutrients. These include carbohydrates, proteins, fats, vitamins, minerals, and water. All of these are essential for good health.

Carbohydrates

Carbohydrates constitute the majority of energy for people across the world. Carbohydrates also represent the preferred source of energy for the body, particularly the brain, and are categorized as being either simple or complex. Simple carbohydrates are foods that are high in sugar. In general, they are high in calories and low in nutrients. They also tend to provide a short, rapid burst of energy. These include foods such as cakes, candies, sodas, table sugar, and juices (figure 4.2*a*).

Complex carbohydrates include foods such as pasta, cereals, breads, and grains (figure 4.2*b*). In general, complex carbohydrates provide a longer, sustained supply of energy, which is optimal for physical activity. Whole grains are the preferred type of complex carbohydrate. Whole grains are higher in nutrients as well as fiber. Fiber may help to reduce the risk of colon diseases and possibly help to lower blood cholesterol levels. All carbohydrates contain four kilocalories per gram. Current recommendations are that 45 to 65 percent of the diet should consist of carbohydrates, primarily complex carbohydrates.

TABLE 4.1   Common Food Values

Food	Kilocalories	Protein*	Fat*	Vitamin C~	Calcium~	Fiber*
American cheese (2 oz)	213	13	18	0	349	0
Reduced fat Monterey cheese (1 1/2 oz)	120	12	8	0	360	0
Turkey pot pie (1)	410	16	24	0	80	0
Roasted turkey, white meat (3 oz)	134	25	3	0	16	0
White corn (1/2 cup)	66	2	1	5	2	5
Corn chips (13 chips)	160	2	11	0	72	1

*Indicates grams

~Indicates milligrams

Note the difference in nutrient density between the foods.

Wardlaw, *Perspectives in Nutrition*, 1999.

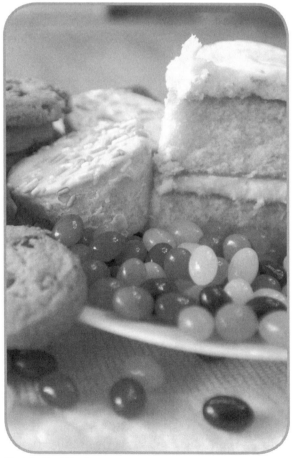

Photo by Dan Wendt

a

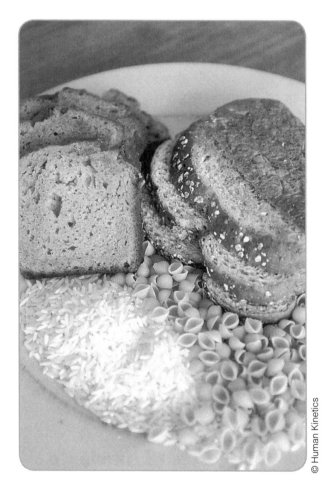

© Human Kinetics

b

■ **Figure 4.2** Foods containing *(a)* simple carbohydrates and *(b)* complex carbohydrates.

Protein

Protein is a constituent of vital body parts. Every cell contains proteins—muscles, blood-clotting factors, immune cells, and so on. The body's preferred use for protein is growth and cell replacement. The body can use protein for energy if no carbohydrate is available. Protein sources can be either animal or plant based. Examples of animal sources of protein include meats, cheeses, milk, and eggs (figure 4.3*a*). Examples of plant sources of protein include beans, nuts, and soy products (figure 4.3*b*). In the United States, most protein, approximately 65 percent, comes from animal sources. This is in contrast to the rest of the world, which only gets 35 percent of its protein from animal sources. Unfortunately, animal sources of protein are usually higher in saturated fat than other sources (Wardlaw 2002). Current recommendations are that 10 to 15 percent of the diet should consist of protein. Protein, like carbohydrate, provides four kilocalories per gram.

Fat

The purpose of **fat** in the body is to provide a concentrated supply of calories in a limited volume. Unlike protein or carbohydrate, fat provides nine kilocalories per gram. Fat also gives food some pleasant sensory qualities. Fat makes food tender and also adds a lovely smell when cooking. Think of the savory smell of bacon wafting across the kitchen. Fat can be more or less healthful depending on its level of saturation. Saturated fats tend to be hard at room temperature and come predominantly from animal sources. Examples of saturated fats include lard, butter, and marbling in steaks and meats. Palm oil, palm kernel, and coconut oils represent the only major plant sources of saturated fat (figure 4.4*a*). Unsaturated fats are liquid at room temperature and come from plant sources. Examples of unsaturated fats include olive, soybean, peanut, and canola oils (figure 4.4*b*).

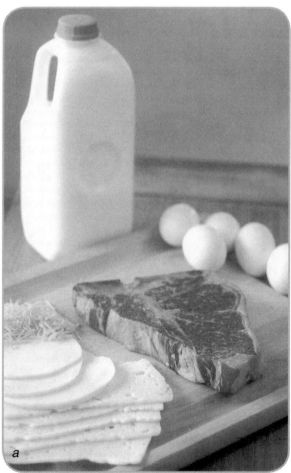

Photo by Dan Wendt

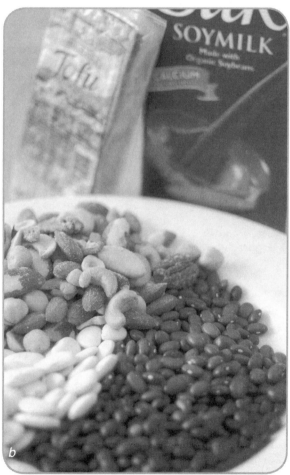

Photo by Dan Wendt

■ **Figure 4.3** Protein from *(a)* animal and *(b)* plant sources.

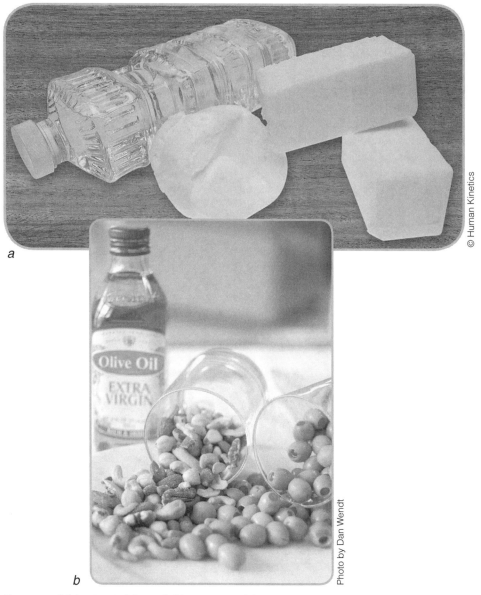

■ **Figure 4.4**   Sources of *(a)* saturated fat and *(b)* unsaturated fat.

Excess intake of saturated fats has been found to contribute to chronic diseases such as heart disease, cancer, stroke, and obesity. The American Heart Association (AHA) does not put a quantitative limit on total fat for the public, only for those trying to maintain or reduce weight, in which case the AHA recommends a level of fat intake of no more than 30 percent of total calories. Current U.S. levels of fat intake range from 30 to 40 percent as compared to European countries where the level of fat intake averages closer to 40 to 45 percent of total calories (Zeigler and Filer 2000). Cultures with diets high in animal products, such as the United States, tend to have higher levels of saturated fat intake. Items high in saturated fat also usually contain cholesterol. Both contribute to high levels of blood cholesterol.

Vitamins

Vitamins are organic substances that contribute to the normal functioning of the body. Vitamins are essential for normal growth and maintenance. Although vitamins contain no calories, they facilitate chemical reactions within the body that often yield energy (Wardlaw 2002). Vitamins can be either fat soluble or water soluble. The fat-soluble vitamins are vitamins A, D, E, and K. Not surprisingly, the fat-soluble vitamins are found in high-fat foods such as fatty fish, oils, and nuts. The water-soluble vitamins are the numerous B vitamins and vitamin C. The water-soluble vitamins are found in enriched and whole grains, fruits, and vegetables. Vitamin supplements are widely available. Multivitamins are a good source of dietary insurance but should never be used as a substitute for a good diet.

Minerals

Minerals are nonorganic substances that are necessary for normal functioning of the body. Minerals are needed for growth and maintenance. Minerals are classified as either major or trace minerals. Major minerals are classified as such if their daily requirement is over 100 milligrams or 1/50 teaspoon (Wardlaw 2002). The risk of mineral toxicity is fairly high when using high doses of supplements, so it's important to know the recommended dietary allowance (RDA). It is best not to exceed the RDA when choosing mineral supplements unless under the supervision of a health care provider.

Major minerals

Sodium

Potassium

Chloride

Calcium

Phosphorus

Magnesium

Sulfur

Trace minerals

Iron

Zinc

Selenium

Iodide

Copper

Fluoride

Chromium

Manganese

Molybdenum

Minerals, like vitamins, contain zero calories. One of the most important minerals to athletes, particularly females, is calcium. Throughout a life, the body continuously builds and breaks down bone. Humans turn over their skeleton every 7 to 10 years. The bone is built from minerals, primarily calcium. In fact, 99 percent of the calcium in the body is found in the skeleton (Zeigler and Filer 2000). Nutritional factors affecting bone density include calcium, vitamin D, and fluoride to build the mineral matrix, which forms the hard interior of the bone. The synthesis of bone is stimulated by weight-bearing exercises and certain hormones. In females with very low body fat,

there is a limited response to female hormones, thus leading to brittle bones and osteoporosis. Maintaining an ideal body weight, including not becoming overly thin, and performing weight-bearing activity will stimulate bone production and will help prevent osteoporosis and brittle bones (see figure 4.5*a* and *b*). Dairy foods are the primary source of calcium for children and adolescents. In instances of low intakes, supplementation is indicated. A health care provider should be consulted for recommendations regarding any needed supplementation.

Water

Many people are surprised that water is an essential nutrient. It makes up 50 to 70 percent of the human body's weight and serves multiple functions in the body:

- Water contributes to temperature regulation (each liter of sweat represents 600 kilocalories of energy lost).
- Water forms lubricants for the joints.
- Water is the basis for saliva and bile.
- Water helps to eliminate wastes via urine. Most people produce one to two quarts of urine per day (Wardlaw 2002).

Water can be obtained from various food and beverage sources; however, the best source is just simple water, be it tap or bottled. Items such as coffee, tea, and soda should not be considered good sources of water. These may contain caffeine, which is a diuretic. A diuretic causes increased fluid loss and an increased urine volume. This becomes especially important during exercise when fluid loss is already high due to perspiration.

In general, people need approximately 1 milliliter of water for every kilocalorie ingested. So, a person who eats 2,000 kilocalories a day needs to consume a minimum of 8 cups (1,920 milliliters) of water per day (1 cup = 240 milliliters). By the time a person loses as little as 1 percent of her body weight in fluids, she is getting thirsty. If she continues to ignore thirst, the body will release antidiuretic hormone (ADH), which will cause the kidneys to conserve water and concentrate the urine. This also triggers the body to release the hormone aldosterone, which causes water and sodium retention. With continued dehydration, the cardiovascular, respiratory, renal, and temperature regulation systems are compromised. With a continued loss of up to 20 percent of body weight in fluids, coma or death is imminent (Kleiner 1999).

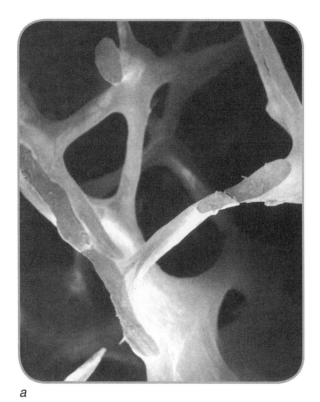 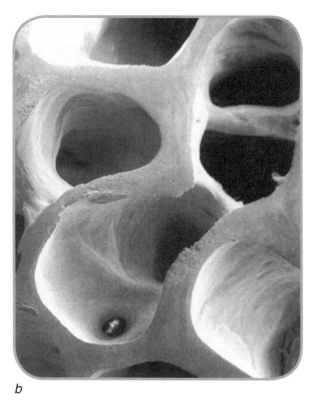

a   *b*

■ **Figure 4.5** View of (*a*) osteoporotic bone and (*b*) healthy bone.

Reprinted, by permission, from the American Society for Bone and Mineral Research, 1986, *Journal of Bone and Mineral Research* 1: 15-21.

Dietary Tools

Tools are available to help people make optimal food choices. These include the food guide pyramid, dietary guidelines, and food labeling regulations. The U.S. government created these tools, and information on each is readily available. Nutrition software programs are also available to help people monitor their nutritional needs and behaviors.

Food Guide Pyramid

The U.S. Department of Agriculture (USDA) developed the food guide pyramid to graphically show the most necessary nutrients within each food group, the number of recommended servings, and the foods within each group categorized by nutrient and density. Figure 4.6 is a modification of the food guide pyramid, with fluids added to emphasize the importance of hydration.

The food guide pyramid should be used as a general guide for healthful eating. In addition, the diet should allow for maintenance of an appropriate weight. Obesity is now at epidemic proportions in the United States. According to the Centers for Disease Control and Pre-

vention, more than 60 percent of adults are overweight or obese, and the percentage of young people who are overweight has more than doubled in the last three decades. For Americans ages 6 to 17, between 10 and 15 percent are overweight (2002). For more details, refer to the "Obesity" section in chapter 8.

Potential contributors to the obesity epidemic include people's difficulty with judging appropriate portion size along with decreased levels of daily activity. For example, according to the National Health and Nutrition Examination Survey III (NHANES III), the average American is eating 14 percent more calories daily than 30 years ago (CDC 1996). The amount of food that counts as a serving in each category is listed in table 4.2. If a person eats a larger amount than what is listed in table 4.2, it counts as more than one serving. For example, an average restaurant portion of spaghetti counts as two to three servings on the food guide pyramid.

Food Labels

The **Food and Drug Administration** (FDA) regulates food labeling (figure 4.7). The Nutrition Labeling and Education Act of 1990 (NLEA) revamped

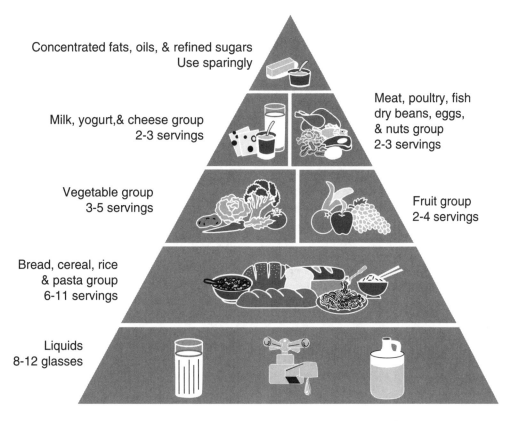

Concentrated fats, oils, & refined sugars
Use sparingly

Milk, yogurt,& cheese group
2-3 servings

Meat, poultry, fish
dry beans, eggs,
& nuts group
2-3 servings

Vegetable group
3-5 servings

Fruit group
2-4 servings

Bread, cereal, rice
& pasta group
6-11 servings

Liquids
8-12 glasses

■ **Figure 4.6** A modified food guide pyramid focusing on daily intake.

Reprinted, by permission, from AAHPERD, 1999, *Physical best activity guide—Elementary level* (Champaign, IL: Human Kinetics), 67.

TABLE 4.2   Serving Sizes to Use With the Food Guide Pyramid

Food group	Amounts that count as one serving
Milk, yogurt, and cheese	1 cup of milk or yogurt
	1.5 oz of natural cheese
	2 oz of processed cheese
Meat, poultry, fish, legumes, eggs, and nuts	2 to 3 oz of cooked lean meat, poultry, or fish
	1/2 cup of cooked dry beans, 1 egg, or 2 tbsp of peanut butter count as 1 oz of lean meat
Vegetables	1 cup of raw leafy vegetables
	1/2 cup of other vegetables, cooked or chopped raw
	3/4 cup of vegetable juice
Fruit	1 medium piece of fruit
	1/2 cup of chopped, cooked, or canned fruit
	3/4 cup of fruit juice
Bread, cereal, pasta, and grain	1 slice of bread
	1 oz of ready-to-eat cereal
	1/2 cup of cooked cereal, rice, or pasta

www.nal.usda.gov:8001/py/pmap.htm

the food label. It also standardized and established criteria for the health claims and nutrient content claims that appear on food labels. Under the NLEA requirements, nutrition labeling is required for most foods. Labeling of meat and poultry products is regulated by the USDA. Voluntary nutrition information is also available for fish and for the 20 most frequently eaten raw fruits and vegetables. In addition, information is available for the 45 best-selling cuts of meat. This information is available to the stores to post through these programs, and a 1996 survey found that more than 70 percent of U.S. foods were in compliance (FDA 1999). Most major grocery chains offer nutrition-based tours for public groups. Contact the local store manager to see if this is available in your area.

Under FDA regulations, food manufacturers are required to provide information on certain nutrients. Information on other nutrients can be provided on a voluntary basis. Figure 4.8 shows a list of each.

RDA amounts can't be used in food labeling because they're written specifically for different age groups and genders. Food labels require something more generic that can be used across populations. The daily values (DV) were established by the FDA just for this purpose. The daily values are based on a 2,000-calorie diet, which is an average intake. Of this 2,000-calorie intake, the daily values represent the following:

- Fat based on 30 percent of calories
- Saturated fat based on 10 percent of calories
- Carbohydrates based on 60 percent of calories
- Protein based on 10 percent of calories
- Fiber based on 11.5 grams of fiber per 1,000 calories

For the DV reference diet of 2,000 calories, this represents less than 65 grams of fat, less than 20 grams of saturated fat, less than 300 milligrams of cholesterol, and less than 2,400 milligrams of sodium (FDA 2003).

The FDA also regulates the claims that food manufacturers can make on their products, such as *low fat* or *light*. Appendix B lists claims and the requirements a food must meet before such claims can be put on product labels.

Food Labels at a Glance

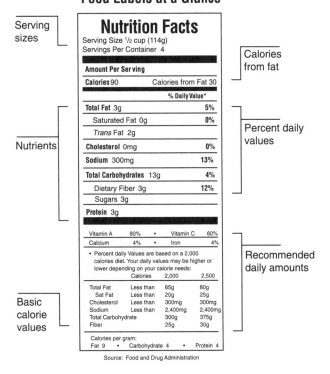

Figure 4.7 The standard format for food labeling, as developed by the Food and Drug Administration.

Mandatory	Optional
Total kcal	Kcal from saturated fat
Kcal from fat	Polyunsaturated fat
Total fat	Monounsaturated fat
Saturated fat	Potassium
Trans fat	Soluble fiber
Cholesterol	Insoluble fiber
Sodium	Sugar alcohol
Total carbohydrate	(includes sweeteners
Dietary fiber	sorbitol, xylitol,
Sugars	mannitol)
Protein	% of vitamin A as beta-
Vitamin A	carotene
Vitamin C	Other essential vitamins
Calcium	and minerals
Iron	

Figure 4.8 Mandatory and optional nutrient listings for a food label.

(FDA Office of Food Labeling, 2003, www.cfscan.fda.gov/~dms/fdnewwlab.html)

Dietary Guidelines

The USDA and USDHHS jointly collaborate to produce the Dietary Guidelines for Americans (figure 4.9), an overall set of guidelines for building a healthy, balanced lifestyle. These dietary guidelines are best used in conjunction with the food guide pyramid. The guidelines encourage moderation as well as variety in the diet. They also strive to moderate intake of fat and cholesterol. Finally, they also recommend moderating intake of sugar, sodium, and alcohol. If followed, these guidelines will minimize the risk of obesity and decrease risk for chronic disease in the future. Visit www.usda.gov for additional information.

Consequences of an Unhealthy Diet

There are no magic pills when it comes to maintaining an ideal diet. At the end of the day, it comes down to calories ingested must equal calories expended. This concept is called **energy balance**. Calorie

Aim for fitness
- Aim for a healthy weight.
- Be physically active each day.

Build a healthy base
- Let the pyramid guide your food choices.
- Choose a variety of grains daily, especially whole grains.
- Choose a variety of fruits and vegetables daily.
- Keep food safe to eat.

Choose sensibly
- Choose a diet that is low in saturated fat and cholesterol and moderate in total fat.
- Choose beverages and foods to moderate your intake of sugars.
- Choose and prepare foods with less salt.
- If you drink alcoholic beverages, do so in moderation.

■ **Figure 4.9** Dietary Guidelines for Americans.
From *Dietary Guidelines for Americans*, 5th ed., 2000, USDA.

requirements will, however, increase during periods of growth, and this must be accommodated as well. But if a person eats more than needed, then that person will gain weight. Period. One pound of fat is equivalent to 3,500 kilocalories. An additional 10 calories per day over a person's daily needs can result in a gain of a pound over a year! Also know that all calories are equal, no matter what food source they come from. Low-fat diets will result in weight gain if they contain excessive calories.

There are plenty of strategies you can use to help youngsters learn good eating habits. Remember, nutrition-related activities with students should emphasize the following:

- Individual eating habits should respect family lifestyles.
- Begin the day with breakfast to provide energy and nutrients.
- Control calorie consumption by spacing meals throughout the course of the day.
- Most nutritional needs should be met with regular meals, supplemented by snacks.
- Find pleasure in food while being aware of the nutrient and caloric content in food.
- Practice balance, variety, and moderation.
- Enjoy food. Enjoy good health. Enjoy life.

Additional Resources

The following Web sites provide additional information on nutrition:

- www.nutrition.gov—Comprehensive online resource for government-based nutrition information, including the Dietary Guidelines for Americans, food labeling information, and the food guide pyramids
- www.eatright.org—Web site for the American Dietetic Association
- www.navigator.tufts.edu—Reliable source for health and nutrition information
- vm.cfsan.fda.gov—Provides FDA information on supplements and food labeling
- www.usda.gov/fnic—Reviews food labeling standards
- www.nal.usda.gov/fnic/Fpr/pyramid.html—Provides information on the food guide pyramid

Other sources include programs such as The Power of Choice, which was developed by the U.S. Department of Health and Human Services, the Food and Drug Administration, and USDA's Food and Nutrition Service in 2003. It is intended for after-school program leaders working with young adolescents. The program includes a Leader's Guide that contains everything you need to know, including most activity materials. It's full of quick, simple things to do with kids; many activities take little or no preplanning. The publication contains 10 interactive sessions based on four posters. Included in the Leader's Guide are a recipe booklet, parent letter, and nutrition facts cards. A CD is also included that contains additional activities, tips for improved communication with adolescents, a training video for the adult leaders, and a song for preteens. The program is available to organizations participating in USDA's Child Nutrition programs. For more information, see www.fns.usda.gov/tn/Resources/power_of_choice.html.

Summary

The most serious consequence of a person's poor diet is an ongoing failure to achieve his or her physical best. The diet provides both energy and building blocks for everyone, regardless of activity level. It's impossible to build aerobic fitness without having the energy to keep the heart rate elevated. Muscular strength and endurance require building new muscle tissue with nutrients. Good flexibility requires a healthy skeleton, also built up from nutrients. An ideal body composition clearly depends on an appropriate diet. Good diet alone cannot create fitness, and neither can activity alone. The interactions of physical activity and nutrition are important in every person's life. People need physical activity as much as they need all 45 nutrients in their diet. A good diet will optimize physical activity and promote health. Use the information in this chapter to teach students these connections.

Components of Health-Related Fitness

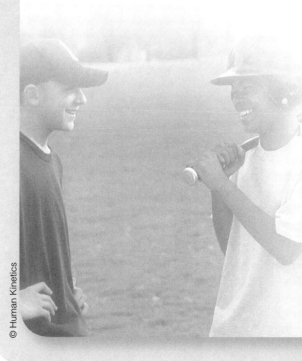

Part II covers the basic concepts and applications related to the components of health-related fitness for K-12 programming. Each chapter defines a component of health-related fitness and provides teaching guidelines and training methods related to that component. Chapter 5 focuses on aerobic fitness. Updated information is provided throughout this part of the book, including a new target heart rate zone formula in this chapter. Chapter 6 focuses on muscular strength and endurance. Muscular fitness is often taught as two separate components with adults, but strength and endurance are combined in the Physical Best program because it is developmentally appropriate to do so with children in a physical education setting. Chapter 7 explores flexibility training for youth, and chapter 8 covers body composition education, measurement, and related issues.

CHAPTER

5

Aerobic Fitness

Aerobic fitness is just one component of health-related fitness, but it is generally considered the most important physiological indicator of good health and physical condition. The many benefits of good aerobic fitness include those outlined in chapter 1. There are a number of other terms frequently used to describe this component of health-related fitness, such as *cardiorespiratory fitness*, *aerobic endurance*, *aerobic capacity*, *aerobic power*, *cardiorespiratory endurance*, *cardiovascular fitness*, and *cardiovascular endurance*. Throughout this chapter and text, we use the simpler term *aerobic fitness*.

The importance of increased physical activity and enhanced fitness in youth cannot be overemphasized. In fact, Healthy People 2010 (USDHHS 2000aa) lists physical activity as one of the nation's 10 leading health indicators, and two of the plan's objectives specifically target increased physical activity for youth. Objective 22-6 targets moderate physical activity, and the goal is to increase the proportion of adolescents who engage in moderate physical activity for at least 30 minutes on five or more days of the week. Objective 22-7 targets vigorous physical activity, striving to increase the proportion of adolescents who engage in vigorous physical activity that promotes aerobic fitness three or more days per week for 20 or more minutes per occasion. **Moderate physical activity** is defined as "activity of an intensity equal to brisk walking . . . and can be performed for relatively long periods of time without fatigue" (NASPE 2004b, 7). **Vigorous physical activity** is defined as "movement that expends more energy or is performed at a higher intensity than brisk walking. Some forms of vigorous activity, such as running, can be done for relatively long periods of time while others may be so vigorous (e.g., sprinting) that frequent rests are necessary" (NASPE 2004b, 8).

Lack of physical activity during adolescence may also have long-term health implications as an adult. There is a known increase in morbidity and mortality in adults attributable to chronic disease and sedentary lifestyles (USDHHS 2000aa). Research (Guo et al. 1994) also shows an association between overweight adolescents and an increased risk of being overweight as an adult; in addition, Janz (2002) states that maintenance of physical fitness through puberty has favorable health benefits in later years. Further rationale for promoting increased physical activity during childhood stems from the *National Health and Nutrition Examination Survey, Phase I, 1988-1991* (McDowell et al. 1994). Data indicate that increased caloric intake is not solely responsible for the increased prevalence of overweight youth, and that lack of physical activity may be a contributing factor. Many organizations, including the National Association for Sport and Physical Education (NASPE 2004b), the Centers for Disease Control and Prevention (CDC 1997; CDC 2000), the American Academy of Pediatrics (AAP 2000b), and the U.S. Department of Health and Human Services (USDHHS 2000bb), advocate increasing childhood physical activity that will carry into adulthood, thereby reducing health problems associated with inactivity. This is where Physical Best can help you provide your students

with the knowledge, skills, values, and confidence they need to engage in physical activity now and in the future through fun and enjoyable activities.

Defining and Measuring Aerobic Fitness

The American College of Sports Medicine defines **aerobic fitness** as the "ability to perform large muscle, dynamic, moderate- to high-intensity exercise for prolonged periods" (ACSM 2000, 68). A person's level of aerobic fitness is contingent upon the ability of the heart and lungs to circulate oxygen-rich blood to the exercising tissues. For a child, this definition may mean the ability to exercise or play for long periods of time without getting tired.

The criterion measure of aerobic fitness is **maximal oxygen consumption** ($\dot{V}O_2$max), a laboratory test measuring the maximal amount of oxygen that can be consumed despite an increase in workload. This test provides information on how efficiently the body uses oxygen during moderate to vigorous physical activity. Many valid and reliable field tests are also available to predict $\dot{V}O_2$max from submaximal aerobic fitness tests. Physical Best exclusively endorses *FITNESSGRAM/ACTIVITYGRAM* (developed by the Cooper Institute) and all related materials and products as the submaximal assessment instrument to estimate $\dot{V}O_2$max and aerobic fitness (see chapter 13). Teachers may choose the mile run, the PACER (progressive aerobic cardiovascular endurance run), or the mile walk test depending on the age and ability of the student. Refer to the *FITNESSGRAM/ACTIVITYGRAM Test Administration Manual* (CIAR 2004) for more information on the administration of these tests. Physical Best also supports the use of the Brockport Physical Fitness Test (BPFT) for individuals with disabilities. The BPFT is also a health-related fitness assessment instrument and may serve as a valuable tool, not only for fitness testing, but also for the development of an individualized education plan for students with disabilities. This test "may be used to identify the present level of performance, identify unique needs, and establish annual goals including short-term objectives" (Winnick 1999, 6). It is beyond the scope of this text to describe the BPFT in detail. For more information, refer to the *Brockport Physical Fitness Test Manual* (Winnick and Short 1999a).

The *FITNESSGRAM* PACER test is recommended for all ages and is preferred for participants in grades K-3. The emphasis in grades K-3 should be on having fun and allowing the students to participate in a pleasant experience. The PACER also serves as an excellent tool for teaching the concept of pacing for the mile run at the elementary, middle, or high school level. An additional feature of *FITNESSGRAM* is the capability to compare results among the three aerobic fitness tests. As you read and use the *FITNESSGRAM/ACTIVITYGRAM* test manual, note that the Cooper Institute (creators of *FITNESSGRAM/ACTIVITYGRAM*) uses the term *aerobic capacity* instead of *aerobic fitness*; however, as previously noted, the terms are synonymous.

Teaching Guidelines for Aerobic Fitness

Fitness concepts should be taught through physical activity, and classroom lessons where the students are inactive should be minimized, especially if the class only meets once or twice per week. Focus on a single concept each day, rather than multiple concepts. You could teach anatomy by presenting a muscle or bone each class period during the warm-up and cool-down, or the circulatory system could be covered using a jogging course where the students act as blood traveling through the heart, arteries, or veins. Cross-discipline lessons and homework may also serve as other avenues to teach fitness concepts.

Children of all ages should develop an understanding of aerobic fitness. When working with children, keep in mind that they are not "little adults." Adult training strategies of continuous exercise, use of the FITT guidelines, and interpretation of test results are not the same for children. A child's score on an aerobic fitness test does not predict performance in endurance activities. Even if adult training guidelines are applied, it is unclear whether the increases in aerobic fitness, as measured by $\dot{V}O_2max$ (ml/kg/min), are due to training or simply due to increases in body size and maturation (Rowland 1996). When teaching children about aerobic fitness, keep in mind that genetics, developmental factors, body composition, and activity levels influence differences in performance on any aerobic fitness assessment. The goal of the Physical Best program is to promote noncompetitive, self-enhancing, and fun activities that encourage students to be physically active now and later, as adults. Even if the relationship is not strong between increased physical activity and aerobic fitness in children (Rowland 1996), the program

aspires to promote active children to become active adults for whom aerobic training (following the FITT guidelines) yields improvements in aerobic fitness and enhanced health benefits. Parents, teachers, and coaches should encourage participation in a wide variety of enjoyable and available activities; they should place less emphasis on activity and exercise at a specified target heart rate and less emphasis on sport-specific training and conditioning (figure 5.1). This is important for two reasons: (1) Participation in a variety of activities during childhood is related to greater sports success later in life while decreasing the physical, physiological, and psychological demands of specializing in a single sport as a child; (2) emphasizing physical activity and fitness skills as opposed to sports training decreases the risk of children's injuries (AAP 2000a; Faigenbaum 2001).

When preparing to teach students about physical activity and fitness, remember that the level and tempo of a child's play activity are characterized by alternating cycles of vigorous activity followed by a recovery period (Bailey et al. 1995; Corbin and Pangrazi 2002). Plan multiple activities with rest periods to provide variety and to parallel a child's natural play pattern. Circuit training provides an excellent challenge where children can independently explore movement, develop fundamental motor skills, and develop areas of health-related fitness. Circuits or station activities also provide opportunities for all children to be successful. Stations may be set up with different challenge levels, and the student may explore and self-select activities to promote success. This type of activity removes the element of competition and the necessity to determine a winner and a loser of the activity. Many Physical Best activities use stations or are designed so that most children are active at the same time.

NASPE (2004b) suggests 11 guidelines for promoting physical activity in schools and physical education. As a physical educator, you can use these guidelines to enhance your lessons and to promote active lifestyles outside of the physical education setting.

- Provide time for activity throughout the school day—include recess and short activity breaks that supplement the allotted time for physical education.
- Encourage self-monitoring of physical activity.
- Individualize activity.
- Expose children to a variety of physical activities.

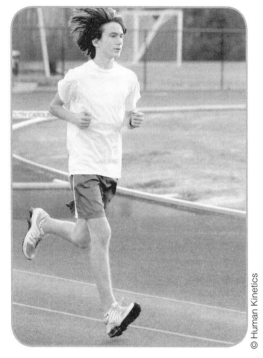
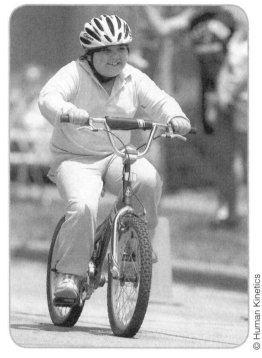
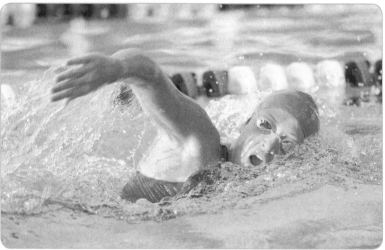

Figure 5.1   Sample activities that can help students improve aerobic fitness.

- Offer feedback that reinforces regular participation and encourages children to give their best effort; avoid giving feedback on how fast the performance was or how many repetitions were completed.

- Do not sacrifice class time for fitness-only activities—include fundamental skill development.

- Be an active role model.

- Care about the attitudes of your students. Help them set goals and then provide achievable challenges to meet those goals.

- Enhance exercise self-efficacy by teaching the value of various activities and how to develop personalized exercise or activity programs that can be achieved.

- Promote activity outside the school environment.

- Consider lifetime activities that will carry into adulthood such as walking, jogging, hiking, or cycling. Physical Best provides an opportunity for students to learn why activities are important and what the benefits of the activity are for today and in the future.

Determining How Much Physical Activity Is Needed

Aerobic fitness activities form a large segment of the physical activity pyramid (see figure 3.3) which parallels activity recommendations by the International Consensus Conference on Physical Activity Guidelines for Adolescents (Sallis and Patrick 1994), NASPE guidelines for elementary school aged children (NASPE 2004b), and Healthy People 2010 recommendations (USDHHS 2000aa). The following is recommended for adolescents (Sallis and Patrick 1994):

1. All adolescents should be physically active daily, or nearly every day, as part of play, games, sports, work, transportation, recreation, physical education, or planned exercise, in the context of family, school, and community activities.

2. Adolescents should engage in three or more sessions per week of activities that last 20 minutes or more at a time and that require moderate to vigorous levels of exertion.

NASPE (2004b) guidelines for elementary school aged children state the following:

1. Children should accumulate at least 60 minutes, and up to several hours, of age-appropriate physical activity on all or most days of the week. This daily accumulation should include moderate and vigorous physical activity with the majority being intermittent in nature.

2. Children should participate in several bouts of physical activity lasting 15 minutes or more each day.

3. Children should participate each day in a variety of age-appropriate physical activities designed to achieve optimal health, wellness, fitness, and performance benefits.

4. Extended periods (periods of two hours or more) of inactivity are discouraged for children, especially during daytime hours (p. 9-10).

To assist teachers in determining what activities are considered moderate, vigorous, or age-appropriate, the following definitions are provided by NASPE (2004b). **Age or developmentally appropriate physical activity** "refers to activity of a frequency, intensity, duration and type that leads to optimal child growth and development and contributes to the development of future physically active lifestyles"

(p. 8). **Moderate physical activity** is described as follows: "Activities of moderate intensity can be performed for relatively long periods of time without fatigue" (p. 7). The authors suggest brisk walking, bike riding, some chores or housework, low-intensity games such as hopscotch or four-square, or playing low-activity positions such as goalie or outfield. Vigorous physical activity "is movement that expends more energy or is performed at a higher intensity than brisk walking. Some forms of vigorous activity, such as running, can be done for relatively long periods of time while others may be so vigorous (e.g., sprinting) that frequent rests are necessary" (p. 7-8).

Aerobic fitness lessons should include teachers helping students to explore practical applications such as logging free-time aerobic fitness activities or lifestyle activities in a journal, learning to take their pulse, or organizing a school fitness night for families and friends.

Be sure that students who are new to aerobic activity start out slowly. It is better to gradually increase one variable (frequency, intensity, or time) at a time rather than increasing all three variables, and for the less-fit individual, it is better to increase time (duration) first instead of intensity. Children are less likely to become discouraged, and they will adhere to an activity or exercise program, if it does not cause extreme fatigue and soreness. You must remember that long periods of continuous vigorous activity are not recommended for children age 6 to 12 unless chosen by the child and not prescribed by an adult (NASPE 2004b).

To reduce the risk of injury or medical complications, work with the school nurse to determine which students have medical conditions that you should be aware of, such as orthopedic problems, asthma, epilepsy, diabetes, or other disabilities. Proper screening of your students will help you develop a well-rounded program that addresses the needs of all students, including those who should use extra caution when engaging in aerobic fitness activities.

Aerobic Fitness Training Principles

The training principles (progression, overload, specificity, individuality, and regularity) outlined in chapter 3 should be followed when developing aerobic fitness. These guidelines are especially helpful for older children; however, Welk and Blair (2002) point out that "just because children CAN adapt to physical training does not mean they should be encouraged or required to do so" (p. 14). Postpubescent children will respond more favorably to training and conditioning in contrast to younger prepubescent and pubescent children (Payne and Morrow 1993). Rather than emphasize the adult exercise prescription model, it is generally agreed that the aim with children should be to foster and maintain a physically active lifestyle, as previously outlined. It is beyond the scope of this text to fully explain the physiological changes affecting aerobic fitness and performance that occur in children during aerobic training. For more information on the trainability of children and endurance performance, refer to *Developmental Exercise Physiology* (Rowland 1996) or *Total Training for Young Champions* (Bompa 2000).

Although the lifetime physical activity model provides guidelines for aerobic fitness training sufficient for good health, you may encounter students who want to achieve higher levels of fitness. It is important to provide accurate and helpful information to assist interested students in reaching their aerobic fitness goals safely; however, the five training principles are only applicable to older, postpubescent children. Table 5.1 provides information on how to apply the FITT guidelines for younger (5 to 12 years old) and adolescent (11 and older) children as well as older youth participating in athletics. Note that table 5.1 includes some overlap in age, allowing for changes in the guidelines based on individual developmental age, not chronological age.

Taking the Pulse

There are some inherent difficulties estimating **maximal heart rate** (MHR) using the common formula (220 minus age) and subsequently calculating an exercise heart rate as a marker of training intensity in children. Children's maximal heart rates are age independent and generally range from 195 to 205 beats per minute; the range for maximal heart rate does not change with age until the late teens (Rowland 1996).

Recent research (Tanaka, Monahan, and Seals 2001) suggests a new formula for estimating maximal heart rate: $208 - (.7 \times age)$. Although children were not used as participants in the development of the new formula, the new formula estimates maximal heart rates in children more in line with the range of 195 to 205 beats per minute reported by Armstrong et al. (1991); Bailey et al. (1978); Cumming, Everatt, and Hastman (1978); and Rowland (1996).

While the old formula was simpler to use, it generally overpredicted MHR in those 20 to 40 years of age and underpredicted MHR in those over 40 years of age (Tanaka, Monahan, and Seals 2001).

More research is needed, especially on children, but the general consensus on the new equation is that it will be adopted in clinical settings, and it is already included in at least one fitness and wellness textbook. Therefore, for high school students, the new formula, MHR = $208 - (.7 \times age)$, should be used to calculate exercise heart rates. Younger children (age 6 to 14 years) should not use exercise heart rate thresholds or zones. Younger children should engage in activity following the previously discussed NASPE (2004b) guidelines for elementary school children or the guidelines for adolescents (Sallis and Patrick 1994).

As mentioned, long periods of vigorous continuous activity are not considered to be age and developmentally appropriate for children 6 to 12 years old unless the child self-selects the activity (NASPE 2004b). High-intensity activity may actually discourage children from being active because it is generally unpleasant to exercise at this level. The emphasis for children should be on having fun and developing the locomotor skills necessary to succeed in more advanced activity or sport later in life. Malina (1996) suggests that activities performed in adulthood are based on locomotor and leisure skills learned early in a child's life. If a child is confident in the skills developed during childhood, he or she is more likely to continue those activities into adulthood. Also, self-perception of competence declines as children get older (Jacobs et al. 2002), and children who underestimate their physical competence may discontinue participation in sport or may have low levels of physical achievement (Weiss and Horn 1990). You should keep this information in mind when working with children. Exercising at specified training heart rates or performing continuous high-intensity activity should be reserved for high school students.

Target Heart Rate Zones

For students beyond age 14, teachers may begin to introduce the calculation of target heart rates using the new maximal heart rate formula or the heart rate reserve (HRR) method. For younger students, you can begin to teach concepts of intensity and heart rate monitoring—providing the student with opportunities to compare resting heart rate with exercise heart rate, to learn basic anatomy of the

TABLE 5.1 FITT Guidelines Applied to Aerobic Fitness

	Children (5-12 years)[a]	Adolescents (11+ years)[b]	Middle and high school youth who participate in athletics[c]
Frequency	• Developmentally appropriate physical activity on all or most days of the week • Several bouts of physical activity lasting 15 min or more daily	• Daily or nearly every day • Three or more sessions per week	5 or 6 days per week
Intensity	• Mixture of moderate and vigorous intermittent activity • Moderate includes low-intensity games (hopscotch, four-square), low-activity positions (goalie, outfielders), some chores, and yard work • Vigorous includes games involving running or chasing and playing sports (level 2 of activity pyramid)	• Moderate to vigorous activity. Maintaining a target heart rate is not expected at this level. • 12-16 rating of perceived exertion (RPE)[d]	• 60-90% heart rate max (MHR) or 50-85% heart rate reserve (HRR) • 12-16 rating of perceived exertion (RPE)[d]
Time	• Accumulation of at least 60 min, and up to several hr, of activity • Up to 50% of accumulated min should be accumulated in bouts of 15 min or more	• 30-60 min daily activity • 20 min or more in a single session	20-60 min
Type	• Variety of activities • Activities should be selected from the first 3 levels of the activity pyramid • Continuous activity should not be expected for most children	• Play, games, sports, work, transportation, recreation, physical education, or planned exercise in the context of family, school, and community activities • Brisk walking, jogging, stair climbing, basketball, racket sports, soccer, dance, lap swimming, skating, lawn mowing, and cycling	Activities that use large muscles and are used in a rhythmical fashion (e.g., brisk walking, jogging, stair climbing, basketball, racket sports, soccer, dance, lap swimming, skating, and cycling)

[a]National Association for Sport and Physical Education (2004). *Physical activity for children: A statement of guidelines for children ages 5-12*, 2nd edition (Reston, VA: Author).

[b]Corbin, C .B., and Pangrazi, R. P. (2002). Physical activity for children: how much is enough? In G. J. Welk, R. J. Morrow, & H. B. Falls (Eds), *Fitnessgram Reference Guide* (p. 7 Internet Resource). Dallas, TX: The Cooper Institute.

[c]American College of Sports Medicine (2000). ACSM's guidelines for exercise testing and prescription. 6th Ed., Lippincott, Williams, and Wilkins: Philadelphia.

[d]Borg, G. (1998). *Borg's perceived exertion and pain scales* (Champaign, IL: Human Kinetics), 47.

cardiovascular and respiratory systems, and to learn how increased physical activity helps children play longer without getting tired. Reserve calculations and goals of meeting a specified target heart rate for high school students (or at least late teen years). Primary grade students can begin to monitor their intensity levels by placing a hand over the heart before, during, and after moderate to vigorous physical activity; they can note the general speed of the heartbeat using terms such as slow, medium, and fast or turtle and race car. Fourth- through sixth-grade students can begin to locate the carotid and radial arteries to count heart rate, but they should not use target heart rate zones. Most students seventh grade and up can be expected to calculate target heart rate values, but you should still avoid the use of target heart rate zones (THRZ) as requirements for participation in physical activities.

High school students can begin to use the THRZ to guide them in monitoring intensity of activity. Refer to tables 5.1 and 5.2 for selecting the appropriate percentage to monitor intensity. Once intensity has been selected, begin by teaching the heart rate max method (Tanaka, Monahan, and Seals 2001), which is the simpler of the two methods of calculating the THRZ. To save class time, students can perform this calculation as a homework assignment. The second method, the Karvonen or heart rate reserve (HRR) method (ACSM 2000; Tanaka, Monahan, and Seals 2001) takes into account the individual's resting heart rate. Refer to "Calculating Maximum Heart Rate and Target Heart Rate Zones for Middle or High School Students" section.

If teachers working with young children (6-14 years old) must make use of a target heart rate, they should use 85 percent heart rate max (HR max = 200 beats per minute) (Rowland 1996). This is equal to approximately 170 beats per minute (T.W. Rowland, personal communication, December 2002). This heart rate provides a goal for students to attain but does not necessarily relate to intensities necessary for fitness improvement. Rowland's *Developmental Exercise Physiology* (1996) provides further explanation of the physiological changes and the high-intensity exercise required to elicit those changes in children. Remember that specifying target heart rates is not recommended for elementary level children.

Two common sites used to count heart rate are the carotid artery (on the neck) and the radial artery (wrist, thumb side). Teach students to first locate the pulse by placing their first two fingers of the right hand lightly on the right side of their neck, below and to the right of the Adam's apple (figure 5.2a). The Adam's apple is not prominent in children, especially for girls. In an alternate method, the children look straight ahead and place two fingers on the bone behind the bottom earlobe (mastoid process), and then gently press and slowly slide the fingers down and forward until the heartbeat is felt. The fingers will naturally follow the angle of the jaw and end up to the right of the Adam's apple. (K-3 children may place their hand over the left side of the chest to feel the heartbeat.) Be sure each student is capable of feeling his or her heart beating. Make sure students do not press

TABLE 5.2   Progression of Activity Frequency, Intensity, and Time Based on Fitness Level

	Low Fitness	Marginal Fitness	Good Fitness
Frequency	3 days a week	3 to 5 days a week	3 to 6 days a week
Intensity			
Heart rate reserve (HRR)	40-50%	50-60%	60-85%
Maximum heart rate (max HR)	55-65%	65-75%	75-90%
Relative perceived exertion (RPE)	12-13	13-14	14-16
Time	10-30 min	20-40 min	30-60 min

Reprinted from C. Corbin et al., 2004, *Concepts of Fitness and Wellness,* 5th ed. (New York, NY: McGraw-Hill Companies). Reproduced with permission of The McGraw-Hill Companies.

Calculating Maximum Heart Rate and Target Heart Rate Zones for Middle or High School Students

Heart Rate Max Method

The first step when using this method is to calculate the maximal heart rate (MHR) using the new formula: $208 - (.7 \times age)$. Then, to calculate a target heart rate zone (THRZ), select a percentage between 55/60 to 90 percent. This becomes the threshold percentage for the calculation of target heart rate. Next, select a second percentage 10 percent higher than the threshold percentage. For example, a student who is 16 years old seeking a basic level of fitness (at 65-75 percent MHR) would find his or her THRZ as follows:

$$MHR = 208 - (.7 \times 16) = 196.8 \text{ or } 197$$

Calculate the THRZ by changing the selected percentages to decimals and multiplying them by the MHR:

$$.65 \times 197 = 128.05 \text{ or } 128$$

$$.75 \times 197 = 147.75 \text{ or } 148$$

Rounded to the nearest whole number, this student's THRZ for maintaining or improving basic aerobic fitness is 128 to 148 heartbeats per minute.

Karvonen Method

This method takes into account an individual's fitness level and resting heart rate. For high school students, this method can be taught and used to demonstrate how intensity can be modified as fitness levels improve and resting heart rate decreases. This is also known as the **heart rate reserve** (HRR) method and involves multiple steps. HRR is calculated by subtracting resting heart rate from maximal heart rate. Once this is completed, the student follows the same procedures in selecting two percentages; however, the range of possible percentages is slightly different (50-85 percent) and the final step is to add back in resting heart rate. For example, the same 16-year-old student, with a resting heart rate of 70, seeking a basic level of fitness (at 65-75 percent MHR) would find his or her THRZ as follows:

$$MHR = 208 - (.7 \times 16) = 196.8 \text{ or } 197$$

Calculate the THRZ by subtracting resting heart rate from maximal heart rate, and complete the following formula where HRR is heart rate reserve and RHR is resting heart rate. In this example, resting heart rate is 70 beats per minute. $HRR = [208 - (.7 \times AGE) - RHR]$ and THRZ is $[[[208 - (.7 \times AGE)] - RHR] \times \%] + RHR$

$$HRR = [208 - (.7 \times 16) - 70] = 127$$

$$THRZ = [[[208 - (.7 \times 16)] - 70] \times .65] + 70 = 152.55 \text{ or } 153$$

$$THRZ = [[[208 - (.7 \times 16)] - 70] \times .75] + 70 = 165.25 \text{ or } 165$$

Rounded to the nearest whole number, this student's THRZ for maintaining or improving basic aerobic fitness is 153 to 165 heartbeats per minute.

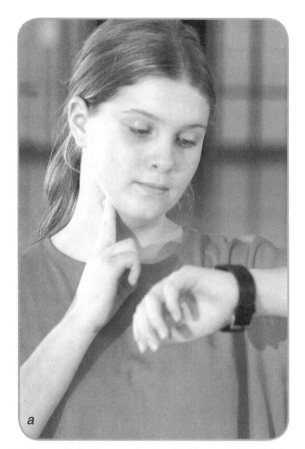

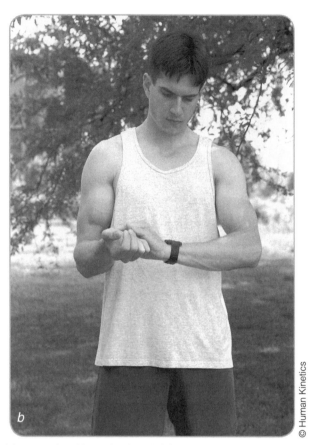

■ **Figure 5.2** Two methods of taking a pulse: *(a)* the carotid artery (neck) method and *(b)* the radial artery (wrist) method.

too hard or massage the neck because this will slow the heart rate; they should never palpate both arteries at the same time because reduced blood flow to the brain may cause the student to faint. Teach older students to use the radial artery at the wrist by placing their first two fingers of either hand on the opposite wrist (palm facing up), just below the base of the thumb (figure 5.2*b*). Students should move their fingers around until they locate the pulse.

Heartbeat is often counted for one minute when measuring resting heart rate; shorter time intervals are used to measure exercise heart rate. If the first heartbeat is counted while simultaneously starting the stopwatch, the first beat should be counted as zero. If the stopwatch is running, the first beat should be counted as one (ACSM 2001). Students may either count their pulse for 6 seconds and multiply by 10 (simply add a zero to the number they counted), count for 10 seconds and multiply by 6 (see table 5.3), or count for 15 seconds and multiply by 4.

Using Heart Rate Monitors

Although heart rate monitors are not necessary, they are a popular and exciting way to teach students about

TABLE 5.3 Heart Rate Based on a 10-Second Count

Beats	Heart rate	Beats	Heart rate
10	60	22	132
11	66	23	138
12	72	24	144
13	78	25	150
14	84	26	156
15	90	27	162
16	96	28	168
17	102	29	174
18	108	30	180
19	114	31	186
20	120	32	192
21	126	33	198

© Human Kinetics

TEACHING TIP: Teaching About Aerobic Fitness

Many students, particularly young children, will understand and monitor their heart rates more effectively when you provide some extra context. For example, you might use a metronome for teaching about heart rate. Students will better understand what 200 beats per minute sounds like.

Another fun method to reinforce how hard the heart works is to ask the students to calculate how many beats their hearts have made since birth. Figure out how many heartbeats per minute, then per hour, per day, per week, per year, and then years since birth. Encourage students to be as exact as their ages and abilities allow.

Carolyn Masterson, Associate Professor
Montclair State University
Upper Montclair, New Jersey

aerobic fitness concepts. Heart rate monitors provide accurate information, whereas some students may have difficulty manually palpating the pulse, especially children below the fourth grade. If using heart rate monitors at the elementary level, make sure they are used for fun and for teaching aerobic fitness concepts, and not for attaining a specified target heart rate. You may try activities such as asking students, "Who can get their heart rate to 140 beats per minute?" "150 beats per minute?" and so on, followed by a rest period. Then repeat the sequence using different heart rate goals. This provides short bursts of activity, is considered vigorous activity when higher heart rates are used, and provides a goal for elementary students to attain for brief periods. At the middle and high school levels, these monitors can be used to check calculated target heart rate or exercise intensity and to help teach students about individualizing aerobic fitness programs.

Cross-Discipline Ideas

There are many opportunities to use a cross-disciplinary approach when teaching aerobic fitness concepts. Coordinate activities with math, science, and language arts. Examples of cross-discipline activities might include calculating target heart rates (at the middle or high school level) or adding up the number of minutes of physical activity during physical education class, recess, and at home (at the elementary level). Language arts teachers may have children write about what they did in physical education today. Science teachers may help students follow a drop of blood through the heart, lungs, and to the exercising muscles.

Pulse Math

To promote interdisciplinary learning, you can easily create math problems based on calculating heart rate by having students count their pulse for different intervals. To add interest, make up problems such as the following:

1. Sam counted 35 heartbeats in 30 seconds. What is Sam's heart rate?

   60 seconds ÷ 30 seconds = 2

   So you multiply 35 heartbeats by 2:

   35 heartbeats × 2 = 70 heartbeats per minute

2. Lan counted 27 heartbeats in 10 seconds. What is Lan's heart rate?

   60 seconds ÷ 10 seconds = 6

   So you multiply 27 heartbeats by 6:

   27 heartbeats × 6 = 162 heartbeats per minute

3. Which person is more likely to be jogging, Sam or Lan? (Lan) Which person is more likely to be sitting in class? (Sam)

Because this is a practical way to integrate math across the curriculum, fourth-, fifth-, and sixth-grade classroom teachers may be willing to help you construct similar problems or may provide time in math class for students to learn and complete this type of work. Some students may also be able to design problems for themselves or peers to complete.

Training Methods for Aerobic Fitness

Three main training methods are used to maintain or increase aerobic fitness: continuous, interval, and circuit training. You must adjust application of these methods depending on the age, ability, and fitness level of each student. Building personal choice into each activity can do some of this individualizing for you. For example, offer a longer rest option during interval training, or allow students to assist in the development of aerobic fitness circuits. Remember that students can monitor heart rates, but calculations and target heart rate zones should only be used for older students, as previously discussed.

Continuous Training

Continuous training is performing the same activity or exercise over an extended time period. This style of activity is not common for children. **Continuous activity** is defined as "movement that lasts at least several minutes without rest periods" (NASPE 2004b, 6). As stated previously, vigorous continuous activity is not recommended for children 6 to 12 years old; however, some continuous moderate activity is appropriate (NASPE 2004b). If using continuous activity at the elementary level, build plenty of rest periods in the activity. Three to five minutes of continuous activity at a moderate intensity level may be the limit for primary grades or low-fit students, whereas 10 minutes may be a good limit for older (grades three to five) elementary students. Twenty minutes or more of continuous activity, depending on fitness level and goals, is appropriate for middle school through high school. Table 5.1 provides information on using the FITT guidelines for youth of various ages.

For students at the high school level, calculating and monitoring exercise heart rate becomes important. At the middle school level, students can calculate heart rate, but should not be required to maintain a set range. Activity at high intensities can become discouraging, so limit the time spent performing high-intensity activity, which is often more appropriate for training and conditioning athletes. Middle and high school students may use the adult model and calculate target heart rates or simply perform the activity at a pace where a conversation can comfortably occur.

To apply the principles of overload and progression, increase the frequency, intensity, or duration of the activity to provide positive health benefits to your more-fit students, but do not lose the enjoyment factor by increasing these variables too quickly. Also, frequency, intensity, and duration should not be increased at the same time in any single workout, nor should the weekly training volume be increased by more than 10 percent (ACSM 2001). Active, low-organization games are fun ways to provide continuous physical activity. Teach games and activities that students will want to play in their free time. Middle and high school students may find that a mix of aerobic activities that sustain a target elevated heart rate for a designated period of time will be more enjoyable and therefore more beneficial to their overall fitness level.

Fartlek training is a modification of continuous training where periods of increased intensity are interspersed with continuous activity over varying and natural terrain. The word *fartlek* comes from the Swedish word for "speed play," and the bursts of higher intensity exercise are not systematically controlled as in interval training. True fartlek training should be reserved for coaches and athletes and should not be used in physical education classes. This type of training (traversing over hills) develops technique, strength, muscular endurance, general aerobic endurance, and mental fitness (Greene and Pate 1997); these benefits are not attributes that physical educators are trying to develop in the classroom. This training should only be used by coaches working with serious athletes who want to increase speed in a particular sport such as basketball. Despite the negative aspects of true fartlek training, a modified version of it may be used at the elementary level by placing stress on different muscle groups, changing levels and direction frequently (Virgilio 1997). Figure 5.3 shows a sample fartlek training course appropriate for older, reasonably well-conditioned elementary students.

Circuit Training

Circuit training involves several different exercises or activities, allowing you to vary the intensity or type of activity as children move from station to station. Children naturally engage in this intermittent type of activity. Bailey et al. (1995) suggest that intermittent activity mixed with short rest periods is necessary for normal growth and development. You can also adjust

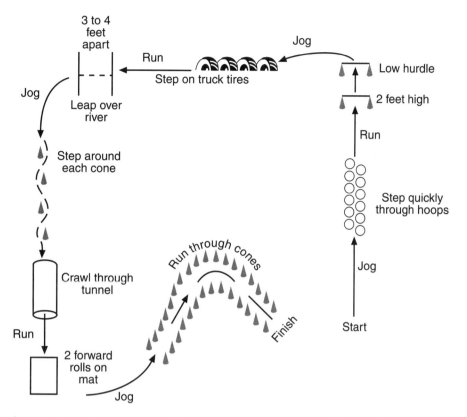

Line Change

Virgilio (1997) offers a continuous aerobic fitness activity. This could also be considered a fartlek training activity (see the "Continuous Training" section) because students may have to speed up temporarily to take over the lead.

Arrange students in straight lines of seven or eight, facing the same direction. Have them begin jogging or walking in any direction, staying in lines. At the signal, the last student in line jogs to the front to become the leader. Continue until everyone has had a chance to lead the line.

intensity by changing the amount of time each group spends at each station or the amount of rest or activity between stations (for instance, stretching between stations versus running once around the activity area). An example of circuit training appropriate for elementary age children is shown in figure 5.4. Middle and high school students might use the weight room and lift weights to music, changing the exercise station every 30 seconds. Circuit training is an excellent way to create variety in aerobic fitness activity because the possible station combinations are endless. Older elementary students and middle and high school students can even design the stations as a practical application of the fitness knowledge they are learning. Like continuous training, circuit training should be aerobic in nature, and the individual's fitness level will dictate the intensity and duration of the activity. To keep the activity organized and moving quickly, consider using task cards and arrow signs to help facilitate the movement direction of the activities.

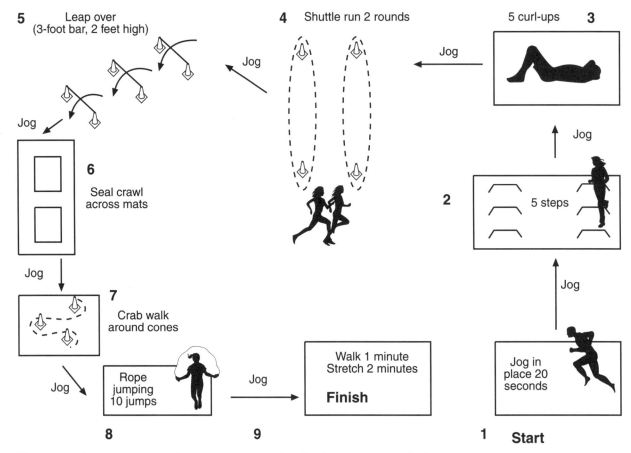

Figure 5.4 Sample circuit training plan appropriate for elementary age children.

Reprinted, by permission, from S. Virgilio, 1997, *Fitness education for children* (Champaign, IL: Human Kinetics), 149.

Interval Training

Interval training is based on the concept that more activity can be performed at higher exercise intensities with the same or even less fatigue compared to continuous training (figure 5.5). This type of training involves alternating short bursts of activity with rest periods. Young children naturally engage in this type of activity; you must simply ensure that the students have a rest period between activity bursts. This may also serve as an opportunity for older students to have a choice of how quickly the work period begins. Once middle and high school students know how to palpate heart rate, you can have them count their preexercise heart rate and use this number to determine when the next activity begins. For this to be effective, you will want to limit the maximum number of students at any one station. So even if a student's heart rate has decreased, signaling it is time to move on, the student must wait until a spot opens for him at the next station. Start each station with the same number of students, and plan equipment and space for three or four extra students per station. Most students will naturally want to move to the next station, especially if the activities are fun. Older students are capable of engaging in more structured interval training, but this should not be part of your physical education lesson. The trick is to make this type of training interesting. Leave running wind sprints for the track coach and have your students, for example, pass a soccer ball between partners, running as fast as they can downfield. Interval training can be designed to develop aerobic fitness by matching activity time (generally three to four minutes) with the equivalent rest interval (three to four minutes rest) or by using one-half the work period as the time interval for the rest period (one and a half to two minutes rest).

Station Learning and Equipment

Stations arranged on a circuit are a good way to stretch the equipment you have a little further while also providing variety. For example, if you only have four stationary bikes, you can place these in one station on a circuit and divide the class into groups of four. The other stations can also feature aerobic fitness activities, such as rope jumping, step routines, and aerobic dance. If you have plenty of steps and jump ropes, arrange more than one station using each of these so that groups alternate activities. Here are some other tips for using stations effectively:

- Use stations as a review of previously learned skills.
- Design task cards that are grade and age appropriate—they are good motivators.
- Have students design the stations based on a particular theme or fitness component.
- Alternate intensity levels at the stations, and alternate fitness components.

From Mosston and Ashworth, 2002; and from S. Grineski, 1996.

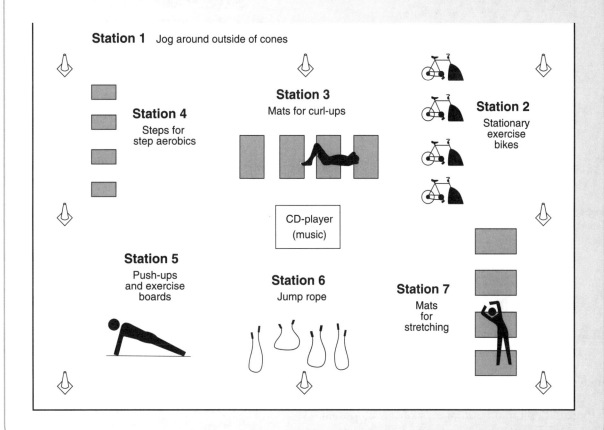

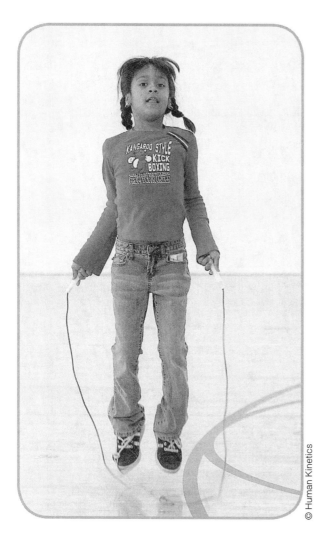

© Human Kinetics

Figure 5.5 Interval training is more than wind sprints. Here a student jumps rope to an audiotape that alternates faster and slower music.

Addressing Motor Skills Through Aerobic Fitness Activities

The importance of skill development should not be underestimated, especially at the elementary level. The *Physical Best Activity Guides* provide many opportunities to address motor skill development during aerobic fitness training to help make fitness activities more enjoyable and interesting. For example, "Catch the Thrill of the Skill" in the *Physical Best Activity Guide: Elementary Level* rotates students through a variety of stations using sport skills or lifestyle activities.

Many activities could be modified to include a manipulative object or to vary the form of locomo-tion while developing aerobic fitness and sport skills. This approach demonstrates to students how aerobic fitness applies in the real world of physical activity. Address both health-related fitness and skill-related fitness whenever possible. Here are several specific ways to integrate motor skills with aerobic fitness activities:

- Aerobic circuit training using sport-specific skills at each station
- Obstacle courses
- Soccer keep-away
- Activities in the *Physical Best Activity Guides*— modified to include sport skills
- In-line skating
- Swimming relays

Safety Guidelines for Aerobic Fitness Activities

Research has shown that children respond to exercise differently than adults (Bar-Or 1993, 1994; Zwiren 1988; Rowland 1996), and there are many issues to consider when helping children increase their aerobic fitness. As a teacher, you should keep the following information regarding physiological differences between adults and children in mind when manipulating the principles of training (Bar-Or 1984; Rowland 1996):

- Children produce more heat, relative to body size, at rest and during exercise (equal absolute workloads) than adults.
- Children sweat less than adults and therefore have difficulty using evaporation as a method of heat dissipation.
- Prepubertal children cannot sustain exercise in very hot environments as compared to adults.
- Children fatigue sooner than adults when exercising in the heat.
- Children are less economical and use more oxygen than adults at any given submaximal exercise intensity.
- Children's heart rates are generally higher than adults at rest and across all levels of exercise.
- Children's maximal heart rates vary from 195 to 205, with large variability between individual subjects.

- Children have less efficient **ventilation** (volume of air moved) compared to adults.

- Children have higher breathing frequencies (bf) and lower **tidal volumes** (V_t), or volume of air either inhaled or exhaled in a normal resting breath, compared to adults.

- Children have higher pulmonary ventilation (breathing frequency × tidal volume) per liter of oxygen consumed during submaximal and maximal exercise.

- Children hyperventilate during exercise more than adults.

Because of these physiological factors, you should build in frequent rest periods, especially for younger students, and provide water before, during, and after physical activity. Emphasize lifestyle activities and limit highly organized sport with high-intensity training to avoid injury. Avoid very hot and humid weather conditions with elementary children, and, using your best judgment, slow down or cancel the activity with middle and high school students. Although most students in your classes will handle aerobic fitness activities safely, you will encounter a few who will need special guidance and modified activities. Be sure you know which students have any form of asthma, orthopedic concerns, heart anomalies, and the like. Not all of these conditions will be obvious, so review school records, talk to the school nurse or classroom teachers, survey parents, and carefully follow school or district policies to ensure you are fully informed. Ask for input on what each child in question can handle, and seek advice on how to apply the overload and progression principles and FITT guidelines safely. If in doubt, obtain written parental permission to talk to the student's health care provider (see also chapter 11).

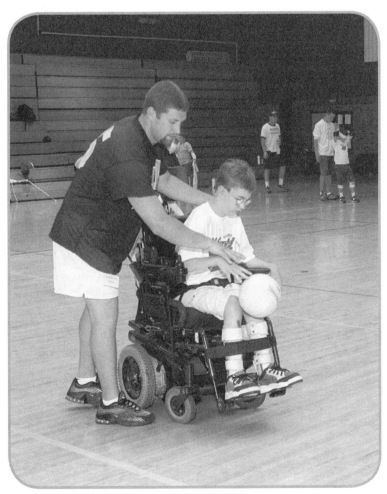

© Human Kinetics

Teach the overload and progression principles and FITT guidelines to students with special needs through carefully planned and modified activities.

Alaskan Teacher Takes Physical Education to Heart

Teaching quality middle school physical education can often be frustrating. Despite the long hours spent designing meaningful assignments, some students—and even some parents—still consider "gym" to be a waste of time, a bother. But Alaska physical education teacher Martin Niemi has never let frustration get in the way of his dedication to providing quality programs, and at least one student and her parents couldn't be happier about that fact.

Martin has been teaching physical education for the past 10 years at the State Department of Education's Alyeska Central School in Juneau, a correspondence school for students who live in isolated areas of the state ("out in the bush"), take part in high-level training (as did Olympian Tommy Moe), or are home-schooled.

The five or six courses Martin teaches each semester (by mail, phone, and computer) allow 415 students in grades 6 through 12 to increase their knowledge and skills about fitness and physical activities relative to their specific lifestyles and circumstances. His duties typically include creating and sending out assignments, grading them, and then determining if students have met the requirements of their particular class.

Molly Meeham, 12, of Eagle River is one of Martin's students. Molly, a seventh grader who is being home-schooled, has always been a normal and active kid: hiking, biking, swimming, horseback riding, jumping on the backyard trampoline with her friends. She had never shown any sign that might lead one to think she had a potentially fatal heart condition. That is, until she met up with Martin. That's right, Martin Niemi, her physical education teacher.

Molly was enrolled in Martin's physical education contract course, the purpose of which, Martin says, is "to get students participating in activities that enhance their lifestyles and help them develop proper exercise habits." As part of the course Molly had to participate in at least 65 hours of approved activities (most students, Martin says, end up with 90 to 200 hours). Students also complete such assignments as fitness challenges, a written paper on the benefits of health-related fitness, a pulse graph activity, and a daily log of participation time.

Molly's mom, Sandy, thought doing all this would be "a bother. After all, my husband [Mike] and I knew she was physically fit. Why did we have to document it for someone else?" Although they didn't know it at the time, Molly's pulse graph would not just help her pass the class—it would save her life.

For the pulse-graph activity, students take their pulses on seven different occasions over a given period (for example, while completely rested, after doing chores, and after aerobic and anaerobic exercising); then they graph them and send them in. When he looked at Molly's graph in March, Martin saw that all seven of her heart rates were between 100 and 125 beats a minute—making "the strangest pulse graph I had ever seen."

Given that Molly had completed her assignment, Martin could have stopped right there. Instead, he drew in red on her graph what a "normal" pattern should look like and sent it back to Sandy, expressing his concern that either the assignment had not been completed properly or that there was possibly "some sort of a health problem."

Upon receiving the assignment back, Sandy Meeham was a little peeved at first, she recalls. "We were just getting ready to go on a family vacation; the PE course was the last one Molly had to finish. We had figured that because it was just PE, the class would be a piece of cake—no big deal. And here we were getting an assignment back because it may not have been completed properly?" Once Sandy thought about it over the course of the day, however, she felt that perhaps there really was something to Martin's comments. "I started thinking, how could we have counted that many pulses wrong?"

Now concerned, Sandy contacted her pediatrician, who assigned her to take Molly's pulse that night while Molly was sleeping. It turned out to be 120 beats a minute, compared with a normal rate of 80 beats or less. The next day, with the help of an EKG, it was determined that something was indeed wrong with the electrical impulses of Molly's heart. She was taken immediately to a specialist in Portland, OR, for testing, and a few weeks later, after 5 hours of exploratory surgery, Molly's condition was diagnosed—she was born with an extra pacemaker in her heart, which caused it to beat much faster than normal.

Sandy credits Martin with alerting their family to Molly's condition. "Had Martin not been so thorough and adamant in his concern over her graph, it is likely I wouldn't have paid it immediate attention. If I hadn't, there is no doubt Molly would be one sick little girl right now. I can only say, I believe it's all part of a big plan. We are thankful that Martin has been part of that plan."

Martin, who received a commendation from Alaska's Governor Walter Hickel for his action, says, "I feel really proud and happy that I got to play a part in Molly's having a chance to live a healthy, happy life. This has helped remind me that we as physical educators do a lot of things day in and day out, and it's important not to trivialize them. Each child we teach is important and has important things to say."

And what about Molly? A week after her surgery, she was playing the piano at church. She's recently completed a 12-mile hike; a 27-miler is in the works. Thanks to the dedication and persistence of her physical education teacher, Molly can again be just like her friends. "We will be forever grateful," says Sandy. "The bottom line of this all is that I saw the PE course as the least significant class Molly had, but it turned out to be, literally, a lifesaver."

Reprinted, by permission, from Scott Wikgren, 1995, "Alaskan Teacher Takes Physical Education to Heart," *Teaching Elementary Physical Education* 1(1):17.

Summary

Use the information in this chapter as a quick reference when teaching aerobic fitness concepts. In addition, refer to the aerobic fitness activities in the *Physical Best Activity Guide: Elementary Level* and the *Physical Best Activity Guide: Middle School and High School Levels* to show students how to apply the concepts in practical ways. Review the teaching guidelines outlined in this chapter periodically to ensure that your expectations are reasonably based on your students' ages, abilities, fitness levels, and interests. Always adjust your program to meet individual needs.

CHAPTER

6

Chapter Contents

- Definitions of Muscular Strength and Endurance Concepts

- Benefits of Resistance Training

- Resistance Training Cautions

- Teaching Guidelines for Muscular Strength and Endurance

- Principles of Training

  Overload, Progression, Specificity, Individuality, and Regularity

  FITT Guidelines

  Estimating 1RM

  Manipulating the Intensity of the Workout

- Training Methods for Muscular Strength and Endurance

  Body Weight Training

  Partner-Resisted Training

  Resistance Band and Medicine Ball Training

  Weight Training

- Addressing Motor Skills Through Muscular Strength and Endurance Activities

- Safety Guidelines for Muscular Strength and Endurance Activities

- Summary

Muscular Strength and Endurance

For the development of total fitness, a well-rounded health-related fitness program must include muscular strength and muscular endurance. The health benefits of muscular strength and endurance programs for adults are well documented; however, little research is available on the health benefits for children. This lack of documented health-related benefits does not mean that children cannot improve muscular strength and endurance. When developing muscular fitness programs, it is important to remember that children are not little adults and that the adult model of weightlifting is not applicable to children. Many adults lift weights for reasons other than improved weightlifting performance, such as enhanced sports performance or prevention of muscular injury, but there is inconsistency in the research supporting these same benefits for children. Youth strength-training experts (Faigenbaum and Westcott 2000) suggest that children participating in youth sports programs do need strength developing activities prior to participation, much like adult preseason conditioning, to prevent injury and enhance skill development. Although these training and conditioning recommendations may be true, the emphasis of physical education classes should be on creating positive experiences that focus on technique (see figure 6.1). This will enable children to carry these skills into their leisure (sport participation) activities.

83

Children should set realistic goals based on their individual needs and should be thoroughly educated in the techniques and safety issues of resistance training. This chapter covers basic definitions, potential health benefits, and teaching guidelines for safe and effective programs. In this chapter, our goal is to provide an overview of a solid, scientifically proven approach to teaching the principles of muscular strength and endurance to students.

Definitions of Muscular Strength and Endurance Concepts

To safely and effectively administer a resistance training program for children, you must understand a variety of terms related to the development of muscular strength and muscular endurance. **Muscular strength** is the ability of a muscle or muscle group to exert a maximal force against a resistance one time through the full range of motion. It is important to emphasize "through the full range of motion" because any movement less than full range is counterproductive—strength or endurance gains occur only in the range of motion exercised. Muscular strength is often denoted as **1RM,** which stands for **"one-repetition maximum." Muscular endurance** is the ability of a muscle or muscle group to exert a submaximal force repeatedly over a period of time.

In the Physical Best program, muscular strength and muscular endurance are combined together as **muscular fitness,** because in practical application of activities and exercises, they are difficult to separate, especially at the primary grade level. You will find that many Physical Best activities use the weight of the child's body as the resistance (see "Teaching Tip: Teaching About Muscular Strength").

It is sound weight-training practice, for children and adults, to focus on good form and multiple repetitions (muscular endurance) prior to engaging in lifting heavier weights and fewer repetitions (muscular strength). No participant, child or adult, should engage in rapid repetitions where momentum assists in the lifting process. Use a six-second count where the participant takes two or three seconds to lift the weight and three or four seconds to lower the weight, focusing on technique. Furthermore, children should not engage in lifting heavy weights (fewer than 6 repetitions). The general guideline is for children to perform 6 to 15 reps of an exercise to see strength changes. Studies indicate that single-set programs of 8 to 10 exercises, using the 6 to 15 repetition guideline, maximizes strength increases in youth (AAP 2001; Faigenbaum and Westcott 2000). You may choose to label your lessons as muscular fitness instead of specifying muscular strength or muscular endurance.

Resistance training or strength training is a systematic, preplanned program using a variety of methods (e.g., a person's own body weight or tension bands) or equipment (e.g., machines or free weights) that progressively stresses the musculoskeletal system to improve muscular strength (ACSM 1998; Faigenbaum and Westcott 2000; Faigenbaum 2003). On

TEACHING TIP: Teaching About Muscular Strength

Elementary students need to learn how different weights feel. You should have different types and sizes (2 to 10 pounds) of weights available at a station so the students can learn about using different weights and learn how each weight feels.

There is more than one way to do a push-up, but they all require keeping the back stable. Place a beanbag or tennis ball on the backs of students to help them understand the correct form of a push-up. Challenge the students to keep the beanbag or tennis ball on their backs, which will indicate good technique.

Carolyn Masterson, Associate Professor
Montclair State University
Upper Montclair, New Jersey

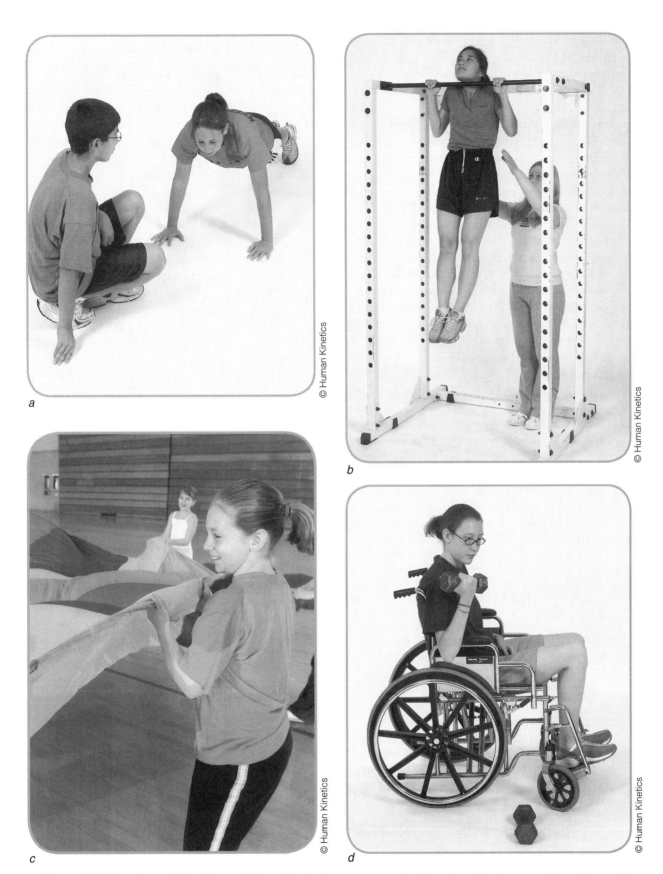

Figure 6.1 Sample activities that can help students improve muscular strength and endurance: *(a)* push-ups, *(b)* pull-ups, *(c)* shaking a parachute, and *(d)* hand weights.

the other hand, **weightlifting** is considered a competitive sport involving maximal lifts, and further specification includes Olympic weightlifting using the snatch and the clean and jerk lifts (AAP 2001). It is also ill-advised for children to participate in **power lifting** (a competitive sport involving the dead lift, the squat, and the bench press) or **body building,** where muscle size, symmetry, and definition are judged (AAP 2001). Children are not physiologically mature enough to see changes in muscle size, symmetry, or definition. The medical concerns about resistance training often stem from the confusion in terminology. Many people follow the adult model of training and conditioning, focusing on lifting as much weight as possible (1RM) and on weightlifting competitions. These practices are inappropriate for children. Multiple recommendations or position statements on resistance training exist that provide guidance in developing children's resistance training programs (ACSM 1998, 2000; AAP 2001; Faigenbaum 2003; Hass, Feigenbaum, and Franklin 2001; NSCA 2000). It is generally agreed that resistance training or weight training is safe for children, but weightlifting, body building, and other competitions where the focus is on maximal lifts are not recommended. Throughout this text, the term *resistance training* will be used when referring to activities that develop muscular strength and muscular endurance because it encompasses a greater variety of activities and does not require the use of weights only.

CAUTION!

Safety is a concern in any aspect of physical education and health-related physical fitness, but it is especially critical to closely follow the safety guidelines outlined later in this chapter. You should also seek additional training specific to working with children and adolescents in developing muscular strength and endurance in a safe and effective manner. Furthermore, use common sense when designing and implementing curricula and activities in this area, paying careful attention to the ages, developmental readiness, abilities, maturity levels, past experiences, and fitness levels of your students.

Benefits of Resistance Training

A variety of benefits are associated with resistance training, and many of these benefits are age related, with greater sport performance benefits associated with postpubescent adolescents. Potential benefits of resistance training include the following:

- Increased muscular strength (AAP 2001; Falk and Tenenbaum 1996; Faigenbaum, Zaichkowsky, et al. 1993; Faigenbaum 2003; NSCA 2000).
- Increased **muscular power,** or ability to exert a force rapidly (Faigenbaum 2003).
- Increased muscular endurance (AAP 2001; Faigenbaum and Westcott 2000; Faigenbaum 2003; NSCA 2000).
- Improvement in aerobic fitness using circuit weight training (Fleck 1988; Faigenbaum 2003).
- Prevention of musculoskeletal injury (Faigenbaum and Westcott 2000; Faigenbaum 2003).
- Improved sports performance (Faigenbaum 2003; Faigenbaum and Westcott 2000).
- Reduced risk of fractures in adulthood (Karlsson et al. 2002).
- Exercise during the skeletal growth period is better for bone development, increasing bone strength and bone growth (Faigenbaum 2003; Turner and Robling 2003).

Postpubescent children achieve these benefits, plus many of the health benefits associated with adult resistance training programs, including the following:

- improved blood lipid profile;
- improved body composition;
- improved mental health and well-being; and
- a more positive attitude toward lifetime physical activity (Faigenbaum 2003).

Position of the National Strength and Conditioning Association on Youth Resistance Training

This is the current position of the NSCA:

1. A properly designed and supervised resistance training program is safe for children.
2. A properly designed and supervised resistance training program can increase the strength of children.
3. A properly designed and supervised resistance training program can help to enhance the motor fitness skills and sports performance of children.
4. A properly designed and supervised resistance training program can help to prevent injuries in youth sports and recreational activities.
5. A properly designed and supervised resistance training program can help to improve the psycho-social well-being of children.
6. A properly designed and supervised resistance training program can enhance the overall health of children.

Reprinted, by permission, from A. Faigenbaum and W. Kraemer, 1996, "A position paper and literature review of youth resistance training," *Strength and Conditioning* 18(16): 62-75.

Resistance Training Cautions

Before they consider equipment and teaching ideas, physical educators must understand some of the cautions involved with resistance training, especially for the prepubescent child. The following program considerations should be reviewed before developing children's resistance training programs (Faigenbaum and Westcott 2000).

- The child must be psychologically and physically ready to accept teaching or coaching instruction.
- There must be adequate supervision (1:5 teacher/student ratio or 1:10 with experienced teenage participants) by instructors who know resistance training concerns for children and special problems of prepubescent children.
- Proper technique and safety for each lift must be emphasized.
- Caution must be used with machines that are not designed to fit children.
- Resistance training should not be an isolated component—it should be part of a comprehensive program to increase motor skills and fitness.
- The resistance training program should be preceded by a warm-up and followed by a cool-down.

- Both **concentric** (muscle shortens) and **eccentric contractions** (dynamic, muscle lengthens) should be included in the program.
- Full range of motion must be emphasized.

In addition to these program considerations, the American Academy of Pediatrics also recommends that children and adolescents receive a medical evaluation to determine any underlying medical condition or orthopedic problem that may limit or prohibit participation in resistance training. Do not let these cautions deter you from incorporating resistance training in your physical education class. With proper instruction and supervision, resistance training can be a fun and safe activity for all ages.

Age-specific training guidelines, program variations, and competent supervision will make resistance training programs safe, effective, and fun for children. Instructors must understand the physical and emotional uniqueness of children and, in turn, children must appreciate the potential benefits and risks associated with resistance training. Although the needs, goals, and interests of children will continually change, resistance training should be considered a safe and effective component of youth fitness programs (Faigenbaum et al. 1996).

Although age-specific guidelines have been provided (table 6.1), with resistance indicated by light to heavy weights, your program should accommodate the "training age" (i.e., resistance training experience) of the child when developing resistance programs. This will allow younger, more experienced children to challenge themselves safely under proper instruction and supervision (using the progression and overload principles). Use the number of repetitions to determine the weight lifted, such that a child is performing 6 to 15 reps. This eliminates the ambiguity of the "light" or "heavy" weight recommendations. When a child can lift 15 reps, then increase the weight by no more than one to three pounds (Faigenbaum and Westcott 2000).

Teaching Guidelines for Muscular Strength and Endurance

You can teach muscular fitness concepts and conduct resistance training sessions whether or not you have state-of-the-art equipment. Surgical tubing or other resistance band material is inexpensive and readily available. In the primary grades, most children will be challenged using the weight of their own body, and for some children, this challenge carries through to the middle and high school level. Another idea is to collect cans of food and use them as small weights (you can later donate them to a local food bank). If

Youth Resistance Training Guidelines

- Each child should understand the benefits and risks associated with resistance training.
- Competent and caring fitness professionals should supervise training sessions.
- The exercise environment should be safe and free of potential hazards, and the equipment should be in good repair and properly sized to fit each child.
- Warm-up and stretching exercises should be performed before resistance training.
- Each child's tolerance to the exercise stress should be carefully monitored.
- Children should begin with light loads to allow appropriate adjustments to be made.
- Resistance should be increased gradually (e.g., 5 to 10 percent) as strength improves.
- Depending on individual needs and goals, one to three sets of 6 to 15 repetitions on a variety of single- and multi-joint exercises can be performed.
- Advanced multi-joint exercises, such as modified cleans, pulls, and presses, may be incorporated into the program, provided that appropriate loads are used and the focus remains on proper form.
- Two or three nonconsecutive training sessions per week are recommended.
- When necessary, adult spotters should be nearby to actively assist the child in the event of a failed repetition.
- The resistance training program should be systematically varied throughout the year.
- Children should be encouraged to drink plenty of water before, during, and after exercise.

Adapted by permission, from A. Faigenbaum et al., 1996, "A position paper and literature review of youth resistance training," *Strength and Conditioning* 18(16): 62-75.

you or a parent is handy with a sewing machine, you can make small saddlebags to hold small weights, cans of food, or other items used for resistance training. The saddlebags can be draped over the extremities, and a child can individualize the program by selecting appropriate weights at each station. You can also use balls that incorporate balance and strength. Partner-resistance exercises can be used if equipment is lacking. Many children at the elementary level lack the emotional maturity to engage in formal resistance training, but they can perform the muscular strength and endurance activities from the *Physical Best Activity Guide–Elementary Level*. This guide provides appropriate muscular fitness activities for this level. Late elementary may be the first opportunity to introduce a more formal or comprehensive resistance training program (Faigenbaum 2003). Always take into account the participant's psychological and physical maturity when implementing resistance training programs, even though most guidelines utilize chronological age.

If you are planning to purchase equipment, focus on buying items that will meet the primary needs of your students. Most machine weights are not designed for the small size of children; therefore, resistance bands, dumbbells, medicine balls, or free weights may be a better choice of equipment. This recommendation does not come without caution, because the use of free weights poses additional safety concerns regarding proper form and spotting techniques. Most injuries involving youth resistance training activities are related to improper lifting techniques, maximal lifts, or lack of qualified adult supervision (Faigenbaum 2003); also, injury often occurs in exercise involving dead lifts, the bench press, or the overhead press. Remember that using traditional weight-training equipment represents only a small segment of exercises and activities. It's important for students to first manage their own body weight before lifting heavier weights. We have included many activities and exercises in the *Physical Best Activity Guides* that teach muscular strength and endurance concepts without requiring the use of a weight room.

Principles of Training

The basic training principles presented in chapter 3 apply to resistance training, and teachers may use a variety of activities to improve muscular strength or endurance as long as these training principles are

followed. Manipulating the mode of exercise, number of sets, number of repetitions, and the amount of weight lifted is critical in the adult model, but recent research (Faigenbaum, Westcott, Loud, and Long 1999) indicates that greater gains in strength occur in preadolescent youth (boys and girls) when doing approximately 14 reps (lifting moderate weight) in contrast to doing 7 reps (lifting heavier weight). As previously indicated, one **set** of 8 to 15 **repetitions** is appropriate for youth, and more sets may be added as youth improve and the goal moves from learning techniques to increasing **volume** as needed for training and conditioning for sport. This section provides a review of how the training principles from chapter 3 are specifically applied to resistance training.

Overload, Progression, Specificity, Individuality, and Regularity

The **overload principle**—placing greater-than-normal demands on the musculature of the body—suggests that individuals involved with activities designed to improve muscular strength or muscular endurance must increase their workload periodically throughout the course of the program. Specifically, overload requires increasing the resistance against the exercising muscles to a level greater than that used before. Increasing the number of repetitions provides another avenue to overload the muscle, but this type of overload does not develop muscular strength; it does provide the overload needed to develop muscular endurance. You can also choose to decrease the rest interval between activities, or you can use a combination of these methods. Keep in mind that the increase must be appropriate for the age and fitness level of the students (table 6.1), and that chronological age may not always be the best indicator for determining the amount of weight to be lifted or the number of repetitions to perform. These recommendations are slightly different than the exercise prescription for adults, and they yield a safe and effective method of increasing strength in children. Therefore, one to three sets of 6 to 15 repetitions is recommended. This protocol provides opportunities for children to succeed and appreciate what they have accomplished (Faigenbaum, Westcott, Loud, and Long 1999; Faigenbaum and Westcott 2000; Faigenbaum 2003).

The principle of **progression** refers to a gradual increase. It is a systematic approach to increasing the resistance and intensity of the activity. To avoid injury,

TABLE 6.1　FITT Guidelines Applied to Muscular Fitness

Ages	9-11 years[a, b]	12-14 years[a, b]	15-16 years[a]	17+ years[b]
Frequency	2 or 3 days/wk	2 or 3 days/wk	2 or 3 days/wk	2 days/wk
Intensity	Very light weight	Light weight	Moderate weight	Light to heavy weight (based on type selected)
Time	At least 1 set (may do 2 sets), 6-15 reps, at least 20-30 min	At least 1 set (may do 3 sets), 6-15 reps, at least 20-30 min	At least 1 set (may do 3 or 4 sets), 6-15 reps, at least 20-30 min	Minimum 1 set, 8-12 reps
Type	Major muscle groups, 1 exercise/muscle or muscle group	Major muscle groups, 1 exercise/muscle or muscle group	Major muscle groups, 2 exercises/muscle or muscle group	Major muscle groups, 8-10 exercises; select muscular strength, power, or endurance

[a]Modified from AAP (2001). "Strength training by children and adolescents (RE0048)". Pediatrics, 107(6): 1470-1472.

[b]Modified from Faigenbaum, A.D., et al. 1996. Youth resistance training: Position statement paper and literature review. *Strength and Conditioning* 18(6):62-75.

[c]Modified from American College of Sports Medicine, 2000, *ACSM's guidelines for exercise testing and prescription*, 6th ed. (Baltimore, MD: Lippincott, Williams, and Wilkins).

however, students must understand appropriate progression and set goals accordingly. For example, as beginners, they should know that developing a good base for muscular fitness often entails using the weight of their own body first, followed by one to three sets of 6 to 15 repetitions. The resistance lifted begins with a weight that can be lifted 6 to 10 times (and not 11), and the number of repetitions is gradually increased to 15. Point out that adding only one to three pounds at a time is safer and more realistic than increasing by an excessive amount (more than three pounds). Avoid increasing the load by more than five pounds under any circumstances. There may be instances in which one component is increased, while the other components are actually decreased. For example, as intensity increases, volume will decrease, and vice versa. Make sure that you develop a plan of health-related fitness activities that will lead the student to an improved level of fitness in a safe but progressive manner. The *Physical Best Activity Guides* provide many activities that have been developed with this principle in mind.

The **specificity principle** states that the "training effects derived from an exercise program are specific to the exercise performed and muscles involved" (ACSM 2000). For resistance training, specificity

suggests that the activities selected should provide the outcome represented by the day's class objectives (see the *Physical Best Activity Guides* for examples). The previously described principles of overload and progression provide the foundation for establishing specificity in your teaching plan.

The **regularity principle** states that activity must be performed on a regular basis to be effective, and that long periods of inactivity can lead to loss of benefits achieved during the training session. Engaging in muscular strength and endurance training two or three times per week is sufficient for a lifetime of good muscular health. Yet, as mentioned in chapter 5, you will most likely encounter students who want to achieve higher levels of fitness. It is your job to provide accurate and helpful information to assist interested students in reaching their muscular strength and endurance goals safely. Table 6.1 summarizes the FITT (frequency, intensity, time, and type) guidelines based on age and current recommendations by the American Academy of Pediatrics, the American College of Sports Medicine, and the National Strength and Conditioning Association.

The **individuality principle** takes into account that each child has different goals for physical activity and muscular fitness, as well as different initial muscular fitness levels. For children, a variety of activities should be incorporated into a program, facilitating a broad range of skill development, including muscular fitness activities. This variety provides opportunity for all children to be successful and provides a baseline of motor skills for future development as the child matures and shows interest in specific sport activities.

FITT Guidelines

Guidelines for muscular fitness are based on policy statements or position statements from the American Academy of Pediatrics (2001) and the National Strength and Conditioning Association (2000). It is generally agreed that the *frequency* of resistance training should be two or three times per week. In examining exercise *intensity*, the recommendations are more complex and are related to stages of maturation (table 6.1). The emphasis during childhood (prepubescent) is generally thought of as a period where students should learn proper technique and use the weight of their own body. They then progress through to the postpubescent stage, where the adult model may be applied. Weight should always be added in small increments (one to three pounds), and a range of 6 to 15 repetitions should be performed. The *time* or duration of resistance training should be at least 20 to 30 minutes or the time it takes to lift one to three sets, 6 to 15 repetitions, with rest periods based on the goal of the activity session. A rest period of 2 or 3 minutes should be used for a strength session, whereas shorter periods of 90 seconds may be used for a muscular endurance or power session. Keep in mind that developmentally, the child's anaerobic system is not fully developed, and feelings of light-headedness or nausea may result if the child is not allowed short rest periods while progressing through an endurance session.

Type refers to the kind of resistance training performed during the session, such as muscular strength, power, or endurance (see table 6.1). It may also refer to the variety of weight-training methods available such as tension bands, free weights, body weight, machine weights, or partner-resistance exercises.

Estimating 1RM

Extreme caution must be applied when discussing the concept of a one-repetition maximum (1RM). Children will naturally want to know how much weight they can lift and will want to challenge classmates to determine who is the strongest. Remember that safety precautions must be taught first and foremost, and the lifting of a 1RM should *absolutely not* be used to obtain a training intensity. The National Strength and Conditioning Association (Faigenbaum et al. 1996) indicates that the use of a 1RM in a supervised laboratory setting for research purposes could be philosophically supported, but children should never be subjected to this technique due to the risk of injury. Children should not be exposed to loads greater than 70 to 80 percent of an estimated 1RM or to explosive lifts using free weights during prepuberty, puberty, and early postpuberty (Bompa 2000). Keep in mind that these suggestions apply to most children and most educational programs. There may be instances in late postpubescent youth where, with proper training and supervision, explosive lifting techniques may be taught. A variety of methods are used to estimate the 1RM, such as performing a 10RM and using a table to predict the 1RM (Baechle and Earle 2000) or calculating a 1RM from a weight that is lifted no less than 6 and no more than 12 repetitions. For children, it is much simpler to use the range of 6 to 12 repetitions to estimate the 1RM versus determining a precise 10RM. Estimating a 1RM should be reserved for the postpubescent child (girls 13 to 18 years; boys 14 to 18 years) or those at the high school level.

To estimate a student's 1RM, consult table 6.2. In the "Max reps (RM): 10/75% 1RM" column, first find the tested 10RM load; then read across the row to the "Max reps (RM): 1/100% 1RM" column to find the student's projected 1RM. For example, if a student's 10RM is 75 pounds, the estimated 1RM is 100 pounds (Baechle and Earle 2000).

Manipulating the Intensity of the Workout

An individual can develop either muscular strength or muscular endurance with the same total load by manipulating the intensity of the workout. To develop muscular strength, increase intensity by increasing the weight lifted and reducing the number of reps (e.g., a student leg presses 100 pounds for 6 reps; total load is 600 pounds). To develop muscular endurance, increase intensity by decreasing the weight lifted and increasing the number of reps (e.g., the student leg presses 50 pounds for 12 reps; total load is 600 pounds).

TABLE 6.2 Estimating 1RM and Training Loads

Max reps (RM)	1	2	3	4	5	6	7	8	9	10	12	15
% 1 RM	100	95	93	90	87	85	83	80	77	75	67	65
Load (lb or kg)	10	10	9	9	9	9	8	8	8	8	7	7
	20	19	19	18	17	17	17	16	15	15	13	13
	30	29	28	27	26	26	25	24	23	23	20	20
	40	38	37	36	35	34	33	32	31	30	27	26
	50	48	47	45	44	43	42	40	39	38	34	33
	60	57	56	54	52	51	50	48	46	45	40	39
	70	67	65	63	61	60	58	56	54	53	47	46
	80	76	74	72	70	68	66	64	62	60	54	52
	90	86	84	81	78	77	75	72	69	68	60	59
	100	95	93	90	87	85	83	80	77	75	67	65
	110	105	102	99	96	94	91	88	85	83	74	72
	120	114	112	108	104	102	100	96	92	90	80	78
	130	124	121	117	113	111	108	104	100	98	87	85
	140	133	130	126	122	119	116	112	108	105	94	91
	150	143	140	135	131	128	125	120	116	113	101	98
	160	152	149	144	139	136	133	128	123	120	107	104
	170	162	158	153	148	145	141	136	131	128	114	111
	180	171	167	162	157	153	149	144	139	135	121	117
	190	181	177	171	165	162	158	152	146	143	127	124
	200	190	186	180	174	170	166	160	154	150	134	130
	210	200	195	189	183	179	174	168	162	158	141	137
	220	209	205	198	191	187	183	176	169	165	147	143
	230	219	214	207	200	196	191	184	177	173	154	150
	240	228	223	216	209	204	199	192	185	180	161	156
	250	238	233	225	218	213	208	200	193	188	168	163
	260	247	242	234	226	221	206	208	200	195	174	169
	270	257	251	243	235	230	224	216	208	203	181	176
	280	266	260	252	244	238	232	224	216	210	188	182
	290	276	270	261	252	247	241	232	223	218	194	189

Speed of lifting also influences intensity (Griffin 1998), and speed should not be introduced to children. Circuit training that involves multiple repetitions in a specified time period should include activities that use the weight of the body, such as push-ups, curl-ups, or other activities not performed on machine weights or free weights. It is better to specify the number of repetitions to perform slowly and in the correct form rather than emphasize how many repetitions to complete in a 30-second time span (Bompa 2000). Be aware, especially with weight machines, that lifting too fast creates momentum that aids the lifting, thereby reducing intensity. The focus of resistance training for children should be on developing form and technique, and not on changing the intensity by varying the speed at which the weight is lifted. Lifting too fast (4 seconds or faster per rep) also increases the likelihood of injury. Faigenbaum and Westcott (2000) recommend 6-second reps (2 seconds lifting and 4 seconds lowering) but assert that 8-second reps (4 lifting and 4 lowering) to 14-second reps (10 lifting and 4 lowering) are also effective. Moderate to slow exercise speeds are recommended over fast lifting speeds for a variety of reasons, including longer periods of muscle tension, higher levels of muscle force, decreased levels of momentum, and decreased risk of injury (Faigenbaum and Westcott 2000).

Training Methods for Muscular Strength and Endurance

According to the National Strength and Conditioning Association (NSCA 2000; Baechle and Earle 2000), when guiding a student to progress from base development to intermediate to advanced development, a 5 to 10 percent increase in overall load is appropriate for most children. Beginning students, especially elementary students, should primarily engage in circuit training using their own body weight, partners, or light medicine balls, and the volume should be low and intensity very low (Bompa 2000). Help each child begin slowly, then gradually increase frequency, intensity, or time according to individual needs and goals. Table 6.1 offers general progression guidelines based on age group. A training log such as the one shown in figure 6.2 can help a child see individual progress and feel a sense of accomplishment (see appendix A for a reproducible example).

Kids Workout Log

Name: Sue Ramsden **Age:** 9 **Class:** M, W 3:15 pm

Comments: Injured Shoulder Fall '04 **Telephone:** 479-8500

Exercise:	Seat Position:	Date: 3/20 Wt: / Reps:	Date: 3/22 Wt: / Reps:	Date: Wt: / Reps:	Date: Wt: / Reps:	Date: Wt: / Reps:	Date: Wt: / Reps:	Date: Wt: / Reps
(1) DB SQUAT		8 / 10	8 / 11					
(2) LEG CURL	2	10 / 10	10 / 11					
(3) DB HEEL RAISE		10 / 10	10 / 11					
(4) CHEST PRESS	2	20 / 10	20 / 11					
(5) SEATED ROW	1	15 / 10	15 / 11					
(6) DB LATERAL RAISE		3 / 10	3 / 11					
(7) DB BICEPS CURL		5 / 10	5 / 11					
(8) TRICEPS PRESSDOWN		10 / 10	10 / 11					
(9) PRONE BACK RAISE		Reps: 10	Reps: 11	Reps:	Reps:	Reps:	Reps:	Reps:
(10) CURL-UPS		Reps: 10	Reps: 11	Reps:	Reps:	Reps:	Reps:	Reps:

■ **Figure 6.2** Sample training log.

Adapted, by permission, from A. Faigenbaum and W. Westcott, 2000, *Strength and power for young athletes* (Champaign, IL: Human Kinetics), 20.

Training Recommendations

If a child of any age begins a program with no previous experience, you should start the child at lower levels and move him or her to more advanced levels as exercise tolerance, skill, amount of training time, and understanding permit.

- Start slowly—single set, 10 to 15 repetitions, twice per week—allowing students to gain confidence.
- Gradually increase the overload to performing one to three sets, 6 to 15 repetitions, two or three times per week.
- Use 5 to 10 percent increases in training load (two to five pounds); this is appropriate for most exercises.
- Emphasize full range of motion.
- Emphasize intrinsic enjoyment.
- Have students use personalized logs.
- Share personal success stories.
- Emphasize having fun.
- Incorporate variety in your classroom activities.
- Introduce new exercises.
- Change the training mode.
- Vary the number of sets and repetitions.
- Use multiple goals.
- Do not limit the goals to increasing muscular strength or endurance.
- Teach students about their bodies and safe lifting techniques; aim for development of positive attitudes toward physical activity.

Faigenbaum (2003); Faigenbaum and Westcott (2000).

Body Weight Training

Although it is difficult to quantify intensity, curl-ups, push-ups, and other body weight exercises all help build muscular strength and endurance with little or no equipment. This type of resistance training is appropriate for the very young student (K-4) or the student who is just beginning resistance training activity. Primary grade students or those having difficulty with the curl-up or push-up should perform reverse curl-ups or simply perform the lowering phase of the push-up, holding this position. These activities can be presented in a fun and safe way, and they provide very positive health-related benefits to the student. Add interest to them by playing music or creating games such as Around the World from

Right Fielders Are People Too (Hichwa 1998). (See the "Around the World" text box.)

Body weight training is not only for young children. It has the advantage of not requiring equipment, which means it is an inexpensive part of a muscular fitness training program throughout adulthood. Body weight training is also less likely to cause injury—and it is the easiest program to take along on vacation! So teach proper form for a variety of body weight alternatives to students of all ages, even if your high school is lucky enough to have a state-of-the-art weight room.

Your ultimate goal is that your students will take personal responsibility for health-related fitness, so give them opportunities to practice planning and implementing their own programs.

Around the World

Build upper body strength and reinforce math skills with this activity. Divide students into groups of four to six students. Have them each get into push-up position and form a circle with their feet in the center and their heads facing outward. Direct the students in each group to pass a beanbag from one person to the next around the circle. Have each group count the number of passes they can make in 30 seconds, then rest for 30 seconds. Conduct up to three 30-second rounds.

Reprinted, by permission, from J. Hichwa, 1998, *Right fielders are people too* (Champaign, IL: Human Kinetics), 106.

Partner-Resisted Training

The partner-resisted training method is an extension of basic body weight exercises. Although it is difficult to gauge the intensity of this type of training, this method is helpful when starting a program or living within a tight budget. Using either no equipment or simple equipment such as a towel, cords, or elastic bands, partner-resistance exercises better isolate individual muscles or muscle groups than solo body weight exercises. Partner-resistance exercises are useful for all age groups from upper elementary grades through adulthood, but especially for those too small to fit standard weight machines (see figures 6.3 and 6.4 in the "Partners as Resistance" sections for examples). When selecting partners, match height, weight, and strength levels as closely as possible to ensure safety and ease of working together. Encourage good communication and demand mature, safe behavior. Partners should also help each other maintain correct technique and high motivation by monitoring and encouraging each other.

Partners as Resistance: Elbow, Flex and Extend

- **Position:** Partners stand facing each other, arms at sides, elbows bent to right angles, palms down.
- **Part 1:** Partner B places hands on top of A's hands and presses down. Partner A resists, but allows elbows to extend until arm is straight. Rest for 10 seconds.
- **Return motion:** Partner A flexes elbow while Partner B resists, but allows elbows to bend to right angle in 10 counts. Rest for 10 seconds.
- **Reverse:** Partner B flexes elbows while Partner A's hands are on top. Repeat the exercise.

Text is reprinted, by permission, from K. McConnell, C.B. Corbin, and D. Dale, 2005. *Fitness for life activity and vocabulary cards*, 5th edition (Champaign, IL: Human Kinetics).

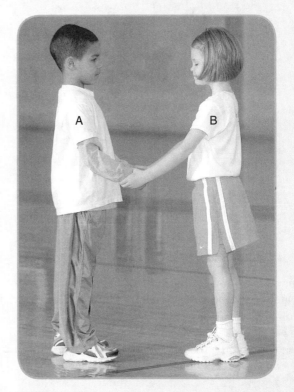

■ Figure 6.3

Partners as Resistance: Knee Flex

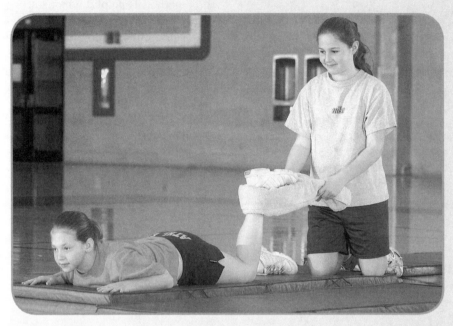

■ **Figure 6.4**

- ■ **Position:** Partner B lies face down on a bench or mat, with knees hanging over the edge. If on a mat, B's left knee should be bent to a 45-degree angle. Partner A kneels at B's feet, looping a towel over B's left ankle, with the ends downward. Keep towel pull perpendicular to the leg.

- ■ **Part 1:** Partner A maintains resistance on the towel as B flexes the left knee as far as possible. Rest for 10 seconds and lower the leg.

- ■ **Part 2:** Repeat with the right leg. Repeat again on each leg and rest again.

- ■ **Reverse:** Change places and repeat all knee exercises.

Text is reprinted, by permission, from K. McConnell, C.B. Corbin, and D. Dale, 2005. *Fitness for life activity and vocabulary cards*, 5th edition (Champaign, IL: Human Kinetics).

Resistance Band and Medicine Ball Training

Resistance band training is appropriate for upper elementary and older students, while medicine ball training can be adapted to all ages, including primary grade children using a variety of weighted balls. Band training involves using surgical tubing, rubber cords, or bands manufactured specifically for muscular strength and endurance training, such as the Exertube, Dyna Band, Flexi-Cord, or Thera-Band.

Use thicker tubing for greater resistance and thinner tubing for less resistance. In addition, a student can adjust resistance by pre-stretching the cord more or less. Although a user cannot measure intensity precisely, this is an inexpensive, effective way to expand your muscular fitness training program. An added advantage is that spotting is rarely required for such exercises. Figure 6.5 in the "Rubber Cord Standing Chest Press" section shows an example of resistance band exercises.

Rubber Cord Standing Chest Press

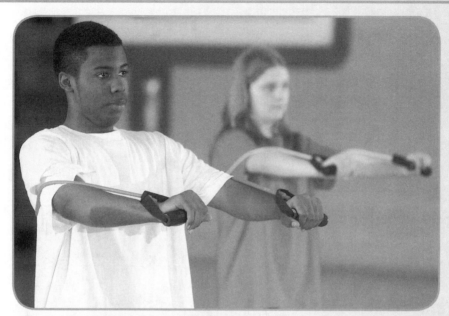

■ **Figure 6.5** Rubber cord standing chest press

Muscles

■ Pectoralis major, anterior deltoid, triceps

Procedure

■ Stand with your feet about shoulder-width apart and the rubber cord wrapped around the back of your shoulders.

■ Grasp the ends of the cord firmly, and place both hands (palms facing the floor) in front of your shoulders with your elbows flexed.

■ Slowly straighten your elbows until you fully extend both arms. Then return to starting position and repeat.

Technique Tips

■ Exhale during the pushing phase of the exercise and inhale during the return phase.

■ Do not twist or arch your body.

Reprinted, by permission, from A. Faigenbaum and W. Westcott, 2000, *Strength and power for young athletes* (Champaign, IL: Human Kinetics), 97.

Medicine balls can be purchased in various weights and sizes. Faigenbaum and Westcott (2000) suggest three benefits in using medicine balls in your program. First, this type of training uses dynamic movements that can be performed either slowly or rapidly. Second, the balls can be used to develop the upper body, lower body and trunk using catching and throwing movements. The most important reason listed is to develop the core which includes the abdominal muscles, and the hip and lower-back musculature. Besides being an effective avenue of increasing muscular fitness in children, these methods of conditioning involve multiple students simultaneously participating and are relatively cheap to purchase (Westcott 1996). Figure 6.6 in the "Medicine Ball Chest Pass" section shows an example of an exercise that can be performed with a medicine ball.

Medicine Ball Chest Pass

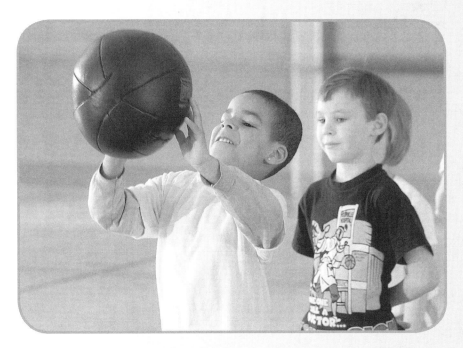

▩ **Figure 6.6**   Medicine Ball Chest Pass

Muscles

▩ Chest, arms

Procedure

▩ Stand erect while holding a medicine ball at chest level with both hands.

▩ Step forward and press the ball off your chest.

Technique Tips

▩ Exhale as you push the ball off your chest.

▩ Keep your torso erect after you release the ball. Do not lean forward.

▩ A partner can stand about 10 feet away and catch the ball. Over time the students can increase the distance between partners. The farther the distance, the greater the effort that is required.

▩ For variety, you can perform this exercise while kneeling on the floor. Keep your body straight as you push the ball off your chest.

Weight Training

A program may use free or machine weights or both, depending on goals, equipment availability, and space in which to safely conduct a weight-training program. Introduce exercises one at a time by discussing each one's purpose, demonstrating correct technique, and outlining ranges of appropriate weight loads, repetitions, and speed. In addition, relate these factors to intensity, program goals, and individual goals. Follow the safety and health guidelines provided earlier in this chapter to ensure a safe and effective weight-training program. While you may opt to use weight training in addition to or in place of other forms of training, as discussed in the body weight training section, teach students alternative exercises that target the same muscle or muscle group. Likewise, if your program relies heavily on machine use, demonstrate the corresponding free weight exercises to broaden the chances that students will use the exercises outside of and after your program. Figure 6.7a shows the biceps curl as performed on a machine, and Figure 6.7b shows its free weight alternative. Most weight training using machine weights and barbells should be reserved for postpubescent children. Table 6.3 provides suggestions that are appropriate exercises for the prepubescent child (Bompa 2000). Appendix C contains illustrations of these exercises.

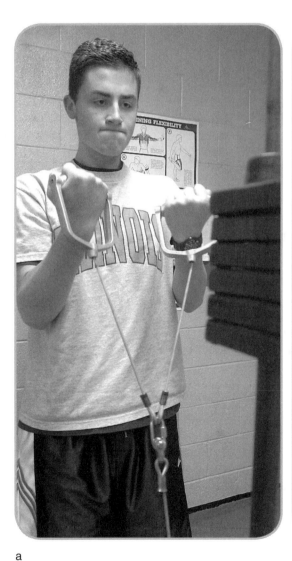

a

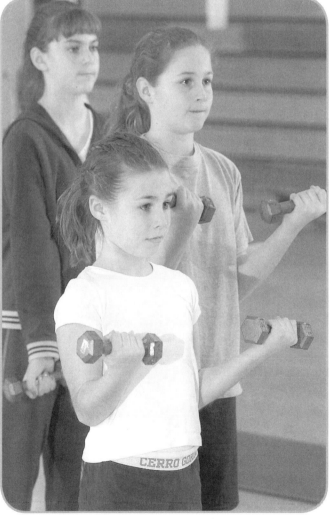

b

■ **Figure 6.7** Biceps curl performed (a) on a machine and (b) with free weights.

TABLE 6.3 Muscular Fitness Exercises*

Exercise	Muscles worked
Dumbbell side raise	Shoulders
Dumbbell curl	Biceps
Dumbbell shoulder press	Shoulders, trapezius
Dumbbell overhead raise	Shoulders
Dumbbell fly	Chest, shoulders
Medicine ball chest throw	Shoulders, triceps
Medicine ball zigzag throw	Arms, shoulders
Medicine ball twist throw	Arms, trunk, oblique abdominals
Medicine ball forward overhead throw	Chest, shoulders, arms, abdominals
Medicine ball scoop throw	Ankles, knees, hip extensors, arms, shoulders, back
Abdominal crunch	Abdominals, hip flexors
Medicine ball back roll	Abdominals, hip flexors
Medicine ball side pass relay	Oblique abdominals, shoulders
Trunk twist	Oblique abdominals
Single-leg back raise	Hip extensors, spine
Chest raise and clap	Lower back
Seated back extension	Back, shoulders
Two-leg skip	Calves, knee extensors
Loop skip	Calves, knee extensors
Dodge the rope	Calves, knee extensors

*See appendix C for descriptions and photos of these exercises.

Bompa, (2000), p.115-123.

Addressing Motor Skills Through Muscular Strength and Endurance Activities

Simply put, a strong, more-enduring muscle can do what it's called on to do reliably and accurately. Therefore increasing muscular strength and endurance can enhance performance. The National Strength and Conditioning Association (Faigenbaum et al. 1996) states that children cannot "play" themselves into shape, and that preseason and in-season training time should be supplemented with a resistance training program to enhance sports and recreational activities. Most research in this area indicates that training adaptations are specific to the movement pattern, velocity of movement, contraction type, and contraction force (Faigenbaum 2003). These fast movements (power) are generally contraindicated when weightlifting; however, children can engage in plyometric exercises (hops, jumps, and throws) if intensity and volume are carefully monitored. Faigenbaum and Chu (2001) also suggest caution when using plyometric training. They strongly suggest a solid base of strength training prior to plyometric training and suggest beginning **plyometrics** using low-intensity drills.

You can have students perform motor skills to increase muscular strength and endurance. For example, young children enjoy playing tag games using various locomotor skills. These games increase the muscular endurance of the leg muscles. Students fourth grade and up may enjoy team-building activities that require arm strength to conquer, such as the "circle of teamwork." This activity requires a group of students to stand in a circle, interlock their arms, stretch the circle out by walking backward, then at the tightest point, the students simultaneously lean backward. Such activities help students see how specific strength-building activities (e.g., calisthenics and weightlifting) help a person enjoy real life. Students also see the practical ways that enjoyable activities build muscular strength and endurance. You should help students see the connections among the many physical activities in your program as well as among community-based physical activities.

Safety Guidelines for Muscular Strength and Endurance Activities

In the past, many fitness and health experts, as well as parents, have feared that strength training is dangerous for children. They pointed to the possibility of harming bone development or stunting growth; however, research does not support these fears—as long as the child strength-trains in a developmentally appropriate program that emphasizes safe limits and includes adequate adult supervision. The American Academy of Pediatrics (2001), the American College of Sports Medicine (1998), and the National Strength and Conditioning Association (2000) have all taken the position that weight training can benefit children provided that it is properly prescribed and supervised. Specifically, the NSCA asserts that even in the very young child, strength can be improved through training, and strength training can begin at any age (NSCA 2000). This includes using the child's body weight in calisthenics (such as sit-ups, push-ups, and the like) or high repetitions with light weights or resistance bands. Lifting maximal weights, however, should be delayed until all the long bones have finished growing at about 17 years of age (older in boys).

To determine the number of reps a child should do per set, have the child count how many total reps (up to 15) he or she can do with correct form, then use half of that number as the set size. As this becomes easy, work up to two sets, then three, conscientiously applying the principles of progression and overload. Retest for maximum reps when performing three sets becomes too easy. Kraemer and Fleck (1993) recommend no less than two minutes rest between weightlifting sets if strength is the goal, unless an older student (middle school and above) is ready for more specialized training, depending on maturity and fitness levels.

As previously stated, elementary prepubescent children should engage in circuit training using their own body weight, partners, or light medicine balls, and the volume should be low and intensity very low (Bompa 2000). If properly instructed and supervised, older elementary level children can use resistance bands and light free weights safely. Examples of exercises using resistance bands, medicine balls, and free weights are shown in figure 6.8 *a* through *c*. Make sure students understand the safety issues involved in partner exercises and that no "horse play" will be tolerated. Students must also understand that

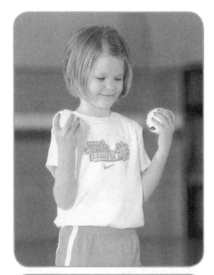

a

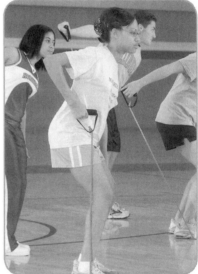

b

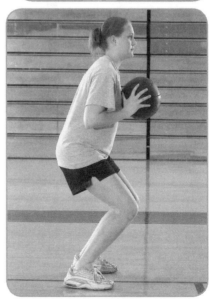

c

■ **Figure 6.8** *(a)* Biceps curl using light free weights, *(b)* triceps curl using a resistance band, and *(c)* front squat using a medicine ball.

they will not build the large muscles that some older postpubescent students and adults are capable of building. Physiologically speaking, this is simply not a realistic goal. Middle and high school students can and should participate in resistive muscular strength and endurance activities that involve the use of free weights if they are able to do so. You do not, however, need to limit these activities to dumbbell and barbell weight room activities. Resistance bands, body weight exercises, homemade equipment (e.g., plastic milk jugs filled with sand), and so on, may actually provide more opportunities for greater simultaneous participation.

One of the most important safety considerations is to individualize the resistance training program. In addition, encourage children to compete against themselves and not each other in terms of how much they can lift. The emphasis should be on the amount of weight lifted 6 to 15 times and not on how much weight can be lifted in a single lift. For all children—kindergarten through high school seniors—setting realistic goals and focusing on correct technique are important safety precautions. To satisfy the competitive spirit in some children, Kraemer and Fleck

(1993) suggest holding correct technique contests in which weight load plays no role in the final calculations (figure 6.9).

Finally, if your school has a weight room, ensure that it is set up so that traffic flows through it efficiently and there is enough room between stations. Kraemer and Fleck (1993) recommend a minimum of five feet between machines and adequate room for free weights to be dropped suddenly if need be. If possible, use machines instead of free weights for overhead movements such as those required in the bench press; reserve the bench press for older high school students. Always use spotters for all free weight exercises, even though some light exercises may not require a spotter. It is a good habit for students to develop, leaving no room for incorrect decisions regarding spotting. Students can work in pairs, spotting each other and monitoring correct technique.

Above all, to provide a safe and beneficial muscular fitness program for children, do *not* use a program designed for adults—even with adolescents. Modify and individualize, progress slowly, and reassess your program's safety and effectiveness frequently.

Training a Student to Spot a Partner

The **spotting** techniques recommended by experts vary, but there is one very important point that everyone in the weight-training community agrees on: Proper spotting is vital to the overall safety of the individual lifting the weight and the effectiveness of incorporating the FITT guidelines. Although this chapter is not geared specifically to weight training, but rather to health-related physical activity that suggests weight training merely as one of many methods, suffice it to say that proper spotting must be used when training your students with resistive weights. Several good books exist on weight training that incorporate spotting techniques, in particular, *Weight Training: Steps to Success, Second Edition*, by Thomas Baechle and Barney Groves.

Bench Press Technique

Resistance used

40 to 50 percent of body weight

Starting position

Elbows are straight; feet are flat on the floor or flat on the end of bench or platform; buttocks and shoulders touch bench; back is not excessively arched; bar is over upper chest; bar is horizontal.

Points available: 0-6

Points earned: _____

Lowering (eccentric) phase

Descent of bar is controlled; elbows are out to side; forearms are perpendicular to the floor; bar touches chest at nipple level; there is no bounce on chest touch; bar is horizontal; feet stay flat on floor; back is not excessively arched; head stays still.

Points available: 0-7

Points earned: _____

Up (concentric) phase

Back is not excessively arched; elbows are out to sides; bar is horizontal; both arms straighten at same speed; motion is smooth and continuous; head stays still; feet stay flat on floor.

Points available: 0-9

Points earned: _____

Finishing position

Same position as starting position.

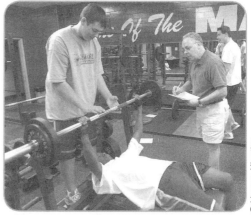

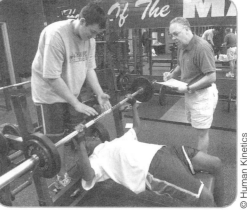

Points available: 0-3

Points earned: _____

Total points available: 0-25

Total points earned:_____

Technique tips

- Inhale as you lower the weight and exhale as you lift it.
- A spotter should be behind the lifter's head and should assist the lifter with getting the barbell into the starting position and returning the barbell to the rack when finished. Impress on young weight trainers the importance of a spotter during the exercise because the bar is pressed over the lifter's face, neck, and chest.
- Learn this exercise with an unloaded barbell or long stick.
- Do not bounce the barbell off the chest, and do not lift your buttocks off the bench during this exercise.
- Avoid hitting the upright supports by positioning your body about three inches from the supports before you start.

Figure 6.9 Correct technique is vital for weight training, so focus on technique during instruction and during assessment. A reproducible version of this form is available in appendix A.

Reprinted, by permission, from W. Kraemer and S. Fleck, 1993, *Strength training for young athletes* (Champaign, IL: Human Kinetics), 30.

Summary

By following the guidelines outlined in this chapter, you can teach students the importance of muscular strength and endurance training in safe and effective ways. You must remember that the best way to keep each child safe is to build in individual choices and help each child set realistic goals. Never push a child to lift a heavier weight than he or she has trained for or to perform "just one more rep." Instead, motivate children to participate and progress through your program by creating an enjoyable and supportive class atmosphere, rewarding effort and correct technique rather than physical prowess. The *Physical Best Activity Guides* offer a variety of age-appropriate muscular strength and endurance activities. Resistance training can be extremely interesting and rewarding, so keep in mind as you select and adapt activities that suit your students' needs that the ultimate goal of health-related physical fitness education is to produce graduates who take personal responsibility for each area of health-related fitness as a way of life.

Flexibility

Your students may have little or no knowledge of safe flexibility training. They may have learned much of what they do know (correct and incorrect knowledge) by mimicking role models at home or in sport or recreation settings. Thus, your task may be either to educate or reeducate students in safe and correct stretching techniques, as well as to inform them about the many health-related benefits associated with good flexibility. Specifically, a well-designed flexibility program (following the principles of training described in chapter 3) aids in muscle relaxation; improves overall health-related fitness, posture, and body symmetry; relieves muscle cramps and soreness; and reduces the risk of injury—all of which make physical activity of all types easier and safer to do (figure 7.1). In addition, stretching relieves emotional stress, increases feelings of well-being, and can help prepare the body to move from resting to exercising more smoothly. This chapter covers basic information regarding flexibility and stretching techniques that your students should know before leaving your program. They can apply this information to achieve and maintain good flexibility for life.

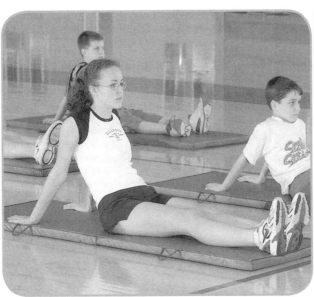
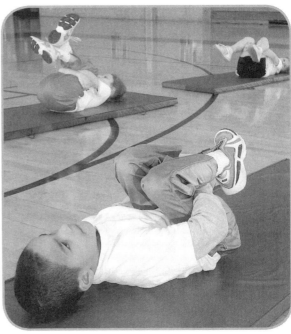

■ **Figure 7.1**   Sample stretches that can help students improve flexibility.

Definitions of Flexibility Concepts

Flexibility is the ability to move a joint through its complete ROM, or range of motion (ACSM 2000). Children may not understand the concept of joint movement through a full ROM, but they will understand "how well they bend and twist." Ask your students how many of them can touch their knees, how many can touch their toes, and how many can perform the *FITNESSGRAM* shoulder stretch with both the right and left hand. An activity such as "head, shoulders, knees, and toes" may be used to demonstrate bending and twisting at different levels. Also, you can use a Tootsie Roll to demonstrate flexibility by showing the children how it does not bend and stretch when it is cold in contrast to how the Tootsie Roll stretches and elongates (like muscles) when it is warm.

Optimal flexibility allows a joint or group of joints to move freely and efficiently; however, too much laxity in a joint is not healthy and may lead to injury. **Laxity** refers to the degree of abnormal motion of a given joint. Abnormal joint laxity means the ligaments connecting bone to bone can no longer provide stability to the joint. **Hypermobility** refers to excess ROM at a joint (Heyward 2002). Both of these conditions may predispose an individual to injury. Individuals with hypermobility should not be allowed to stretch into the extremes of ROM and should try to maintain as much joint stability as possible (ACSM 2001).

Types of Stretching

There are two types of flexibility—static and dynamic—and from a safety perspective, static stretching should be emphasized in the classroom. Dynamic flexibility testing is no longer performed because this type of stretching involves ballistic (bouncy, jerky, momentum-assisted) movements, and Knudson, Magnusson, and McHugh (2000) state that the ballistic movements may be related more to speed, coordination, and strength, and not to flexibility. **Static flexibility** is defined as the range of motion at a joint or group of joints (Knudson, Magnusson, and McHugh 2000). The limits of an individual's static flexibility are determined by his or her tolerance to the stretched position (Halbertson and Goeken 1994; Knudson, Magnusson, and McHugh 2000). **Dynamic flexibility** is "the rate of increase in tension in relaxed muscle as it is stretched. The mechanical variable that represents dynamic flexibility is stiffness" (Knudson, Magnusson, and McHugh 2000). **Stiffness** refers to the force needed to stretch and is related to the amount of elasticity in the musculotendinous unit. Dynamic flexibility exercises are more commonly used in sport-specific movements and physical therapy or rehabilitation settings. Another way to view dynamic flexibility is to examine the available ROM during active movements such as sport movements. Dynamic flexibility requires voluntary muscle contraction and poses limits on an individual's flexibility, because the contraction phase and ROM that the joint moves through do not stress the muscle as effectively as static stretching. So dynamic flexibility may have its place in preparing athletes for sport competition, but people still must use static stretching to prepare the muscles and joints for dynamic flexibility activities. It is best not to engage in dynamic flexibility exercises in physical education classes, but if you use this type of activity, you must be aware of the safety issues. These safety issues are discussed later in this chapter.

The types of stretching that foster flexibility are classified as follows (ACSM 2000):

- In the **active stretch,** the person stretching provides the force of the stretch (e.g., hamstring stretch, as shown in figure 7.2). In the **passive stretch,** a partner provides the force of the stretch (figure 7.3).

- A **static stretch** is a slow sustained stretch that is held for 10 to 30 seconds. The person stretches the muscle-tendon unit to the point where mild discomfort is felt and then backs off slightly, holding the stretch at a point just prior to discomfort. This is generally considered a safe stretch and does not rely on cooperation from a partner. In physical education classes, especially at the elementary level, this type of stretching is preferred. The advantages of static stretching include decreased possibility of exceeding the normal ROM, lower energy required, and less muscle soreness (Fredette 2001).

- **PNF (proprioceptive neuromuscular facilitation)** is a static stretch using combinations of the active and passive stretching techniques (see figure 7.4). This is a specialized static stretch that uses a contraction-relaxation combination of movements, "taking advantage

of reflexes and neuromuscular principles to relax the muscles being stretched" (Knudson, Magnusson, and McHugh 2000). PNF often yields the greatest improvements in flexibility. PNF has also been shown to be more difficult to teach, more difficult to perform, and to yield greater muscle soreness (Fredette 2001). This type of stretch should not be performed by children 6 to 10 years old, but it can be performed by pubescent or postpubescent students (Bompa 2000) or those who have developed a solid base of training and are undergoing formal athletic conditioning with help from a qualified coach. A partner is usually required for PNF. Safety, proper instruction, and responsibility are key issues in performing this type of stretch; injury may result when children are not responsible, fail to listen to the cues of their partner (thereby forcing a stretch), or incorrectly perform a stretch.

- Dynamic or **ballistic stretching** involves moving quickly, bouncing, or using momentum to produce the stretch, and like PNF, also elicits muscle soreness (ACSM 2000). This type of stretch is often viewed as necessary for sport movements and should be reserved for postpubescent students (approximately 15 years and older) or those undergoing specialized sport training. If this type is chosen as the mode of stretching, the students *must* perform a good general warm-up, followed by static stretching, prior to initiating dynamic or ballistic stretching. People tend to use the terms *dynamic* and *ballistic* stretching interchangeably, but dynamic stretching is different from ballistic in that it avoids the bouncy, jerky type of movement and commonly uses sport-specific movements. You could think of dynamic stretching as special preparation for movements performed during competition. Reserve this type of stretching for coaching or conditioning activities and not physical education class.

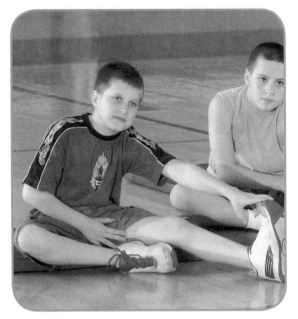

■ **Figure 7.2**   Example of active stretching.

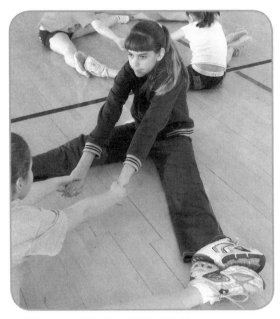

■ **Figure 7.3**   Example of passive stretching.

Physical Best's Position

Many experts caution that participants perform at least five minutes of low-intensity aerobic fitness activity before performing any stretching. Thus, we recommend that you have students take this simple precaution.

Benefits of Flexibility

Remember that flexibility is for everyone, and regardless of ability or disability, everyone can learn to stretch and benefit from improved range of motion. Most people have been taught that increased flexibility reduces the risk of injury and incidence of low back problems; however, research indicates that although this is a logical premise, there is little evidence that greater than normal static flexibility reduces the risk of injury (Corbin and Noble 1980). These findings hold true today as well (Corbin et al. 2004). Moreover, there appears to be more evidence that extreme static flexibility may actually increase the risk of injury (Jones and Knapik 1999; Knudson, Magnusson, and McHugh 2000). Knudson, Magnusson, and McHugh (2000) also indicate that

PNF Hamstring Stretch

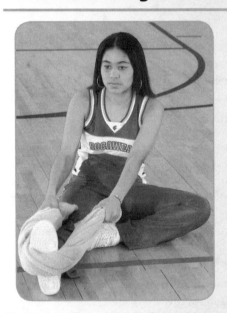

■ **Figure 7.4**   Example of PNF stretching.

■ Pull towel toward you until mild tension is felt

■ Hold towel in position and try to point the toes against the towel resistance.

■ Relax, and then pull towards you again.

a normal level of flexibility is needed to reduce the risk of injury in most vigorous activities. The goal, therefore, is to follow the FITT guidelines and help students maintain normal flexibility and range of motion in all joints.

The specificity principle states that the observed range of motion at each joint is specific to the flexibility exercises performed at each joint; therefore, the benefits that follow apply only to the muscles and joints utilized in a stretching program. Alter (1998) and Fredette (2001) state the following benefits of increased flexibility:

1. Decreased muscle tension and increased relaxation

2. Greater ease of movement

3. Improved coordination

4. Increased range of motion

5. Reduced risk of injury (Remember that it is greater than normal levels of flexibility that fail to show a reduction in the risk of injury and that maintenance of normal flexibility is essential for good muscular fitness.)

6. Better body awareness and postural alignment

7. Improved circulation and air exchange

8. Smoother and easier contractions

9. Decreased muscle soreness

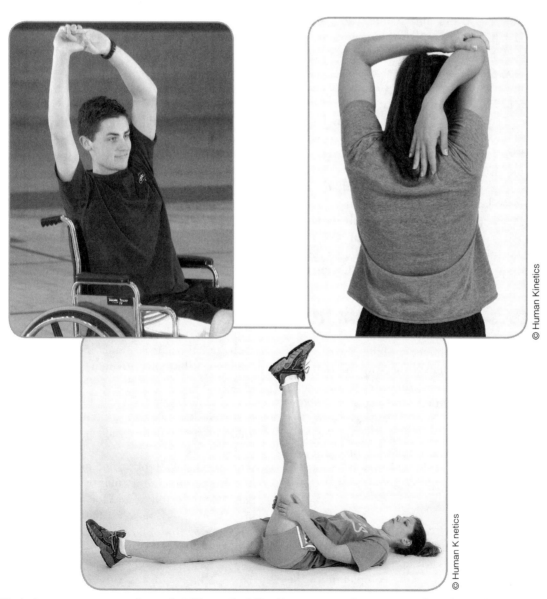

© Human Kinetics

Flexibility is for everyone, regardless of ability or disability. Everyone can learn to stretch and benefit from improved range of motion.

10. Prevention of low back pain and other spinal problems (Again, it is maintenance of normal flexibility that is important.)

11. Improved personal appearance and self-image

12. Improved development and maintenance of motor skills

All of these benefits contribute to the overall health and well-being of the individual and affirm the importance of including flexibility activities in your physical education daily lessons (see the *Physical Best Activity Guides* for specific examples).

Does increased flexibility improve athletic performance? The consensus appears to be that the performance benefits are not as great as once thought (Corbin and Noble 1980; Gleim and McHugh 1997; Knudson, Magnusson, and McHugh 2000). There is also evidence suggesting that less static flexibility may actually benefit performance when it comes to running economy (Craib and Mitchell 1996), and that static stretching prior to some muscular activities may lead to a decrease in strength and muscular performance (Avela, Kyrolainen, and Komi 1999; Kokkonen, Nelson, and Cornwell 1998). Until more research confirms these concerns, teachers should encourage their students to maintain normal flexibility and range of motion and should teach them the importance of a well-rounded fitness program that includes flexibility, especially since students should not be competing and lifting maximal weights.

Factors Affecting Flexibility

No matter what factors affect flexibility, most people can improve their flexibility through appropriate and regular stretching (at least three days per week); however, keep in mind that there are many factors that influence the amount of flexibility observed or measured at each joint. Emphasize to students that irregular participation in a flexibility program also yields poor results. It is the old "use it or lose it" adage. The following are some factors that affect flexibility:

- *Muscle temperature* affects muscle elasticity, or the muscle's ability to stretch beyond its normal resting length and then return to its prestretched length at the completion of the exercise.

- *Age and gender* also affect flexibility. Children are generally more flexible than adults. Also, some changes are seen between the primary grades and high school—flexibility remains stable or gradually declines to about age 12 and then increases to peak flexibility at about age 15 to 18 years old (Knudson, Magnusson, and McHugh 2000). Females are generally more flexible than males (Alter 1998). In addition, research shows that maintaining a good flexibility plan across the life span may limit or reduce the natural changes in elasticity and compliance of muscle tissue (ACSM 2000; Knudson, Magnusson, and McHugh 2000).

- *Tissue interference*, such as excess body fat or well-developed musculature, is another factor affecting flexibility. This constraint may also include bone and joint limitations such as in the elbow joint where ROM beyond 180 degrees is limited by bone. Do not allow tissue interference to limit your plans for improving flexibility, because high body fat is generally a result of inactivity, and the student with well-developed musculature as a limiting factor (usually not a factor until late high school, if at all) may simply be lacking a flexibility exercise program. These individuals can develop and maintain adequate flexibility (Heyward 2002).

Other factors that may limit flexibility include pain, poor coordination and strength during active movement, and extensibility of the musculotendinous unit (i.e., tension in muscles). Note that most of these limitations can be reversed and stated as benefits of flexibility (decreased pain as a result of injury, improved coordination, and reduced tension). Take each limitation into account for each individual when designing a flexibility program (Alter 1998; Knudson, Magnusson, and McHugh 2000).

Although most of the limitations can be overcome in a well-designed, appropriately progressive flexibility program, pain should never be ignored, and limitations caused by bone or joint structures may require special attention and individualization. Certain diseases (e.g., muscular dystrophy and cerebral palsy) limit flexibility, and for many of these conditions, you should consult with your adapted physical educator or the child's physician to inquire about appropriate stretching activities. For more information on health-related fitness for children and adults with cerebral palsy, see ACSM's Current Comments (Blanchard 1999).

Genetics and Flexibility

Although, according to Franks and Howley (1998), flexibility is limited by genetics, it is still necessary to use the joints regularly to develop and maintain the flexibility a person is capable of. If this is not done, the person will not be as flexible as he or she could be. For example, if a person breaks an arm at the elbow, when the cast is removed, the person will have to reteach the joint to move through its normal ROM. This is because, while the arm was immobilized in the cast, fibrous connective tissue, called *adhesions*, began to cling to the ligaments, tendons, and bones in the elbow, impeding its ROM. In addition, because the cast held the arm at a fixed angle, the tendons and muscles in the upper arm shortened, preventing the arm from straightening after the cast is removed. Both the condition of the connective tissues at the joint and the ability of the muscle to stretch affect flexibility. This is true even without the problems caused by wearing a cast. Stretching helps maintain the proper muscle-tendon unit length while helping prevent adhesions. Stretching is an important part of both warm-ups and cool-downs because, along with other gentle activities, stretching helps get the joints ready for more strenuous activity. It does this by encouraging the body to release fluids that lubricate the joints and by increasing the size of the soft cartilage around the joint to help absorb the shock of impact.

Teaching Guidelines for Flexibility

The nice thing about flexibility training is that it is the one area of health-related fitness that improves very rapidly. Anyone can learn to stretch and everyone can attain the benefits of improved flexibility. First, select the type of stretch that meets the needs of your lesson. Allow students to participate in selecting the various flexibility exercises that may be completed for a warm-up or cool-down. Once you have a repertoire of exercises for the total body, and have completed proper instruction for each one, you can then use station cards, change the warm-up or cool-down, or have students select the specific exercise to meet their individual goals.

In the physical education setting, the static stretch is generally preferred and considered the safest method for enhancing ROM. A program of static stretches (like those shown in figure 7.5) does not take much class time, and it is generally easy to ensure that each individual in a large group of students is performing them correctly.

Establish a regular schedule of flexibility fitness lessons and stretching in your classes; include definitions and basic concepts regarding the FITT guidelines (discussed later) and safety precautions. This will not only teach your students the importance of stretching, but will also allow for integration of flexibility concepts into all other aspects of health-related fitness. This is also the time to explain the relationship between flexibility exercises performed in class and the back-saver sit-and-reach test performed during the fitness assessment portion of your program.

Just as in weight training, proper form and technique are important for flexibility training. You do not want students stretching improperly and placing excess stress on joints and connective tissues, thereby increasing the risk of injury during activities designed to improve health and well-being. Also, emphasize that flexibility training, either with or without a partner, is no place for "horse play" because injury may result. This is especially important if you are using PNF or partner stretching. Stress safety and slow, gradual, individualized progression when teaching children about flexibility. Never make flexibility training competitive; instead, as with muscular strength training, emphasize correct technique and personal bests.

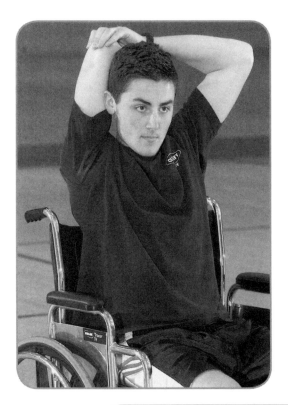
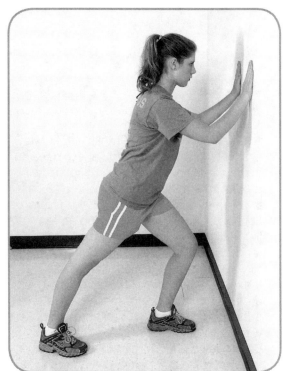
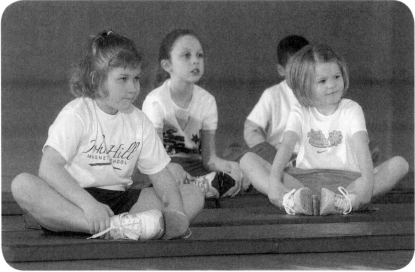
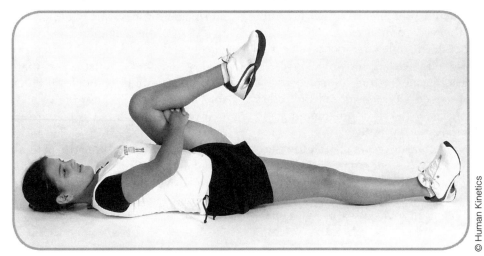

© Human Kinetics

Figure 7.5 Examples of static stretches.

Partner-Resisted Hamstring Stretch

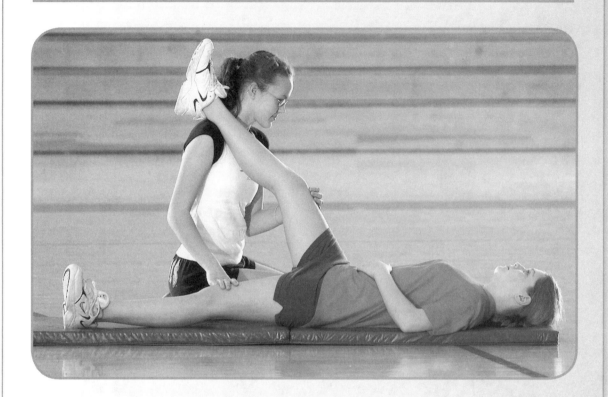

1. The stretcher lies supine and lifts her thigh to flex her hip to 90 degrees, with the knee bent.

2. Partner should stabilize the thigh in this position while the stretcher straightens the raised leg as far as possible, without pain. This lengthens the hamstrings to their pain-free end of range. The straight leg should remain flat on the mat.

3. Partner can offer resistance to the isometric contraction of the hamstrings, at the same time making sure that the stretcher keeps her hips flat on the table. The partner may need to work with the stretcher on body awareness until her is able to stabilize her hips properly before performing this stretch.

4. Partner will direct the stretcher to begin slowly to attempt to push her heel toward the floor, bending the knee, which isometrically contracts the hamstrings.

5. After the isometric push, the stretcher relaxes and inhales deeply. During this time, maintain the leg in the starting position.

Text is adapted, by permission, from R.E. McAtee and J. Charland, 1999, *Facilitated stretching* (Champaign, IL: Human Kinetics), 34.

Safe Stretching

Questionable Exercise

Quadricep stretch
Danger: If the ankle is pulled too hard, muscle, ligament, and cartilage damage may occur.

Safer Alternative Exercise

Opposite leg pull
Description: Grasp one ankle with your opposite hand. Instead of pulling, attempt to straighten the leg you are stretching.

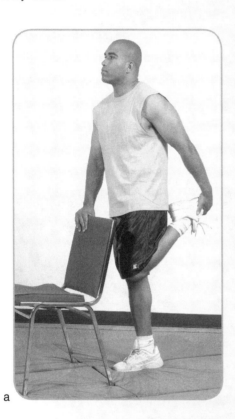

a

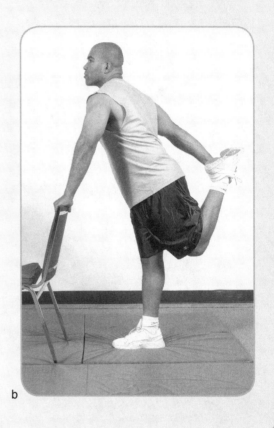

b

■ **Figure 7.4**   Use visual aids to help students understand how to safely perform a stretch. Shown is (*a*) the questionable method for performing a quadriceps stretch and (*b*) the safer alternative for performing a quadriceps stretch. See appendix D for more questionable exercises and their safer alternatives.

Figures and text adapted, by permission, from J.S. Greenberg, G.V. Dintiman, and B. Myers Oakes, 2004. *Physical fitness and wellness: changing the way you look, feel, and perform,* 3rd edition (Champaign, IL: Human Kinetics), 151-153.

Two major advantages of teaching flexibility are that it does not require much equipment and that many different areas provide sufficient space for conducting the program. For example, you can have students stretch in a gymnasium, on a field, on the blacktop, in a classroom, or, if there is little through traffic, in a hallway. Lay mats or parachutes on the ground to protect clothing outdoors. Visual aids such as posters, task cards, and pictures of schoolmates performing stretches help guide students working independently at stations (figure 7.4). As a result of your flexibility unit, students should understand the definition of flexibility, all the methods available to improve and assess flexibility, why flexibility is important across the life span, and how to safely stretch.

Elastic and Plastic and When to Stretch

The argument for warming up indicates that muscles and other tissues are easier to stretch when they are warm. The connective tissues of the **muscle-tendon unit** have both "elastic" and "plastic" properties. The **elastic** property allows the tissue to return to its normal length following stretching; the **plastic** property is what establishes its normal length when at rest. The stretching routine is aimed at changing the plastic property, so that the joint can move through its normal range of motion. It is easier to lengthen the connective tissues while minimizing tissue damage if the muscle-tendon unit is already warm. The contrasting argument suggests that muscles are normally "warm," and light warm-up activities don't increase that very much. We recommend that you have the participants do some light stretching activities at the beginning of an exercise session and a more thorough program of stretching during the cool-down when body temperature is elevated and greater flexibility gains can be made.

Reprinted, by permission, from E.T. Franks and B.D. Howley, 1998, *Fitness leader's handbook*, 2nd ed. (Champaign, IL: Human Kinetics), 92.

Principles of Training

All students should learn how to apply the principles of training to flexibility. These are the same principles discussed in chapter 3, as well as in each chapter on the health-related fitness components. Applying these training principles helps students improve flexibility and implement the FITT guidelines (discussed later in the chapter) in their program.

Overload, Progression, Specificity, Regularity, and Individuality

The principle of overload states that in order to adapt and improve flexibility, the muscle-tendon unit must be stretched until mild tension (point of discomfort) is felt; the person then backs off slightly and holds the stretch at a point just prior to discomfort. The principle of progression calls for gradually increasing the amount of time each stretch is held. Your students should not use the progression principle to increase the load (tension) placed on the muscle, because they only want to stretch a joint through the limits of normal ROM (ACSM 2001). If they always stretch to the point of mild discomfort and then back off slightly, then they will always overload the muscle at the proper tension. The stretch should feel tight, but not painful. Above all, dispel the "no pain, no gain" notion. Flexibility training should not be painful (see "Safety Guidelines for Flexibility Activities" later in this chapter). Specificity and regularity, as in other

areas of health-related fitness, state that to increase flexibility of a particular area, a person must perform exercises for a specific muscle or muscle group, and must do it on a regular basis (flexibility exercises can be done daily). Any improvements in flexibility are lost if the person stops performing flexibility exercises (regularity principle). As stated in other chapters discussing the principles of training, each student should have individual goals based on need, physical limitations, or performance ambition.

FITT Guidelines

The recommended *frequency* for flexibility training is daily (three times per week minimum but preferably daily) to be able to attain the maximum benefits. Increasing the number of flexibility sessions per week from three to daily is also a method to increase the overload placed on the muscle. As previously mentioned, the *intensity* for all flexibility exercises should be to the point just prior to discomfort (stretch to the point of slight discomfort and back off slightly). Intensity is an extremely important factor in a safe and effective flexibility training program. A static stretch that goes beyond the point of mild discomfort (to pain) merely increases the likelihood of injury. *Time* refers to how long the stretch is held, and there is a wide variety of suggestions ranging from 10 seconds through 1 minute. The American College of Sports Medicine (2000) proposes a stretch be held 10 to 30 seconds. (Note that a student should always begin holding a stretch for a short period of time and gradually progress to the 30-second time period.) *Type* refers to the kind of stretching used to develop flexibility, such as static, PNF, partner, or dynamic ballistic stretches (reserved for sport and not physical education classes). Table 7.1 provides information on how to manipulate time and type based on the FITT guidelines when performing stretching exercises.

Before your students begin any flexibility exercise, ensure that proper instruction is provided and that an active warm-up is completed prior to stretching. Younger or less experienced students should learn the basic static stretches that increase flexibility of major muscle groups, while older or more experienced students may be ready for a greater variety of sport-specific stretches and advanced stretching techniques.

Bompa (2000) suggests laying a strong foundation of static stretches when children are 6 to 10 years of age, which he terms the initiation phase of training. He also suggests using various stages of maturation as a guide to indicate when it is appropriate to perform the three basic types of stretching (static, PNF, and ballistic). Remember that PNF and partner stretching require extensive instruction and mature, responsible students; these types of stretches may pose injury problems if not performed correctly.

Teach your students to follow the FITT guidelines using slow, steady, static stretching, holding each stretch only to the point of mild tension, not pain—regardless of what they have been told in the past. They should hold the stretch 10 to

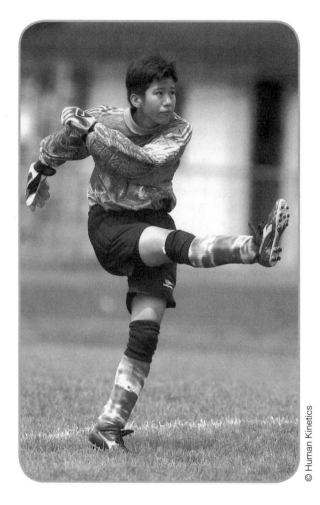

© Human Kinetics

If your students want to be able to punt a football, or perform a high kick in a soccer game, they must have good leg flexibility to be successful.

TABLE 7.1   FITT Guidelines Applied to Flexibility

Frequency	Three times per week, preferably daily and after a warm-up to raise muscle temperature.
Intensity	Slow elongation of the muscle to the point of mild discomfort and back off slightly.
Time	Up to 4-5 stretches per muscle or muscle group. Hold each stretch 10-30 sec. Always warm up properly prior to stretching.
Type	The preferred stretch for the classroom is slow static stretching for all muscles or muscle groups.

Note: Although 10-30 sec is recommended as the length of time to hold a stretch, an advanced student may hold a stretch up to 60 sec.

Modified from Knudson, D.V., P. Magnusson, and M. McHugh. 2000. Current issues in flexibility fitness. In C. Corbin and B. Pangrazi, eds., The president's council on physical fitness and sports digest, 3rd ser., no. 10, Washington, DC: Department of Health and Human Services.

American College of Sports Medicine (ACSM). 2001. *ACSM's Resource Manual for Guidelines for Exercise Testing and Prescription.* 4th ed. Philadelphia: Lippincott, Williams, and Wilkins.

30 seconds, depending on what is comfortable for them, not what a classmate can do. In these ways, you empower students to individualize each stretch—and the flexibility program—for themselves. Teach students that ballistic stretching is only appropriate in certain sport situations and then only if done correctly.

If you believe a student is too flexible (displays hypermobility), has abnormal ROM (laxity), severely lacks flexibility, or has other unusual bone or joint structural limitations, and such an anomaly seems to cause serious performance or safety concerns, refer the student to trained health care professionals, such as a certified athletic trainer, physical therapist, or an orthopedic medical specialist. Then have the student and parents ask this professional for specific recommendations for safe participation in physical education. Meet with the student and parents to discuss and document these recommendations.

Addressing Motor Skills Through Flexibility Activities

Naturally, a student who can move through a full range of motion (ROM) is more likely to be ready to learn to perform motor skills correctly. Likewise, a student with limited ROM will have a more difficult time mastering the same motor skill. The specificity principle applies here: If a person wants to be able to punt a football, or perform a high kick in a soccer game, the person must have good leg flexibility to be successful. Good flexibility, then, enhances motor skill development. Address motor skills through flexibility activities and vice versa by pointing out the connections between the stretches you are teaching and the motor skill activities students practice in class. When students see the connections between flexibility and the physical activities they are engaging in, they are more likely to continue working on enhancing flexibility as a lifestyle choice. In short, you create a deeper awareness of the need for flexibility.

Safety Guidelines for Flexibility Activities

There are many safety issues related to stretching in the physical education setting. Prior to stretching, a general whole-body warm-up should be completed.

If you have students with physical disabilities, you may need to use a longer warm-up period to enhance joint mobility. Remember, all students should use slow, controlled movements (static stretches), holding each stretch at the point just prior to mild discomfort (backing off slightly when discomfort is felt) for 10 to 30 seconds. This allows students to individualize their efforts. Also, be aware of the previously discussed factors that may limit flexibility. Other general rules that apply include making sure that students limit or avoid locking any joint when performing flexibility exercises. "Soft knees" and "soft joints" are often used to describe this important safeguard to prevent any unnecessary overstretching of ligaments. A second rule related to overstretching involves the issue of forcing a stretch. Require students to pay attention to what their body is telling them regarding feelings of discomfort and pain. These feelings are signals that the student is forcing the stretch, going beyond the normal range of motion and possibly damaging ligaments. A third rule is to never allow students to hyperflex (bend from the waist) or hyperextend the spine, because this places undue stress on the intervertebral discs of the spine. It is okay to bend from the hips in a forward flexed position, but not from the waist only. The compression of the discs of the lower back is one of the reasons why the back-saver sit-and-reach test was implemented. The forward flexed position combining both hip flexion and flexion at the waist causes increased pressure on the discs. By doing one leg at a time, this reduces the pressure. Hyperextension is also not recommended for a similar reason of compressing the discs. It is okay to go from a flexed position to extension, but not beyond normal extension into hyperextension (bending backward). Be aware that there may be instances where a physician prescribes hyperextension exercises to rehabilitate the lower back, but this motion should generally be avoided for most of the population. The undue stress on the intervertebral discs is exacerbated if twisting or when rotation is combined with hyperflexion or hyperextension. Although this may not present an immediate concern or injury, over time these actions may contribute to chronic degeneration of the discs and low back pain as a person ages.

Ballistic Stretching

Many exercise scientists, coaches, and personal trainers believe that ballistic stretching, when used appropriately, can help improve a person's skill-related fitness. However, many physical educators believe that ballistic stretching should not be taught in physical education because (1) static stretching is more important to maintaining good health and (2) ballistic stretching is more likely to be harmful if not performed properly. It is the opinion of the Physical Best Steering Committee that ballistic stretching should not be taught in an elementary, middle, or high school physical education program. However, if a student-athlete asks about ballistic stretching to help his or her sport performance, physical educators should provide appropriate information and teach dynamic stretching that uses sport-specific movements, such as the track athlete performing long strides, emphasizing hip extension while maintaining a posterior pelvic tilt (stretches the hip flexors used in competition) (NSCA 2000).

Ballistic stretching can be performed safely to enhance sport-specific movements. Teach older student-athletes (middle and high school level) the following guidelines (Arthur and Bailey 1998):

- Warm up first with a whole-body activity.
- Perform static stretching before ballistic.
- Do quick movements that duplicate specific sport movements.
- Keep movements gentle and controlled despite speed.
- Choose movements that isolate individual muscles or muscle groups needed for the targeted sport-specific movements.
- Avoid overstretching (overloading too aggressively).
- Increase ROM and speed gradually and progressively.

Arguments against ballistic stretching include inadequate time for tissues to adapt to the motion, increased likelihood of soreness, initiation of the stretch reflex, and inadequate time for neurological pathways to adapt to the movement (Alter 1998). In short, some believe that ballistic stretches are too fast and that the stretch reflex will actually cause the tissue involved to contract rather than relax. If choosing to use this type of stretch, make sure that students adequately warm the muscle tissue, perform static stretching prior to this dynamic type of stretch, and perform the dynamic stretch slowly and with caution. The Physical Best program recommends the static stretch as part of a safe and effective lifelong health-related fitness program.

Contraindicated Exercises

Contraindicated exercises are those exercises that have been determined to be unsafe or to have the potential for increasing the risk of injury if individuals continue to incorporate them into their physical activity program. Keep in mind that an injury may not occur every time a contraindicated exercise is performed, but that injury may result over weeks or years of repeated microtrauma to the tissue.

Flexibility training is designed to be an important component of health-related fitness. We have previously discussed hypermobility, joint laxity, and flexibility safety issues. When a student performs an exercise that takes a joint well beyond its normal range of motion, such as in some **hyperflexion** or **hyperextension** exercises, there is an increased risk for the development of joint laxity and possible injury. There are several exercises (see appendix D for examples) that should be avoided so that the risk of joint injury is reduced (Corbin et al. 2004; Lindsey and Corbin 1989).

Provide alternatives when designing your flexibility unit, keeping in mind the specificity principle and the availability of exercise prescriptions by medical personnel. Also, some sports demand extreme ROM, such as gymnastics, dancing, and certain positions such as baseball catcher, which requires the full squat. In these instances, it may be necessary to follow the medically prescribed exercise prescription and to teach dynamic, sport-specific flexibility exercises. If so, use extreme caution, active warm-ups, and static stretching prior to performing the dynamic stretches. Many of the exercises in appendix D are considered questionable or contraindicated for group exercise, such as that used in physical education classes. In many instances, teachers do not have the time, nor the expertise, to individually "prescribe" exercises for special situations. Corbin et al. (2004) suggest that physical educators teach to the needs of the majority and include exercises that have the least negative impact, while providing the most positive benefits. If some exercises possibly cause injury, and there are alternatives to use, it makes sense to use the alternative exercises for a safer, more effective program.

Summary

Flexibility is just as important to health-related fitness as other components, so resist the temptation to always relegate it to warm-ups and cool-downs. When appropriate, feature it as the core activity of a lesson. This will give you the time to demonstrate how important, relaxing, and pleasurable it is. See the *Physical Best Activity Guides* for model flexibility training lessons. Then you can refer to the basic concepts and principles of flexibility as you use it to enhance your students' performance in other areas of the physical education curriculum. Finally, although ballistic stretching can be effective in some circumstances, remember that static stretching is more appropriate in a health-related physical fitness education program.

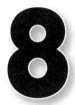

CHAPTER

8

Body Composition

Few physical educators would deny that teaching about body composition is one of the most sensitive areas of health-related fitness education. Cultural, social, and personal beliefs and attitudes make this a difficult topic, so the temptation to avoid the subject is great. But understanding body composition—including what affects it and the benefits of a healthy body composition—is critical to overall health-related fitness. Although it is not important to calculate exact body composition indicators with very young children, these children still need to explore the related concepts and understand how an active lifestyle affects body composition. Older children need this information, too, as well as tools to monitor and positively affect body composition throughout life. This information is also critical for the prevention of chronic disease.

Teaching Guidelines for Body Composition

Body composition is the amount of lean body mass (all tissues other than fat, such as bone, muscle, organs and body fluids) compared to the amount of body fat, usually expressed in terms of percent body fat. There are several common ways to gauge whether or not body composition is healthy, with a range of what constitutes a healthy body composition. Table 8.1 identifies recommended ranges for body fat (CI 2004).

There are four main aspects to teaching students about body composition in a sensitive and professional manner:

- Project an attitude of acceptance toward individual differences and demand that students follow your lead with their peers.
- Respect each individual's privacy.
- Relate body composition to the other components of health-related fitness in meaningful ways.
- Acknowledge whether or not you can help an individual who is over or under an appropriate body composition, and refer the student or parents to professional help if clinically indicated.

Accepting Individual Differences

Teachers should avoid asserting that there are absolute indicators of good and poor health related to body composition. Remember, experts cannot even agree completely on how body composition is best measured. When teaching body composition, it should be approached as an individual and personal topic about which everyone should try to be compassionate. Never use a student as a positive or negative model of composition. Also, explain to students

that genetics plays a role in body composition (this is discussed in greater detail later in the chapter). As a physical educator, you should encourage individuals to find personal satisfaction with their overall health, wellness, and physical activity habits, rather than struggling to measure up to scientific methods of calculating body composition or to cultural expectations. Remind them that "normal" comes in all shapes and sizes.

Respecting Privacy

Never publicize a student's measurements or percent body fat; in addition, be sure to secure the information where it cannot be accessed by other students. Also be aware that students with a less-than-perfect body composition may be reluctant to be measured in front of their more physically fit peers. Conduct skinfold caliper testing or any other measuring in private as a voluntary activity. Ask another adult to help with testing or with conducting the rest of the class while you are occupied with this procedure. Explain to students that body composition is a personal matter and that they should only focus on their own information. Check with your administrator regarding any set guidelines that may be in place for your school; for example, you may need to obtain parental permission for skinfold testing (or at least notify parents of upcoming testing) and have another adult present during testing to prevent harassment issues.

Relating Body Composition to Other Health-Related Fitness Components

As with any other component of health-related fitness, a person's body composition does not happen in isolation from the other components. Indeed, it is perhaps even more important to show students the connections among all health-related fitness components so that they can clearly see how their personal choices affect this area of health-related fitness. Although genetics, environment, and culture play significant roles in body composition, it is in large part a result of the individual's physical activity levels in the other components:

- Aerobic fitness—Aerobic activities burn calories.
- Muscular strength and endurance—Muscle cells burn (metabolize) more calories at rest

TABLE 8.1   Recommended Body Fat

	Males	Females
Minimum healthy body fat	10%	17%
Maximum healthy body fat	25%	32%

than fat cells. Emphasize physical activity that follows the principles of training (chapter 3). This will increase the likelihood of maintaining an appropriate body composition.

■ Flexibility—A flexible body can better tolerate aerobic fitness and muscular strength and endurance activities.

Strive to point out connections among physical activity, diet, and body composition related to daily life, recreational, and physical education activities (see figure 8.1). Emphasize, too, that a student who is overfat because of genetics can still greatly reduce health risks by being physically active. Physical activity, even without calorie restriction, is effective in reducing a person's risk for chronic disease, regardless of the person's level of obesity (Ross, Freeman, and Janssen 2000; USDHHS 1996). In fact, one study revealed that overfat people who exercise regularly are at no greater health risk than thin people who don't exercise (Blair 1995).

Strength Training and Body Composition Management

Strength training can be a valuable adjunct to a body composition management program. A weight reduction program can cause loss of protein tissue (primary muscles) along with body fat. Strength training can prevent significant loss of lean body mass, while also preventing decreases in **resting energy expenditure (REE),** or the energy the body uses at rest. Each additional pound of muscle tissue can raise the REE by 35 kilocalories per day (Campbell et al. 1994), which, over the course of a year, can result in weight loss.

Students need to know that although resistance training does burn calories, the effect is relatively small compared to that of aerobic exercise. They must also understand that it is physiologically impossible for muscle cells to turn into fat in the future, and vice versa. A combination of aerobic exercise and light resistance training is best for body composition management.

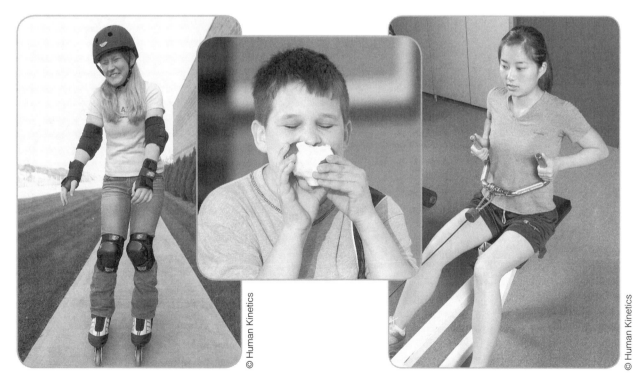

■ **Figure 8.1** A thorough understanding of body composition, what affects it, and the benefits of a healthy body composition is critical to overall health-related fitness.

Percent Body Fat versus Body Mass Index

Body mass index (BMI) does not estimate percent fat, but merely gives an indication of the appropriateness of the weight relative to height (CIAR, 2004). The following example demonstrates how two students fall into the healthy fitness zone (HFZ) through body mass index calculations. However, Jane's percent body fat is 35% and outside the HFZ, while Jeanette's percent body fat is 19%, and in the HFZ.

Jane and Jeanette are both 16 years old, weigh 130 pounds and are 5'6" tall. While both girls have the same body mass index (BMI), body composition tests show that Jane is carrying approximately 45 pounds of fat, while Jeanette has only approximately 25 pounds of fat.

Jane's percent body fat is calculated as follows:

$45 \div 130 = .35$ (round to the nearest 100th)

$.35 \times 100 = 35$ percent body fat

Jane's BMI is calculated as follows:

$$\left(\frac{130}{65^2}\right) \times 703$$

$$\frac{130}{4225} \times 703$$

$$.0308 \times 703 = 21.6$$

Jeanette's percent body fat is as follows:

$25 \div 130 = .19$ (rounded to the nearest 100th)

$.19 \times 100 = 19$ percent body fat

Jeanette's BMI is calculated as follows:

$$\left(\frac{130}{65^2}\right) \times 703$$

$$\frac{130}{4225} \times 703$$

$$.0308 \times 703 = 21.6$$

So although height-weight charts and BMI may provide a general indication of health, they do not provide a measure of percent fat, and therefore do not tell the complete story of body composition.

Methods of Measuring Body Composition

Experts do not agree on what is the best method for measuring body composition. Elementary students should be taught the basic concepts of body composition and what affects it, while middle and high school students should be taught specific methods of assessing body composition and the pros and cons of each method.

Skinfold Caliper Testing

Skinfold caliper testing is a commonly used method for determining body composition in the physical education setting. It involves using **skinfold calipers** to take **skinfold** measurements at specific sites on the body (figure 8.2).

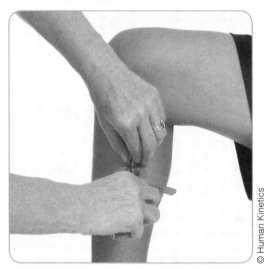

■ **Figure 8.2** Using calipers to take a calf skinfold measurement.

© Human Kinetics

This is the most accurate way of measuring body composition generally available to the physical educator, and it is relatively inexpensive to implement. However, a tester must be well trained to take reliable measurements. Measuring takes a great deal of class time and teacher attention. Because this method involves touching a student, other sensitivities may arise. If you do not feel comfortable with or qualified to perform this testing method, obtain further training or arrange for more qualified personnel to help you (perhaps someone from the physical education or athletic training department of a local university). Specific guidelines for skinfold measurement administration and age-appropriate guidelines are published in the *FITNESSGRAM/ACTIVITYGRAM Test Administration Manual,* Third Edition (CI 2004), see Appendix E.

Tips for Conducting Skinfold Testing

Many teachers feel uncomfortable measuring percent body fat for a variety of reasons, including the following:

- A student may feel embarrassed by his or her test results.
- A teacher may be reluctant to touch students in any manner.
- Students may be reluctant to let teachers touch them in any manner.
- It takes training and practice to measure accurately.

You can take several steps to address these concerns.

1. Get the training and practice you need to take accurate measurements. NASPE/AAHPERD provides workshops and in-services on Physical Best and on *FITNESSGRAM* testing techniques (contact NASPE for details). You may also elect to invite a qualified fitness instructor, university physical education instructor, school nurse, or certified athletic trainer to conduct this testing for you.

2. Teach older students to use the skinfold calipers. This allows them to assume responsibility, ensures the privacy of their results, and gives them the option to peer assess, working with a trusted friend. But be sensitive: If you have overweight children in a class, you may not want to have students measure each other (and possibly expose the overweight children to ridicule). On the other hand, it's also important to teach your class that people come in all different sizes, and that all people should feel welcome and comfortable in physical activity settings. Regardless of positive habits, people are made differently.

3. Focus on making students aware of the personal choices all people make that affect their body composition. This helps students set goals based on the process of a physically active and healthful lifestyle, rather than the product. In addition, teach students that both too much and too little body fat can be harmful. If age appropriate, discuss eating disorders.

4. Conduct skinfold testing in a separate room if possible, testing one student at a time. This may relieve some of a student's discomfort with the situation.

5. If you are especially concerned that you may be accused of touching a student improperly, arrange to have a knowledgeable second adult attend the testing. Also, Physical Best provides options for calculating body composition. You can easily calculate body mass index instead.

Body Mass Index

Although attention paid by the media to **body mass index (BMI)** has recently risen, this method of determining body composition is nothing new. BMI has been used as a measure of obesity in population studies for years. This is generally the measure used by federal agencies when reporting obesity statistics:

BMI Measures

Less than 18.5	Underweight
18.5–25	Optimal
25.1–29.9	Overweight
Over 30	Obese
Over 40	Morbidly obese

The health risk (from weight) increases greatly with BMIs over 30. As BMI continues to rise, so does the health risk.

BMI is a ratio of height to weight. It is a mathematical formula that correlates with body fat in the general population. BMI is a measure best used for postpubescent students. In children, BMI is age and gender specific. Girls and boys mature at different ages and in different ways. As a result, the Centers for Disease Control and Prevention (CDC) has created age-specific BMI tables that allow for gender differences, growth spurts, and changes in growth. These charts exist for children ages 2 through 20 (see Figures E.1 and E.2 in appendix E). The CDC also has a pediatric BMI calculator that is available at www.cdc.gov/nccdphp/dnpa/bmi/bmi-for-age.htm.

BMI provides a quick body composition check that a person can self-administer. This method takes little class time and teacher attention and is easy for a student to use outside of a physical education program. Its primary disadvantage, however, is that it is a vast oversimplification of the body composition picture, because it does not take into account percent body fat. For example, any two individuals at the same BMI and fitness level may have different fat-to-lean mass ratios (based on genetic and nutritional factors such as bone size and density). Or any two people with the same BMI may have vastly different percents body fat (see % fat vs BMI section on p. 124). In short, a person can be fit and healthy or unfit and unhealthy at any of the BMIs within the extremes of clinical obesity and severe underfatness. Even so, BMI gives people one indicator of health and wellness, and it has been used widely in epidemiological studies. When indicated, help students with BMIs at the extremes look for causes and solutions.

Calculating BMI

To calculate an individual's BMI, simply divide weight in pounds by height in inches squared, and multiply that by 703.

$$BMI = \frac{\text{weight in pounds} \times 703}{(\text{height in inches}) \times (\text{height in inches})}$$

For example, a boy who weighs 150 pounds and is 5 feet 5 inches tall would calculate his BMI as follows:

$$BMI = 150 \div 65^{\prime\prime 2} \times 703$$

$$= (150 \div 4,225) \times 703 = 25$$

$$= 25$$

To have postpubescent students calculate their own body mass index, use the "Calculating BMI" information that follows.

Height-Weight Chart

Height-weight charts were originally the creation of Louis Dublin, an actuary for the Metropolitan Life Insurance Company. These charts arose because insurance companies attempted to scientifically predict which clients were lower or higher risks to insure. As with BMI, height-weight charts are oversimplifications of body composition data because they do not take into account percent body fat. They should be used only as guidelines for appropriate weight ranges. Although using wall charts may make teaching progression simpler, it does not provide accurate results, and it has often led to public posting of comparisons of students' body compositions (something that must be avoided at all costs). For examples of the Metropolitan Height/Weight charts, see www.nutritionclassroom.com/metropolitan_life_weight_tables.htm.

Waist-to-Hip Ratio

Because some research shows that where body fat is distributed may affect how unhealthful it is, scientists have investigated the correlation between waist-to-hip ratios and health risks. The findings indicate that it is better to be pear-shaped than apple-shaped; that is, it may be better to have excess weight on the hips and thighs than around the waist (Wickelgren 1998). In fact, research indicates that abdominal fat or having an apple shape increases the risk for heart disease and diabetes later in life (Ziegler and Filer 2000). Waist-to-hip ratio is a simple way to evaluate how pear- or apple-shaped a person is. For example, a person with a waist measurement of 28 inches and a hip measurement of 38 inches would have a waist-to-hip ratio of .74 (28 ÷ 38 = .736, rounded to the nearest hundredth). Ratios above .86 in women and .95 in men indicate a waist-to-hip ratio associated with higher levels of heart disease and cancer (and an apple shape).

These numbers have not been adjusted or validated for children, however, so the usefulness of this test is limited in the health-related physical fitness education program.

Bioelectrical Impedance Analyzers

Bioelectrical impedance is an alternative, noninvasive technique requiring little skill to administer. It is becoming a popular alternative to skinfold measures in the public schools for assessing body composition. Research has shown that fat free mass (FFM) or percent body fat can be accurately predicted in children and adults using impedance, provided that population-specific equations are used (Deurenberg et al. 1991; Houtkeeper et al. 1989; Segal et al. 1988; Van Loan and Mayclin 1987). A low-level electrical current (50 kilohertz) of different amplitudes (800 or 500 microamperes) is introduced into the body through four electrodes placed on the wrists and ankles. Alternative impedance instruments use a handheld device or a bathroom scale type instrument whereby the subject stands on two metal footpads to estimate body composition. Impedance is based on a fairly simple premise that tissues containing a lot of water and electrolytes conduct electricity, whereas tissues such as fat are poor conductors of electricity. However, this method's rapid administration and ease of use does not come without some precautions. It is generally recommended that the manufacturer's general equations not be used, unless the population you are testing is a subgroup of the population in which the equation was validated and then cross-validated.

If you decide to use impedance instead of skinfold tests to assess body composition, use the following recommendations:

- Purchase an impedance instrument with multiple equations, including equations for children.
- The alternative is to purchase an instrument that provides the user with the resistance, reactance, and impedance readings, and you select the appropriate equation (Heyward and Stolarczyk 1996) based on the age, gender, and population you are testing.
- Standardize your measurement protocol according to the manufacturer's recommendations.
- Avoid metal tables or other conductive surfaces.
- Ensure that the student's arms and legs are abducted slightly away from the trunk.
- Require the student to remove metal jewelry.
- Make sure the student is well hydrated

Here are some suggested references to help select an equation:

- The best equation to use for white boys and girls age 10 to 19 years is one developed by Houtkeeper et al. (1992).
- For children under 10 years, use the equations of Lohman (1992) or Kushner et al. (1992).
- Race-specific equations have been developed for native Japanese boys (9 to 14 years) and girls (9 to 15 years) (Kim et al. 1993; Watanabe et al. 1993).
- Presently, there are no cross-validated impedance equations for American Indian, Asian American, black, or Hispanic children.

Helping the Overfat or Underfat Student

Either through formal testing or informal observations, you will likely identify students who appear to be over or under an appropriate percent body fat. It is beyond the scope of a physical educator to treat serious problems such as eating disorders or extreme obesity, but you may be able to point these students or their parents toward professional help. The following sections discuss the symptoms and causes of obesity and eating disorders to help you better identify contributing factors.

Obesity

According to the Centers for Disease Control and Prevention, approximately 65 percent of all adults in the United States are overweight or obese. In addition, the percentage of youth who are overweight or obese has more than doubled in the last three decades. Current estimates are that between 10 and 15 percent of U.S. children aged 6 to 17 are overweight (www.cdc.gov, 2002). Given these statistics, it is likely that physical educators will have overweight children in their classes. **Obesity** is defined as 120 percent of ideal body weight or greater and has three main contributing factors: genetics, diet, and physical activity. Be sure to keep this in mind when preparing lesson plans.

■ Genetics—Research suggests that genetics contributes about 30 percent to a person's body weight (Zeigler and Filer 1996). The genetic component is multiple: It determines placement of excess fat (hips, arms, stomach, and so on), effectiveness of the gastrointestinal tract, level of appetite, and preferences for certain types of food such as sweets and salty snacks. The entire picture of how the gene is inherited and its exact biochemical mechanism is still being researched and developed.

■ Diet—The average American diet contains 14 percent more calories than 30 years ago (McDowell et al. 1994). Eating as few as nine and a half additional calories per day will result in one pound of additional fat over a year. Americans are eating more meals away from home, as well as more fast food and fries. The typical on-the-run American lifestyle leads to long days of snacking and lots of take-out. According to the CDC (2003), more than 60 percent of youth eat too much fat, and fewer than 20 percent eat the recommended five or more servings of fruits and vegetables on a daily basis. These poor eating habits developed during childhood may continue to be established throughout adulthood.

■ Physical Activity—Physical activity increases the body's use of calories, which aids in maintaining a normal weight and optimizing overall health. The level of physical activity continues to decrease in the

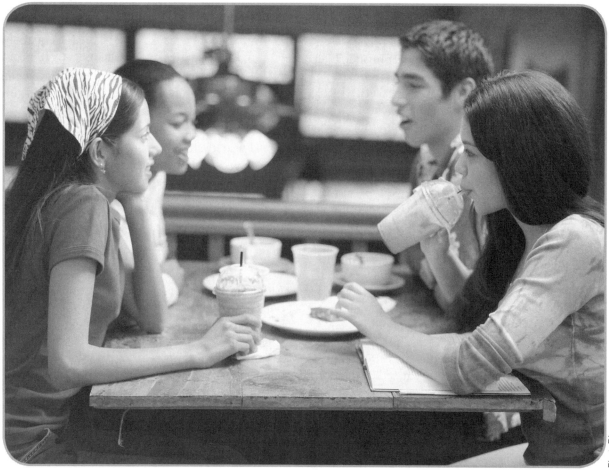

TEACHING TIP

In addition to the many activities in the *Physical Best Activity Guides*, you can use the following class application ideas for teaching nutritional concepts related to body composition.

Lipid Loot

Create play money called "lipid loot" in one-dollar amounts only. Display pictures or models of different types of foods and fast-food items. Each of these items has a **lipid** loot price based on its fat gram content. Based on the students' caloric intake, give them a certain number of fat bucks to spend for a meal. (An appropriate fat content per meal is ideally between 15 and 25 grams.) This is a great way to emphasize fat content in food as well as a way to reinforce making change and using money for younger students.

Use Teaching Models

Create class fat models to supplement lectures and stimulate class discussion. Obtain nutritional analysis information from local fast-food chains. The following Web site also contains extensive information on fast-food nutritional content: www.fatcalories.com. Note that five grams of fat is equivalent to one teaspoon of Crisco or margarine. Label clear plastic cups with food type, and add the proper amount of fat. This helps students to visualize the actual fat content in their favorite fast-food items (see table 8.2).

Journaling

Have students complete a dietary journal of all foods eaten in the last 24 hours. Students should record how they felt (emotions) when they ate and the specific reason they ate that particular item. The objective is to demonstrate how often individuals eat for reasons other than hunger and why they choose the foods they do. (Food choices are often more about convenience and availability rather than healthy choices. Although younger children may not get to choose their food daily, they do get some choice with school lunches and at restaurants.)

Find a Menu

Many restaurants will donate a menu if asked, and many more print take-out menus. Select the healthiest food items from local restaurants. These can then be used to have class discussions regarding the best menu choices.

United States. Despite the widely documented benefits of exercise, including better long-term health, improved body image, and less depression, more than 60 percent of American adults are sedentary. This inactivity is not limited to adults. More than 30 percent of youth aged 9 to 12 don't regularly engage in physical activity. Video games and television have replaced much of the after-school yard play. In addition, daily participation in high school physical education classes dropped from 42 percent in 1991 to 29 percent in 1999 (NCCDPHP 2003).

Eating Disorders

At the opposite end of the spectrum are eating disorders. While obesity is now the biggest nutritional problem among youths, in our complex society, physical educators cannot focus only on obesity. In fact, psychological and social pressures to look thin have driven many youngsters to the extremes of eating disorders, all of which pose serious health risks.

There are two eating disorders that are most common in the school age population: anorexia nervosa and

TABLE 8.2 Nutritive Value of Popular Fast Foods

Food item	Calories	% calories from fat	Total fat (g)	Saturated fat (g)	Cholesterol (mg)	Protein (g)	Total carbohydrate (g)	Fiber (g)	Sugars (g)	Sodium (mg)	Calcium (% RDI)
MCDONALD'S											
Hamburger	280	32%	10	4	30	12	35	2	7	560	20%
Cheeseburger	330	39%	14	6	45	15	35	2	7	800	25%
Quarter Pounder	420	45%	21	8	70	23	36	2	8	780	20%
Quarter Pounder with Cheese	530	51%	30	13	95	28	38	2	9	1,250	35%
Big Mac	580	52%	33	11	85	24	47	3	7	1,050	35%
Filet-O-Fish	470	51%	26	5	50	15	45	1	5	730	20%
McChicken	430	49%	23	4.5	45	14	41	3	6	840	20%
Chicken McNuggets (6 pieces)	310	58%	20	4	50	15	18	2	0	680	2%
French Fries (large)	540	43%	26	4.5	0	8	68	6	0	350	2%
Side Salad (no dressing)	15	0	0	0	0	1	3	1	1	10	2%
Grilled Chicken Bacon Ranch Salad (no dressing)	270	44%	13	5	75	28	11	3	4	830	15%
Ranch Dressing (1 pkg)	290	93%	30	4.5	20	1	4	0	3	530	4%
Low-Fat Balsamic Vinaigrette (1 pkg)	40	63%	3	0	0	0	4	0	3	730	*
Chocolate Triple Thick Shake (small)	430	26%	12	8	50	11	70	1	61	210	35%
Egg McMuffin	300	37%	12	5	235	18	29	2	3	840	30%
Bacon, Egg, & Cheese Biscuit	480	58%	31	10	250	21	31	1	3	1,360	15%
Ham, Egg, & Cheese Bagel	550	36%	23	8	255	26	58	2	10	1,500	20%

Food item	Calories	% calories from fat	Total fat (g)	Saturated fat (g)	Cholesterol (mg)	Protein (g)	Total carbohydrate (g)	Fiber (g)	Sugars (g)	Sodium (mg)	Calcium (% RDI)
Hot Cakes w/margarine & syrup	600	25%	17	3	20	9	104	0	40	770	10%
Hash Browns	130	54%	8	1.5	0	1	14	1	0	330	*

*Contains less than 2% of the daily value.

Additional food items listed at www.mcdonalds.com/countries/usa/food/nutrition/categories/nutrition/index.html.

PIZZA HUT

Food item	Calories	% calories from fat	Total fat (g)	Saturated fat (g)	Cholesterol (mg)	Protein (g)	Total carbohydrate (g)	Fiber (g)	Sugars (g)	Sodium (mg)	Calcium (% RDI)
Hand-Tossed Pizza, cheese, 1 slice	240	38%	10	5	10	12	28	2	1	650	20%
Personal Pan Pizza, pepperoni	620	40%	28	11	30	26	70	5	<2	1,430	30%
Meat Lover's Stuffed Crust, 1 slice	470	49%	25	11	50	22	40	3	2	1,430	25%
Veggie Lover's The Big New Yorker, 1 slice	480	42%	22	6	10	19	57	10	<10	1,410	25%
Thin 'N Crispy Pizza, cheese, 1 slice	200	80	9	5	10	10	22	2	1	590	20%
Mild Buffalo Wings, 5 pcs.	200	110	12	3.5	150	23	<1	0	0	510	2%
Breadstick	130	35	4	1	0	3	20	1	1	170	N/A
Breadstick Dipping Sauce	30	5	0.5	0	0	<1	5	<1	2	170	N/A
Supreme Sandwich	640	250	28	10	28	34	62	4	7	2,150	30%

N/A = not available

Additional food items listed at www.pizzahut.com (click on "Nutritional Info").

bulimia. Physical educators and coaches must be on the lookout for the warning signs of each. To help your students achieve and maintain an ideal body composition, you must teach them the right combination of caloric intake, caloric expenditure, and behavior modification. Behavior modification includes the frequency of eating, the portion size of food, and commitment to an active lifestyle. If you suspect an eating disorder, you should discuss this with the school nurse and decide how to proceed with intervention.

■ **Anorexia nervosa** (see figure 8.3) is a serious and potentially fatal disease that is characterized by self-induced starvation and extreme weight loss. According to the National Eating Disorders Association (2003), anorexia nervosa has five primary symptoms:

■ Refusal to maintain a normal body weight (While there is no clinically established

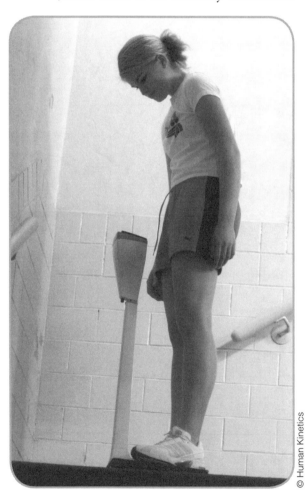

Appearance and body image are important to most teenagers.

cutoff, a weight loss to less than 85 percent of ideal body weight is considered at risk.)

■ An intense fear of weight and of getting "fat"

■ Feeling "fat" despite dramatic weight loss

■ Loss of periods

■ Extreme concern with body weight and appearance

Approximately 95 percent of people with anorexia nervosa are female. Anorexia nervosa has some very negative health consequences. These include an abnormally slow heart rate, a reduction in bone mass, hair loss, dry hair, and severe dehydration (which can result in kidney failure). People with anorexia nervosa will also experience growth of a downy layer of hair called **lanugo.** Its purpose is to help the body to keep warm. Of those individuals with anorexia nervosa, statistics indicate that 5 to 20 percent will die.

■ **Bulimia** (see figure 8.4) is a serious, potentially fatal eating disorder that is characterized by a destructive cycle of **bingeing** and **purging.** According to the National Eating Disorders Association, bulimia has three primary symptoms:

■ Eating large quantities of food in short periods of time, or bingeing, typically in secret.

■ Following these binges, a compensatory behavior is performed to account for the caloric intake. This may include vomiting, laxative abuse, diuretic abuse, fasting, or compulsive exercise.

■ Extreme concern with body weight and shape.

Estimates of bulimia vary, but between 1 and 5 percent of the U.S. population is affected. Estimates vary because bulimia can go undetected for long periods. Approximately 80 percent of bulimics are female. Unlike those with anorexia nervosa, most bulimics are at normal weight or even slightly above. Health consequences of bulimia include tooth decay, ulcers, electrolyte disturbances, and potential for gastric rupture.

Warning Signs of Anorexia

- Dramatic weight loss
- Preoccupation with weight, calories, and fat grams
- Refusal to eat certain foods, progressing to restrictions against whole categories of food
- Frequent comments about feeling fat or overweight despite dramatic weight loss
- Anxiety about getting fat
- Denial of hunger
- Development of food rituals (i.e., eating foods in certain orders, excessive chewing, rearranging food on a plate)
- Consistent excuses to avoid mealtimes or situations involving food
- Excessive, rigid exercise regimen (despite weather, fatigue, illness, or injury)—the need to burn off calories taken in
- Withdrawal from usual friends and activity
- In general, behaviors and attitudes indicating that weight loss, dieting, and control of food are becoming primary concerns

Figure 8.3 You can watch your students for these warning signs of anorexia.

Reprinted, by permission, from the National Eating Disorders Foundation, "Warning signs of anorexia nervosa." [Online]. Available: http://www.nationa leatingdisorders.org [December 1, 2003].

Warning Signs of Bulimia

- Evidence of binge eating, such as the existence of wrappers and containers indicating the consumption of large amounts of food
- Evidence of purging behaviors, including frequent trips to the bathroom after meals, signs/smells of vomiting, presence of wrappers or packages of laxatives or diuretics
- Excessive, rigid exercise regimen (despite weather, fatigue, illness, or injury)—the need to "burn off" calories taken in
- Calluses on the back of the hands and knuckles from self-induced vomiting
- Discoloration or staining of the teeth (from stomach acid in vomit)
- Creation of complex lifestyle schedules or rituals to make time for binge-and-purge sessions
- Withdrawal from usual friends and activities
- In general, behaviors and attitudes indicating that weight loss, dieting, and control of food are becoming primary concerns

Figure 8.4 If you suspect an eating disorder, check these warning signs for bulimia.

Reprinted, by permission, from the National Eating Disorders Foundation, "Warning signs of bulimia nervosa." [Online]. Available: http://www.nationale atingdisorders.org [December 1, 2003].

> ## CAUTION!
>
> Although extreme **underweight** (less than 90 percent of ideal body weight) is a symptom of disordered eating, some children are simply genetically thin. Diagnosis of an eating disorder requires disordered body image perception in addition to unhealthy and dangerous eating habits.

Addressing the Problem

If you are concerned about a particular student, use the following guidelines to approach the situation in a professional manner.

- Always maintain student and family privacy.

- Approach the student and parents diplomatically. Be sure to avoid statements that may be perceived as accusatory.

- Respect parental wishes unless you believe, as in the case of suspected anorexia nervosa, the child is in danger.

- Work with other school personnel, such as the school nurse, and seek written permission to share your observations with the child's health care worker. At the same time, seek advice on how you can tailor your program to meet the child's needs. School districts also have access to registered dietitians who may be able to tailor a meal plan for students with weight problems or eating disorders.

- Ensure that your program is interesting and promotes physical activity as a lifestyle choice for all students. NEVER put overweight children in the position to be last chosen for teams or activities. Avoid unreasonable expectations. For example, obese children are more likely to maintain and therefore benefit from mild physical activity than moderate to vigorous physical activity (USDHHS 1999).

- Deal with less serious problems only; know when you are in over your head, and refer such students to a professional who is qualified to treat the problem.

Summary

Although approaching body composition in the physical education setting can be a delicate matter, it is just as important as any other health-related component of physical fitness. Handle body composition instruction professionally and effectively by focusing on how an active lifestyle positively affects body composition rather than overemphasizing test results. This is where connecting this material to the other components of health-related fitness comes in. Remember, make testing voluntary and respect each student's privacy. Finally, learn to recognize when a student's body composition is a serious health concern and refer such children to qualified health care professionals. You will also find the chapter on nutrition helpful in teaching about body composition.

PART III

Curriculum and Teaching Methods

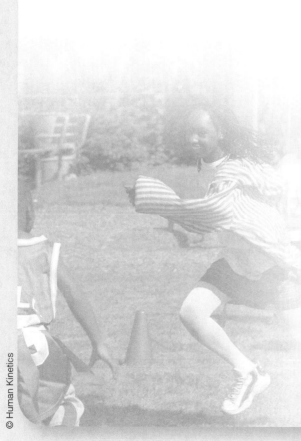

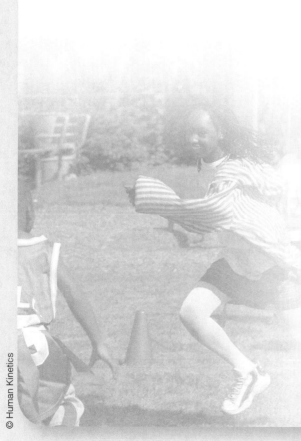

Part III provides an overview of curriculum development and teaching methods relevant to health-related fitness education, as well as information on including children of all abilities and backgrounds in the health-related fitness curriculum. Chapter 9 discusses the relationship of health-related fitness education to national educational standards. It covers basic program design principles, recommended core content, and activity selection. Chapter 10 explores teaching styles, including utilizing multiple intelligences, cooperative learning, and the classroom approach. Teaching strategies are also included in this chapter, such as scheduling and considerations for the teaching environment and teaching tools. Part III concludes with chapter 11, which focuses on the topic of inclusion from a broad perspective, with basic information and practical tips for including students with special needs, as well as addressing gender, cultural, and ability inclusion.

CHAPTER

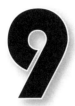

Chapter Contents

■ Philosophy of Health-Related Physical Fitness Education

■ Integrating Skill Development

■ Designing a Program

■ Exit Outcomes and National Standards

■ Basic Design Principles

Curriculum Model Guidelines

Developmentally Appropriate Applications

Cross-Curricular Implementation

■ Recommended Core Content for a Health-Related Fitness Education Model

■ Personal Lifetime Health-Related Fitness Courses

Determine Unit Outcomes

Identify Lesson Outcomes

■ Activity Selection

Sequential

Enjoyable

Variety

Inclusive

Connected

Individualized

■ Summary

Curriculum Development for Health-Related Physical Fitness Education

A well-written health-related physical fitness education curriculum provides the framework within which students learn the necessary health-related physical fitness concepts so they can apply them in real life. It integrates these concepts with motor skills and actual physical activity in a developmentally appropriate K-12 progression. The progression reinforces prerequisite skills and knowledge through their use and application.

For example, you might have first graders put their hand on their chest to feel their heart beating fast and talk about how being active causes this to happen. Third graders might practice counting how many times they feel their heart beat and discuss more specifically how this relates to physical activity. Fifth graders can be taught to find their pulse two different ways (wrist and carotid artery) or can use a heart rate monitor and then graph their rates based on different activities. Seventh graders might be asked to monitor their heart rates for a week doing different activities, graph the results, and write a paper that compares the various rates and offers reasons for the differences. High school students might be asked to develop an exercise plan based on their target heart rates, carry out the plan, and record the results (which requires knowing how to take their own pulse). They might also write a paper or do research regarding the heart's response to stress on the body. Unfortunately, however, there are still some physical education programs in which students do the same lesson year after year, with no applications or extensions. For example, asking third graders, fifth graders, seventh graders, and high school students to simply find their pulse without asking them to apply this information in a progressively more complex or varied manner does little to prepare students for managing personal lifelong physical activity plans.

Of course, at every level you will have students who lack the prerequisite skills, knowledge, and motivation to move forward. In these cases, the use of peer tutors, stations, teaching assistants (including volunteers), and other teaching strategies will allow you to "catch up" some students while not boring the rest of the class. Chapter 10 outlines some excellent ideas for incorporating particular teaching strategies.

Philosophy of Health-Related Physical Fitness Education

Health-related physical fitness education seeks to produce individuals who view physical activity as a worthwhile, pleasurable, and lifelong endeavor—people who have discovered where their physical activity interests lie through experiencing an individualized and varied curriculum. These individuals will know how to design and implement a personal health-related fitness plan, given the opportunities and constraints faced (such as individual abilities, available community facilities and activities, and cultural interests). In short, the quality physical education program includes fitness education that teaches students how and why to engage in lifelong, individualized, health-related physical activity and inspires them to do so. Physical educators can accomplish this by teaching health and wellness through games and activities that are enjoyed by all. This is the essence of the Physical Best philosophy and program (refer to chapter 1 for details).

Although Physical Best is not a complete curriculum in and of itself, the concept of health-related physical fitness education has been described as a curriculum model. This curricular approach is the most consistent with today's focus on developing and maintaining a healthy, active lifestyle, and it teaches both conceptual and practical application to the students. The tenets of this model start with introducing students to the concept of being physically active in a direct style of instruction. The teacher designs the activities and explains to the students the important concepts or the "how" and "why" of the lesson. As the students gain experience and knowledge, the model shifts to a more indirect style of teaching, with the teacher serving more as a facilitator. The students now begin to design their own fitness program and monitor their own fitness levels, thus allowing the students to take more personal responsibility for their learning (Darst and Pangrazi 2002). Naturally, when it comes to children assuming total responsibility for their own health, they will have to "crawl" before they can "run." Health-related physical fitness education focuses on this process of having students assume progressively more responsibility for their own health, fitness, and well-being. For example, it is more appropriate to integrate the teaching of basic motor skills (particularly gross motor) at the elementary level. Middle school students should concentrate on combining skills and strategies that enhance physical activity performance. High school students should be developing a detailed personal fitness plan. Overall, the K-12 program should build progressively toward the ultimate goal: producing members of society who take lifelong personal responsibility for engaging in health-related physical activity, not only because they know it's good for the body, but also because they know how intrinsically rewarding it is to move in ways they enjoy.

With their well-known **"Stairway to Lifetime Fitness,"** Corbin and Lindsey (2004) succinctly outline the process through which teachers must guide their students (see figure 9.1). The younger the student, the more likely that student is to be on a lower, more dependent step. Conversely, the older the student, the more that student needs to be operating on a higher step—and the more responsible you are for facilitating this.

The Stairway to Lifetime Fitness

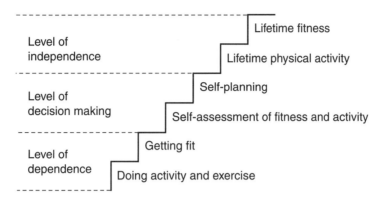

■ **Figure 9.1** The Stairway to Lifetime Fitness outlines the steps teachers can use to guide students toward a lifetime of fitness.

Reprinted, by permission, from C. Corbin and R. Lindsey, 2005, *Fitness for life,* 5th ed. (Champaign, IL: Human Kinetics).

The CDC, in collaboration with experts from federal and state agencies, schools, and voluntary and professional organizations, has printed numerous publications promoting the importance of lifelong physical activity. They suggest implementing physical education programs that emphasize enjoyable participation in physical activity and that help students develop the knowledge, attitudes, skills, and confidence needed to adopt and maintain physically active lifestyles (USDHHS, 2000). This includes the following:

■ Providing planned, sequential physical education curricula for all grades that encourage enjoyable, lifelong physical activity. These curricula should emphasize settings and activity parameters for lifetime activity over those for competitive sport. Physical fitness testing should be integrated into the curricula, but results should not form the basis for report card grades.

■ Using the NASPE national standards for physical education to develop the curricula. These standards are designed to develop the physical, cognitive, and affective domains in children through physical education.

■ Promoting enjoyable participation by using active learning strategies; developing students' knowledge, confidence, motor skills, and behavioral skills; and providing a significant opportunity for regular physical activity.

Integrating Skill Development

In their zeal to focus on health-related physical fitness as the core of their program, physical educators

must not neglect the importance of the development of crucial basic motor skills and concepts (Schmidt and Wrisberg 2000).

Students benefit from skill education in many ways. Performance at adult levels requires higher-order thinking and combinations of basic skills and concepts. Students (and, ultimately, adults) need to be skillful enough to obtain fitness benefits without needless injury or frustration. For example, if a person develops an interest in tennis, the person will not realize health-related or social-emotional benefits from playing it if he is unsuccessful and is picking up the ball most of the time. Another reason to ensure students develop basic skills is that the perception of competence encourages individuals to engage in physical activity. A final reason for skill development is that as students gain in their performance, the activity becomes more enjoyable and less of a task, and the students are more apt to stay active.

As students get older, you should continue to push them toward mastery but offer them choices of the type of skills they focus on. Help them find what they like, and then help them master the skills necessary to enjoy that physical activity. Be careful, however, not to send the message that people who are not highly skilled shouldn't be out there moving. Instead, encourage each student to be the best he or she can, and to keep moving. At the middle school level and beyond, teachers have to begin to loosen their control over student choices and empower students to make personal choices. If a student simply cannot seem to master a physical skill despite repeated instruction, help the student find other ways to stay involved. For example, if a student has trouble performing the steps to a dance correctly, encourage the student not

HELP! A Lot of My Middle Schoolers Never Acquired Basic Skills

Perhaps you teach in a middle school and many of your students never acquired basic skills because your district does not support physical education at the elementary level, or they simply weren't taught in a progressive, developmentally appropriate program. You know they might be insulted and disruptive if you use activities that are too basic, so what can you do? Possible solutions include the following:

- Modify popular games to focus more on basic skills; seeing where they'll need the skills to enjoy the games can be very motivating. Have students use a basic skill in several different ways in various games.

- Review the skills you think will give them what they need to pursue the physical activities they're most interested in (you might survey students to determine this) by asking the students to design their own games to use the skills.

- Occasionally, arrange to have classes of elementary students visit your classes to motivate your students to train as "student teachers." They have to know the basics to teach them. Students learn skills better when they teach the skills to someone else. This has the added benefits of reaching younger students before they come to your program and networking with their teachers.

- Use **peer tutors;** students of equal ability can help each other learn, and highly skilled students will feel more challenged. Give partners critical element checklists to guide their teaching.

The bottom line is that the strategy or activity used to teach the basic skill must be developmentally and age appropriate. Be creative and network with other teachers to brainstorm activity ideas with them.

to give up and emphasize that he or she will still benefit aerobically from the movements. The main goal is movement, not necessarily skill perfection! Thus, such a person can still reach the ultimate goal—that of lifelong, individualized, health-related physical activity—despite lacking a highly developed motor skill.

Designing a Program

To create a quality physical education program that produces students who achieve set standards, work backward from those standards all the way down to day-to-day lesson plans (see figure 9.2). You need to understand where you want to go, and you must know the expected end results for students, before you can design a quality curriculum. In other words, you must understand what you want the students to

know and to be able to do. Unfortunately, in many cases this is not happening. Teachers are drawn to a unique or creative lesson and implement it "just because." When questioned about how it fits into the unit or curriculum or how it helps their students achieve a specific goal or outcome, often there is no logical answer.

Another factor to consider when beginning this process is what, if any, standards are mandated by state or federal agencies and which standards are recommendations. Physical educators have become accustomed to Title IX in their programs, and in most cases this poses no problems, but what about PL 94-142—Education for All Handicapped Children Act? Are you meeting that standard in your program? What about state mandates? Since some states set their own standards, you will need to find out how much flexibility you have to interpret the state standards according to the local student population's needs.

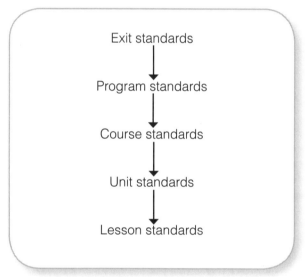

Exit standards

↓

Program standards

↓

Course standards

↓

Unit standards

↓

Lesson standards

■ **Figure 9.2** Designing down helps you create lessons that contribute to your overall curriculum goals.

Adapted, by permission, from C. Hopple, 2005, *Performance based assessment in elementary education*, 2nd ed. (Champaign, IL: Human Kinetics). In press.

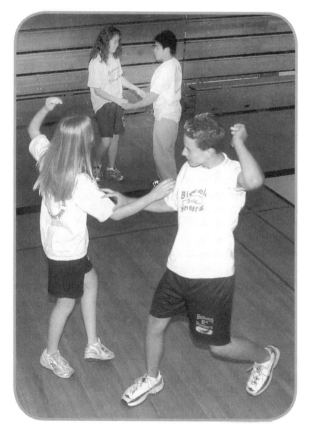

You should take student interest into account when designing courses. If, for example, a version of swing dance is popular with teenagers in your community, it might be a good choice for a dance unit.

Exit Outcomes and National Standards

The term **exit outcomes** refers to the ultimate desired achievements of students who graduate from a K-12 curriculum. The outcomes should specify what you expect students to know, understand, and be able to do by the time they complete high school. National or state standards often provide the guidance for appropriate expectations of achievement by the end of a program. Therefore, first study those expectations and see if they meet your desired outcomes as dictated by your community and student population. If not, modify your approach to them to better fit your situation. Work on a districtwide basis and design down from high school, ensuring appropriate progression and minimizing unnecessary duplication. This allows the elementary and middle school teachers to see what they need to focus on so that students are academically and physically prepared for the high school program. Each "piece of the puzzle" works with the next by examining each level's expectations and ensuring they (elementary, middle, and high school) progressively lead students toward your exit outcomes.

The Physical Best program supports the teaching of the educational standards developed by national associations of AAHPERD, including NASPE for physical education, the American Association for Health Education (AAHE) for health-education, and the National Dance Association (NDA) for dance education. Collectively, these standards help determine exit outcomes and developmentally appropriate curricula that will help students achieve the ultimate goal of becoming adults who value and pursue active lifestyles. Tables 9.1 through 9.3 list the standards set by the national governing bodies for each discipline. The standards that are most strongly correlated with Physical Best are highlighted in bold. These standards are listed in the *Physical Best Activity Guides* to demonstrate the connection of each activity to the applicable standards.

Appendix F also lists the Centers for Disease Control and Prevention's *Guidelines for School and Community Programs to Promote Lifelong Physical Activity Among Young People* (1997). This is another excellent source of information for health-related fitness program design.

Basic Design Principles

Allow several basic principles to guide every curricular decision you and your colleagues make in creating your basic design.

Curriculum designers should take care to (Hopple 2005)

- stay focused on the exit outcomes for each grade level, which are the goals toward which you should teach and assess;

- plan for ample opportunities for students to master the desired outcomes, including ensuring that students have mastered prerequisite skills and knowledge before progressing to higher levels;

- set high expectations within reason, planning how each student will receive the support he or she needs to reach program goals; and

- design down, working backward from exit outcomes so that, ultimately, each unit and lesson enhances each student's chance of achieving those outcomes. For more information, refer to *Moving Into the Future: National Standards for Physical Education*, Second Edition (NASPE 2004a).

Curriculum Model Guidelines

Once you have set your standards, you are ready to choose a **curriculum model.** There are many different approaches that can be used in teaching quality physical education. Examples of different physical education models include sport education, theme/skill based, movement education, activity based, wilderness or adventure education, concept or interdisciplinary based, fitness based, and student centered based. Harrison, Blakemore, and Buck provide a good overview of the different models in their *Instructional Strategies for Secondary School Physical Education* (2001). Many schools today use a more eclectic approach by combining models to meet the needs of their student population. Regardless of the combination of models chosen, the fitness-based model is becoming more accepted as one of the base models in an eclectic approach.

Physical Best's connection to the fitness-based model is obvious, but Physical Best is designed to provide the health-related fitness component in any model chosen.

TABLE 9.1   National Standards for Physical Education

Standard 1	Demonstrates competency in motor skills and movement patterns needed to perform a variety of physical activities.
Standard 2	Demonstrates understanding of movement concepts, principles, strategies, and tactics as they apply to the learning and performance of physical activities.
Standard 3	**Participates regularly in physical activity.**
Standard 4	**Achieves and maintains a health-enhancing level of physical fitness.**
Standard 5	Exhibits responsible personal and social behavior that respects self and others in physical activity settings.
Standard 6	Values physical activity for health, enjoyment, challenge, self-expression, and/or social interaction.

Reprinted from *Moving Into the Future: National Standards for Physical Education* (2004) with permission from the National Association for Sport and Physical Education (NASPE), 1900 Association Drive, Reston, VA 20191-1599.

TABLE 9.2   National Health Education Standards

Standard 1	**Students will comprehend concepts related to health promotion and disease prevention.**
Standard 2	Students will demonstrate the ability to access valid health information and health-promoting products and services.
Standard 3	**Students will demonstrate the ability to practice health-enhancing behaviors and reduce health risks.**
Standard 4	Students will analyze the influence of culture, media, technology, and other factors on health.
Standard 5	Students will demonstrate the ability to use interpersonal communication skills to enhance health.
Standard 6	**Students will demonstrate the ability to use goal-setting and decision-making skills to enhance health.**
Standard 7	Students will demonstrate the ability to advocate for personal, family, and community health.

Reprinted from *Achieving health literacy: National health education standards* (1995) with permission from the American Alliance for Health, Physical Education, Recreation, and Dance (AAHPERD), 1900 Association Drive, Reston, VA 20191-1599.

TABLE 9.3   National Standards for Dance Education

Standard 1	Identifying and demonstrating movement elements and skills in performing dance.
Standard 2	Understanding choreographic principles, processes, and structures.
Standard 3	Understanding dance as a way to create and communicate meaning.
Standard 4	Applying and demonstrating critical and creative thinking skills in dance.
Standard 5	Demonstrating and understanding dance in various cultures and historical periods.
Standard 6	**Making connections between dance and healthful living.**
Standard 7	Making connections between dance and other disciplines.

National Dance Standards 1-7 (pp. 6-9) - These quotes are reprinted from the *National Standards for Arts Education* with permission of the National Dance Association (NDA) an association of the American Alliance for Health, Physical Education, Recreation, and Dance. The source of the National Dance Standards *(National Standards for Dance Education: What every Young American Should Know and Be Able to Do in Dance)* may be purchased from: National Dance Association, 1900 Association Drive, Reston, VA 20191-1599; or telephone (703) 476-3421.

Developmentally Appropriate Applications

In order for any curriculum to be sound, a physical educator must consider the developmental appropriateness of the selected content. **Developmentally appropriate activities** are those that are appropriate based on a student's developmental level, age, ability level, interests, and previous experience and knowledge. You should initially target appropriateness on a grade level basis. First, study the guidelines set by experts in the field such as the Council on Physical Education for Children (COPEC) and the Middle and Secondary School Physical Education Council (MASSPEC) of the National Association for Sport and Physical Education (NASPE). These guidelines include published documents such as the assessment series and the appropriate practices series, available through AAHPERD. Then use experience as the best teacher: Learn by trial and error what each particular group of students can handle. But remember, although developmental appropriateness is important, you must not overlook the age of the student for whom the content is being developed. For example, if a high school student lacks aerobic fitness, tag is not an appropriate activity to offer as a choice, but riding a stationary bike while reading a favorite magazine would be a good alternative based on the student's age and ability. Both activities will accomplish the same goal.

Content selection should occur along a continuum from completely childlike to as adultlike in nature as possible. Figure 9.3 shows a sample continuum for aerobic fitness activities that proceed from very childlike activities in the early grades to very adultlike activities in high school.

Another way to think of designing developmentally appropriate content is to consider a diamond-shaped framework such as that shown figure 9.4. Within the diamond curriculum framework, elementary level students develop the basic skills and knowledge (both fitness and movement related) they need to ultimately be able to enjoy lifetime activities (see "Don't Forget Skills Development"). Middle school students then use these skills to sample a wide variety of physical activities. This gives students the opportunity to form personal opinions about various activities and sports. High school students select a few physical activities in which to specialize and around which they may build personal physical activity plans. The foundation of basic skills in elementary school and development of proficiency in self-selected areas in high school forms a continuum that is likely to lead to positive adult health-related fitness behaviors.

Cross-Curricular Implementation

Regardless of the model chosen, from the earliest stages, your plan should include ways of integrating related disciplines into your program. Coordinate your curriculum concepts with colleagues in other disciplines. A cross-curricular approach helps students see and understand the real-life connections among subject areas, reinforcing their learning in all

TEACHING TIP: Motivating With Knowledge

When I was teaching at the University of Illinois at Chicago in 1967 through 1969, I developed a conceptual approach to teaching fitness, complete with slides, programmed text, and audiotapes. As director of conditioning programs, I selected 8 of 40 classes to which I taught these concepts. Although these 8 classes were not graded on fitness, these students' fitness levels improved more than the students' in the traditional conditioning classes. When I asked why—since they exercised only half the class time the students in the traditional classes did—they said they had exercised at home. It was the first time that they realized they should. When I asked the traditional class students, they said that they were in better condition than they had ever been, they felt great, but now that the class was over, they never wanted to go near a gymnasium again!

Dr. Ron Feingold
Adelphi University, Long Island, New York

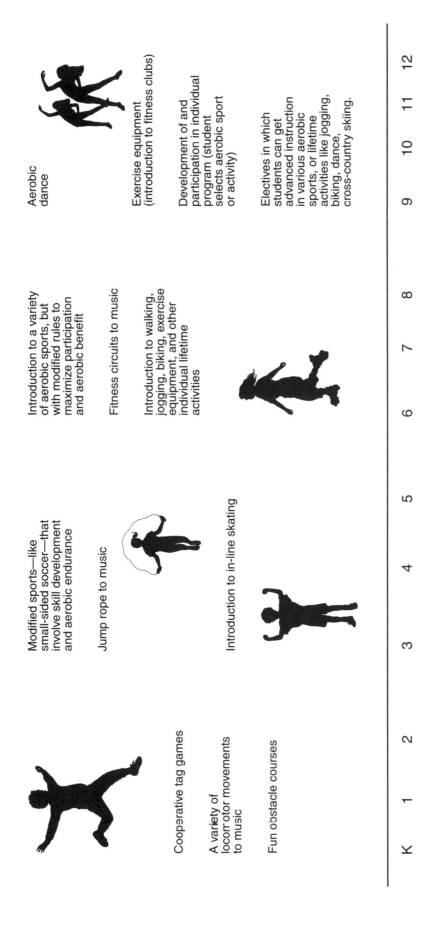

Figure 9.3 Your activity selection should occur along a continuum that moves students from childlike activities. This example describes a possible continuum for teaching aerobic fitness.

145

National Standards and Guidelines

Physically active for life

High school

Middle school

Elementary school

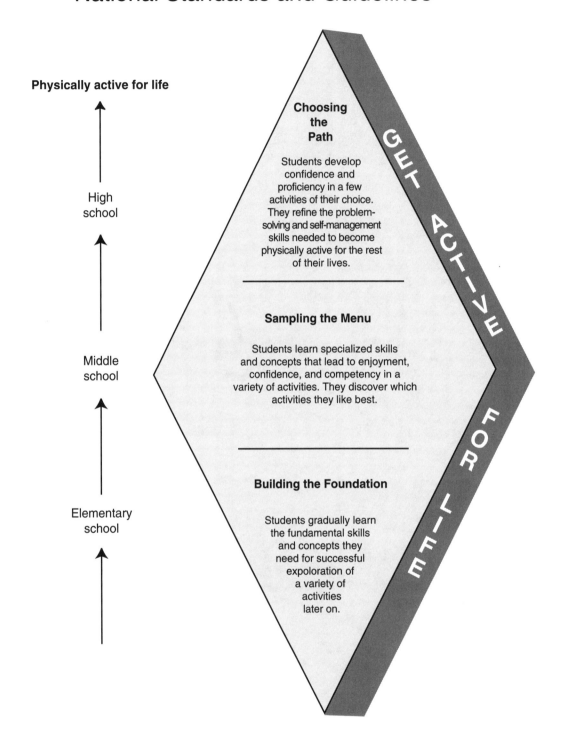

Choosing the Path

Students develop confidence and proficiency in a few activities of their choice. They refine the problem-solving and self-management skills needed to become physically active for the rest of their lives.

Sampling the Menu

Students learn specialized skills and concepts that lead to enjoyment, confidence, and competency in a variety of activities. They discover which activities they like best.

Building the Foundation

Students gradually learn the fundamental skills and concepts they need for successful exploration of a variety of activities later on.

GET ACTIVE FOR LIFE

Figure 9.4 This diamond-shaped framework provides another way of describing a lifetime activity continuum.

Reprinted, by permission, from C. Himberg, 2003, *Teaching secondary physical education in the 21st century* (Champaign, IL: Human Kinetics), 19.

disciplines. It also allows for the health-related fitness concepts to be covered in more depth. Students will ultimately learn more as the various curricular areas reinforce each other. Some examples might include the following:

- Math instructors can teach students to calculate the target heart rate zone.
- Geography classes can use students' mileage or laps to "run" or "walk" across a topographical map while they also study the terrain.

Don't Forget Skills Development

In the past many physical education programs placed their entire focus on the development of sports skills. In this book, we emphasize the need to focus on health-related fitness. However, we want to make it clear that learning skills remains an important part of a quality physical education program. All students can improve their skills to some degree, which is an important factor in preparing them to lead physically active lives. The key is not to overemphasize skill development and therefore discourage those students who, due to any number of factors, will never be as highly skilled as the top athletes in your school. Not all students can be highly successful competitive athletes, but all students can lead physically active, healthy lives.

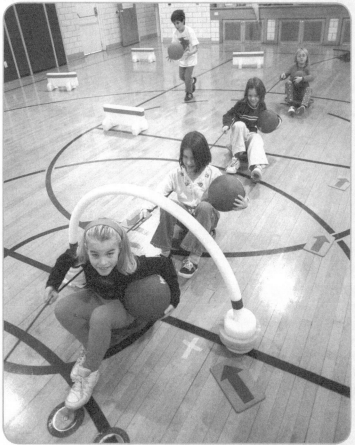

© Human Kinetics

Design developmentally appropriate activities that teach fitness concepts and skill development while making use of available equipment and space.

CAUTION!

Do not sacrifice physical education content or time in the cross-curricular approach. Your main focus still needs to be on ensuring that students leave your program armed with the specific skills and content knowledge they need to design and implement an effective personal health-related fitness plan.

■ English classes could write about the historical sites students are "running" through.

■ Physics instructors can show how Newton's Laws of Motion apply to physical activity.

Another aspect of cross-curricular teaching is to incorporate Gardner's "multiple intelligences" approach to teaching. This is an excellent method that has practical applications in all content areas (see chapter 10 for more specific information). The potential is endless, and the reward is a better learning experience for all involved.

Recommended Core Content for a Health-Related Fitness Education Model

A health-related fitness program teaches the basic training principles of health-related fitness, fitness safety, nutrition, fitness consumer awareness, benefits of physical activity, and that lifelong physical activity is individual and can be enjoyable. Since Physical Best aligns itself predominately with a fitness-based curriculum model, it is only logical that there should be a set of "core" competencies and information that should be included in the curriculum. At a minimum, a program should include the following content information.

■ Basic knowledge of health-related fitness and physical activity principles and skills—Students need concrete knowledge about the principles of progression and overload as applied to each com-

ponent of health-related fitness, including proper nutrition, safety, and how the body adapts to exercise. Include training techniques specific to each component of health-related fitness. Pacing while running, for example, saves precious energy to go the distance. Thus, students need to learn to judge their effort and speed. Students should also master basic running biomechanics and other techniques (e.g., proper stretching and weightlifting safety) to prevent injury, ensuring that they can participate safely and efficiently in the long term. Students must be able to not only identify but also use specific strategies for measuring frequency, intensity, and time of their participation in physical activity. Other relevant health-related fitness skills include the ability to accurately monitor and interpret heart rates and the ability to apply basic injury prevention and treatment strategies. Students should also be required to provide evidence of physical activity participation or, for older students, of employing a self-designed personal fitness plan.

■ Consumer education—Students need to know the truth about fitness, weight control, and nutritional supplements and other products, especially how to discern fact from fiction in advertising. They also need experience comparison shopping for the fitness facilities, equipment, and activity opportunities that suit their interests and resources.

■ Knowledge of the benefits of physical activity—Students need to know how they will benefit from physical activity today (e.g., look and feel better) and in the long term. Remember, youths don't relate well to problems they might have at age 50 or 60. So, although it's vital they know this information, emphasize immediate benefits to maintain their interest.

■ Understanding of the personal nature of fitness—Students need to know they can find what works for them. Not everyone needs to do the same activities, but they do need some sort of physical activity to gain the health benefits. Curriculum should, therefore, emphasize the many choices available to be physically active.

■ Knowledge that physical activity can be fun—The instruction should include lab or physical activity days for students to apply what they're learning in the classroom in an enjoyable learning environment. For example, some schools offer the course as two days per week in the classroom and three days per week in the physical activity setting.

The details of what you include to fulfill each component depend, of course, on your particular curriculum guidelines, student population, and school and community resources. In general, however, select activities that teach students to apply health-related fitness knowledge in real-life settings, that require higher-order thinking and problem solving, and that encourage students to take personal responsibility. This will help them progress up Corbin and Lindsey's Stairway to Lifetime Fitness.

Personal Lifetime Health-Related Fitness Courses

A number of local educational agencies (LEA) and states have begun implementing health-related fitness courses in their curriculums. Other states have developed state standards that can only be met through a concentrated fitness-based curriculum. While their approach might vary, the curriculum for the programs is basically the same, to provide students with the knowledge and tools to allow them to independently develop a personal plan for a lifestyle of active living.

The LEA, Texas, and Fitness for Life courses and programs complement Physical Best. Physical Best sets the foundation leading up to such courses and programs, and reinforces the lifetime fitness skills and concepts after these courses and programs are completed.

LEA Model

In 1998, Lincoln Public Schools (Lincoln, Nebraska) began preparations to reconfigure all junior high schools that included grades 7 through 9 to change them into middle schools with grades 6 through 8. At the time, the junior high physical education curriculum included a semester course known as 9th grade physical education that consisted of short segments of various team and dual sports. Since this course would become part of the high school physical education curriculum, it was the perfect time to examine it in relation to the high school program. The district curriculum specialist presented a proposal to the physical education teachers and school administrators to adopt a "fitness for life" course using the following rationale:

■ The high school physical education graduation requirement had recently been reduced from one

year to three quarters of a year. This introductory course for 9th graders could be used to "sell" the other more specialized high school physical education courses that were essentially viewed as elective courses.

■ The district graduation requirements study committee had recommended combining the health education and physical education graduation requirements. This "fitness for life" course would integrate the physical fitness objectives from health education into a physical education course.

■ The National Standards for Physical Education had been adopted by the district. This course would directly address the two standards related to a physically active lifestyle and physical fitness.

Discussion continued over the next few years; however, implementation was difficult because two of four high schools converted to grades 9 through 12 while the other two high schools remained grades 10 through 12 due to overcrowding. When a bond issue was passed to build two new high schools, it was determined that the transition would be complete in the 2003 to 2004 school year.

In 2002, the district received a PEP grant award to pilot the new course and purchase technology for the existing high schools. The district curriculum specialist requested and received a one-year change of assignment to teach the course, now officially named "Fitness for Life," at the first of the two new high schools. During the 2002 to 2003 school year, the course was piloted. Physical education teachers from the remaining high schools were trained in the summer of 2003. The following fall all six high schools began to offer the course as a foundation course for 9th- and 10th-grade students.

Texas (State Model)

Starting in the early 1980s, when major reforms began in Texas education, TAHPERD members worked with state legislators for quality daily physical education. As a result of this work and many staff hours, the proposal was approved in the early 1990s and implemented in the fall of 1996. Students are encouraged to take the personal fitness course as 9th or 10th graders, although a few students take it as 11th or 12th graders. The course has a threefold purpose: (1) to help students understand the need for physical fitness; (2) to teach students how to assess, develop, demonstrate, and maintain an acceptable level of health-related fitness; and (3) to provide students with the knowledge and tools to allow them to develop a personal plan for a lifestyle of active living.

These programs typically contain both classroom sessions and physical activities, usually in a three-day activity/two-day classroom approach. Comprehensive conceptual information is presented to the students, with topics such as components of health-related fitness, individual fitness assessment methods, nutrition, stress, consumer information, safety, personal attitudes toward staying active, quality of life issues, values of maintaining an active lifestyle, and more. The programs also have homework requirements, parental involvement, and support from their communities.

Fitness for Life

The lifetime personal fitness program that is most used nationwide is Fitness for Life, created by Charles Corbin and Ruth Lindsey. Dr. Corbin has long been recognized as a leader in promoting physical activity and fitness, and he has served as a primary consultant to many of the states that have developed requirements for this course. He is coeditor of the *President's Council on Physical Fitness and Sports Research Digest* and is a long-time member of the *FITNESSGRAM/ACTIVITYGRAM* Scientific Advisory Board.

Ideally offered at the 8th- or 9th-grade level, Fitness for Life is a foundational course in middle and high school physical education. It gives students an overview of the skills, knowledge, motivation, and independent problem-solving skills they need to live physically active, healthy lives. Students can use these skills for participation in all other middle and high school physical education courses. It could also be offered as the final physical education course that students take before graduating. The emphasis of the course is on helping students become responsible for their own activity planning, fitness, and health.

This program, published by Human Kinetics, includes a wide variety of resources. These resources are designed for the many ways in which middle and high school physical education may be scheduled. One- and two-semester outlines are included in the program, as well as block scheduling plans. For more information on Fitness for Life, visit www.fitnessforlife.org or www.HumanKinetics.com or call 800-747-4457.

Determine Unit Outcomes

Units and their outcomes are the "nuts and bolts" of a solid health-related physical fitness education program. **Unit outcomes** are what you expect students to know, understand, and be able to do at the completion of a specified set of lessons. They should be aligned with your exit or program outcomes, taking into consideration your specific teaching environment. When selecting and designing units, take into account the facilities, class scheduling, unit sequencing, equipment, and student ages and interests. Students should learn the requisite psychomotor, cognitive, and affective skills they need to succeed in future courses. Table 9.4 provides one example of such a progression, from the K-12 program in Corvallis, Oregon. Appendix F (table F.1) includes the Olympia, Washington, school district's plan for essential learning goals related to health-related fitness.

You should also take your community resources into consideration. If youth and adult soccer leagues are popular in your area, you might opt to include several progressively advanced units from kindergarten through 12th grade to build student skills so that they can choose to enjoy this physical activity at a proficient level after they leave your program. Plan unit outcomes that make the connections between being fit and enjoying playing soccer more, such as "Students will recognize the value of flexibility to playing soccer and other sports." Meanwhile, introduce students to other physical activities to "broaden their physical activity horizons."

Another example is a locale that offers many winter physical activities such as cross-country skiing and snowshoeing. Here, unit outcomes might include developing an appreciation for each of these lifetime physical activity options. In any case, a learning experience should have the potential to improve health-related fitness or health-related fitness knowledge.

Identify Lesson Outcomes

At the lesson level (**lesson outcomes**), you are planning exactly how students will work toward achieving the unit outcomes, thus leading to meeting the exit or program outcomes. Figure 9.5 demonstrates how a teacher might take a snowshoeing lesson and incorporate a fitness concept, actual physical activity, a psychomotor skill, cognitive development, as well as a practical application all into one integrated package. In this example, it also leads to the achievement of the

TABLE 9.4   Sample K-12 Progressive Scope and Sequence

Beginning grades: K-1 Level 0	Developing grades: 2-3 Level 1	Capable grades: 4-5 Level 2	Fluent grades: 6-8 Level 3	Accomplished grades: 9-10 Level 4	Mastery grades: 11-12 Level 5 EXIT
ACTIVE LIFESTYLE					
Explores moderate to vigorous physical activity in a physical education setting	Demonstrates sustained moderate to vigorous physical activity in a physical education setting	Maintains moderate to vigorous physical activity levels in a variety of activity settings that utilize the skills learned in a physical education setting	Participates regularly in health-enhancing physical activities in both school and nonschool settings	Maintains a consistent pattern of participation in games, sports, dance, outdoor pursuits, and/or other physical activities that contribute to a physically active lifestyle	Continues to maintain a consistent pattern of participation in games, sports, dance, outdoor pursuits, and/or other physical activities that contribute to a physically active lifestyle
FITNESS PRINCIPLES					
Demonstrates awareness of perceived exertion (e.g., "high," "medium," "low" energy output)	Recognizes the physiological indicators that accompany moderate to vigorous physical activity (e.g., sweating, increased heart rate, heavy breathing)	Monitors intensity of exercise (e.g., recognizing target heart rate and recovery time); explores the principles of fitness training (e.g., frequency, intensity, duration, and mode of exercise)	Understands and applies basic principles of training to improve physical fitness (e.g., frequency, intensity, duration, and mode of exercise)	Uses and interprets principles of training for the purpose of modifying levels of fitness (e.g., frequency, intensity, duration, and mode of exercise)	Develops a personal fitness plan that reflects knowledge and application of principles of fitness training (e.g., frequency, intensity, duration, and mode of exercise)

Submitted by Aleita Hass-Holcombe, Corvallis, courtesy of Corvallis School District 509J (Corvallis, Oregon).

program standard: "Develops fundamental physical skills and progresses to complex movement activities as physically able" (Washington State Essential Academic Learning Requirement 1.1; see table F.1).

If you're not sure an activity will enhance this process, think about it, consult with colleagues, and modify it to ensure its value to the overall program. A major advantage of this process is that you can rest assured you're not wasting valuable lesson time going off on a tangent.

Another key to planning lessons that enhance the chances of achieving exit outcomes is to always strive to integrate two or more aspects of physical education into each lesson. When you teach a fitness

concept, for example, you can incorporate moderate to intense physical activity and target a psychomotor skill or concept all in one integrated lesson. You should make the connections among these aspects so that students learn how to do so on their own. In short, you should provide a model for effective real-life approaches to physical activity. Try consciously identifying these aspects in each lesson and activity until this process becomes second nature. Refer to the *Physical Best Activity Guide: Elementary Level* and *Physical Best Activity Guide: Middle and High School Levels* for examples.

A complete lesson plan includes an appropriate introduction, the main activity, and an appropriate

Sample Snowshoeing Objectives and Lesson

Activity: Snowshoeing
Unit outcome: Student will appreciate snowshoeing as both a physical and health-related activity.
Lesson: Snowshoeing field trip
Lesson outcomes:

- Students will calculate how many calories they burned in a half hour of snowshoeing.
- Students will recognize the value of snowshoeing in developing aerobic fitness as evidenced by a journal entry.
- Students will understand how and where to select and purchase snowshoes and appropriate clothing as well as where in the community they can go to snowshoe, as evidenced by completing a shopping list and planning and participating in an outing.

Figure 9.5 You can incorporate many of your teaching goals into one physical activity lesson.

closing. To introduce a lesson, create a set induction, also known as cognitive set or anticipatory set, which involves "priming the pump," or helping students see how and why the current lesson's learning fits into the unit's content. This encourages students to want to learn through today's activities. The core lesson content includes explanations, demonstrations, and the actual activities in which the students will participate.

Remember, each component of the core lesson content must pass the criteria we have outlined, so you don't waste precious instructional time. And just as an entire curriculum builds unit upon unit, course upon course, the activities within a lesson must build one upon another. A closure activity summarizes the day's learning and allows you to quickly assess understanding. It solidifies student learning by reminding students of the lesson's purpose within the context of both the unit and everyday life. You can also use closure time to prepare students for the next lesson, making it a

"pre-set induction." Other closure ideas include having the students be actively involved by either summing up the lesson themselves, doing a reflective writing about their experience in the lesson, or writing a note to their parents about what they learned that day.

Activity Selection

Activity selection is critical for a successful program. This is where it all comes together to form a cohesive lesson, unit, or program. It was mentioned earlier in this chapter that some teachers select activities "just because," but for a program to meet its goal, there must be careful consideration put into each activity chosen. Ask yourself, "Does this activity enhance students' chances of reaching a program goal?" If not, modify it or choose another activity. Remember, the ultimate goal is for students to be physically active for their entire lives. A "boot camp" approach (e.g., regimented calisthenics) does not serve this goal.

Sequential

Doing the same activities with the same students year after year for no clear educational reason will not only bore students, it will also fail to equip them with the tools and experiences they need to be successful in physical activity. Reviewing fitness and movement concepts and skills over the years is important to learning, but the activities should progress in age-appropriate ways. In addition, sequential patterns should take into consideration individual readiness to progress. The key is to build on the topic over the years so that students progress through the program with the knowledge, skills, and experience they need to be physically active adults. Table 9.5 shows examples of topics as they develop from age group to age group.

Enjoyable

What's enjoyable for one individual may not be enjoyable for another individual. Learning is the goal, of course, but enjoyment of an activity will enhance the learning process and is an essential part of a quality health-related physical fitness education program—and a part of what makes Physical Best different (see chapter 1). Pay attention to the psychological makeup of each class as you select activities, because without interesting and enjoy-

TABLE 9.5 Sample Activity Progressions by Topic

	Primary (K-2)	Intermediate (3-5)	Middle school (6-8)	High school (9-12)
Corbin and Lindsey's Stairway to Lifetime Fitness (2004)	Step 1—Doing regular exercise	Step 2—Achieving physical fitness	Step 3—Personal exercise patterns	Step 4—Self-evaluation Step 5—Problem solving and decision making
Heart rate	Place hand on heart before and after vigorous activity and compare speed of HR	Count pulse; learn math to find HR based on partial count	Practice math to find HR based on partial count; graph HR monitor data; assess effort based on graphed data	Design workouts based on knowledge of HR and THRZ
Running	Learn correct stride; run in low-organization games	Analyze running strides of peers using rubric; design low-organization games that incorporate a high amount of running	Teach peers to run more efficiently; report on how running efficiently helps a person succeed in a favorite sport	Design interval workouts that alternate high- and low-intensity effort as determined by HR; make the workout fun for a friend to do
Upper body strength training	Play on the monkey bars on the playground	Play fun push-up games (see Hichwa 1998); learn tubing exercises	Learn more tubing exercises; design games that increase muscular strength without equipment	Learn how to lift weights safely; design a personal weight-training program; explore community options for weight training and do cost analysis
Throwing and catching	Learn basic skills; apply in low-organization, small-sided games	Design low-organization, small-sided games to practice the skills; self-analyze what makes a throw stronger	Modify a physical activity that involves these skills to include a stronger aerobic fitness component	Apply skill in more complex games; analyze similarities in the use of the skills among several sports

able activities, a program lacks one of the greatest intrinsic motivators.

Variety

Variety allows you to show students several different ways they might apply what they learn in real life. For example, different warm-up activities, a change of music, a change of scenery (e.g., walk to a nearby park for the lesson), or a change of leaders (e.g., students or adult volunteers instead of you) can all make your lessons more interesting. An elective course is an example that can be quite effective at the high school level. Design a high school curriculum that offers electives such as aerobic dance, volleyball, fitness walking, softball, and strength training instead of offering 9th-, 10th-, 11th-, and 12th-grade physical education classes. The heart doesn't care if it is getting in shape through in-line skating, swimming, dancing, or whatever. You'll also find that appropriate choices can increase participation and decrease discipline problems.

Inclusive

Although the term **inclusive** is generally used as a philosophical and programmatic descriptor relating to students with special needs or disabilities, we are broadening this to target every student. Simply put, being included in a positive way is fun; being excluded intentionally or by default is not. The Physical Best program sees this as "active participation," and it is one of the foundational practices the program adheres to in its activity design (see "What Makes Physical Best Unique?" in chapter 1). Elimination games and long waits for turns are the opposites of inclusion. Usually the child who most needs to practice the skill is the first to be eliminated. Likewise, the child who waits in a long line gains little or nothing and can even keep slipping to the back of the line to avoid physical activity altogether. See figure 9.6 for some ideas on how to provide for more active participation. Many teachers have worked hard to change games and other physical activities to be more inclusive. Chapter 11 includes information on including students with special needs and game design.

Connected

Another way the Physical Best program guides students toward the ultimate goal of becoming active adults is to connect activities to real life wherever possible. For example, you should let elementary students know that playing small-sided games of soccer now will help them get in better shape and do better in "real" soccer and other physical activities when they are in middle school. Help older students see the connections between being physically active and looking and feeling better.

- Supply enough equipment (e.g., one ball per child).
- Set up small-sided games so turns are more frequent.
- Run several games at once so an eliminated player simply rotates to another group and continues to play.
- Modify rules to keep everyone playing (e.g., in a tag game, have "helpers" who "unfreeze" taggers quickly).
- Have baseball batting teams perform a locomotor task while the base runner runs the bases so all are active.

Figure 9.6 Active participation suggestions.

As students move from middle to high school, it's especially important to select activities that are relevant to them both now and in their futures. Show them what is available in your community for young adults. Are there bike paths, volleyball leagues, cross-country skiing, walking paths, and health clubs? Take field trips to introduce students to the many options available. Have community members (e.g., health fitness instructors, league directors, running club leaders, sport facility owners, and the like) come to class to demonstrate new activities and tell students how they can get involved. Assign homework that relates to the real world, such as consumer education assignments. Have students price ski equipment, lift ticket cost, and other expenses so they can plan a ski trip. Or have them select the health club they would join as an adult and write a paper about why they chose the particular club. In short, the older the students are, the more authentic the activities you choose should be.

Individualized

Try incorporating individualization into each lesson to help ensure developmental appropriateness and, therefore, success and benefits for each child. This may mean making a task easier or more difficult for one individual or small group. For a flexibility task, it may mean you have some students perform the sit-and-reach touching their knees, whereas others reach for their toes or beyond their toes. For an aerobic fitness activity, you might have students use the PACER tape for an activity called Beep and Turn. In this activity, a child runs toward the baseline until she hears a beep; she then turns at whatever point she is on her way to the baseline and travels in the opposite direction until the next beep, at which point she turns and runs toward the opposite baseline again, and so on. This technique is commonly used and known as "task modifications" and it is a way to make a task easier for a lower skilled student or more difficult for a higher skilled student (see figure 9.7). Appropriate adjustments motivate students to keep practicing because the task meets the individual's needs better and is therefore more interesting. Figure 9.8 provides some ideas for individualizing.

Activity selection can be one of the most time-consuming aspects of designing your curriculum, but it is perhaps the most important. The Activity Selection Criteria Checklist provides a list of criteria to consider for your activity selection. Remember, quality activities will be more motivating and help to ensure active student participation and more meaningful learning.

You can offer choices of one or more components of an activity to teach by invitation or designate changes to employ intratask variation.

Equipment—Size, type (e.g., hard or soft ball)

Distances—From target, between bases, of end lines from each other, of sidelines from each other

Rules—Cooperative or competitive, child designed or teacher designed, participate alone or with a group or partner

Movement—Speed, type (e.g., form of locomotion), effort

Time (duration)—Increase or decrease time allowed for a task

■ **Figure 9.7** By offering choices and modifying components of activities, you can create physical activity opportunities inclusive of all students.

- Modify equipment used by changing the size, texture, weight, or type of equipment (larger or smaller racket, harder or softer ball, and so on).
- Modify distance, allowing students to move closer or farther away from the target to increase or decrease difficulty.
- Modify the height of items such as a basket or the angle at which students perform a task.
- Modify the number of repetitions to complete a task.
- Modify the speed or locomotor movement.
- Modify student posture from sitting to standing or even lying down.
- Modify rules to fit your students' ability levels. Add or delete rules as necessary for more or less control.

■ **Figure 9.8** Tips for individualizing and modifying activities.

Adapted from *Teaching physical education,* Mosston & Ashworth, 2002, Chapter 10 – The Inclusion Style.

Activity Selection Criteria Checklist

Look over all the components for selecting appropriate activities for your students.

- ■ _____ Does the activity meet the needs (inclusive) of your student population (age and skill level, gender, special needs, and so forth)?
- ■ _____ Do the objectives for the activity fit (connect) with your program goals and expected outcomes? NASPE outcomes? State standards?
- ■ _____ Do you have the necessary facility and equipment?
- ■ _____ Is the activity developmentally appropriate for your students (this includes complexity of instructions and skills required)?
- ■ _____ Is this activity designed with maximum student participation in mind or can it be modified for greater or lesser student participation? (Use the 80/80 rule: a minimum of 80 percent of your students are engaged in the activity a minimum of 80 percent of the time.)
- ■ _____ Does the activity allow for a variety of difficulty levels (can it be modified for a younger or less skilled student and an older or more skilled student)?
- ■ _____ Can the activity be applied in a setting other than a formal instructional setting?
- ■ _____ Will the activity hold the interest of your students or is boredom likely to set in?
- ■ _____ Is the activity safe?

Why Change?

Making the change from a traditional "skill only" physical education program might seem like a difficult task, but it has proven to be very rewarding for many teachers. Here's what a couple of veteran physical educators from Naperville, Illinois, had to say about their change from a traditional physical education program to a health-related physical fitness education program. These quotes are taken from interviews conducted for the Physical Best Instructor's Video.

To the older physical education teacher, change is not easy . . . nobody likes to change but I guess I would relate it to the medical field . . . would you want me to teach medicine the same way I did 25 years ago, because I feel comfortable doing that? Do you want your children going to that doctor?

Phil Lawler, Middle School Physical Education Teacher
Naperville, Illinois

For a change, I'm glad to see the shift going away from athletics and sports for the elite to involve more kids. I got into this profession to educate kids and for the first time in my life I feel like I'm actually doing it.

Paul Zientarski, High School Physical Education Teacher
Naperville, Illinois

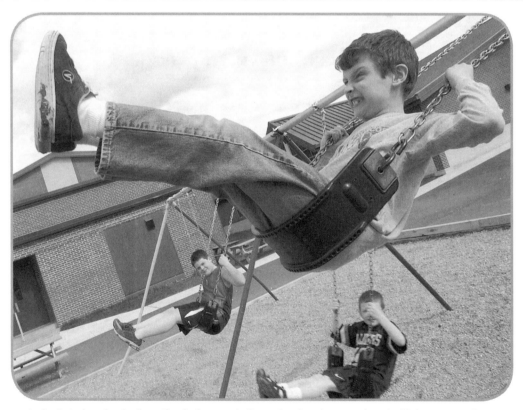

Encourage students to be physically active before and after school and on weekends. Help your students move toward self-responsibility for their personal fitness.

Summary

A quality physical education curriculum provides the framework within which students learn the necessary health-related physical fitness education concepts. It integrates motor skills and actual physical activity in a developmentally appropriate K-12 progression as well as other subject areas to create a well-balanced, meaningful approach. The programs produce individuals who view physical activity as a worthwhile, pleasurable, and lifelong endeavor. Students discover where their physical activity interests lie and learn how to design and implement a personal health-related fitness plan that suits their needs and situations. A well-designed and expertly implemented curriculum will inspire and empower students to lead physically active lives.

Teaching Styles and Strategies

> " Teaching is a process, and because
> it is a process, teaching behavior is
> interactive and, to a large degree,
> context specific. Not only must
> teachers have the technical skills
> of teaching, they must also be able
> to use those skills appropriately for
> particular situations. . . . The goal is
> not the acquisition of discrete, effective
> teaching behavior, but effective,
> context-specific practice. "
>
> **Judith E. Rink (2002)**

No matter how well conceived a curriculum plan is, it is two-dimensional: A plan might look good on paper, but it's flat and lifeless until effective teaching brings the plan to a three-dimensional learning environment. Employing different teaching styles is a great way to provide the diversity that keeps students interested.

Teaching Styles

How you actually teach can greatly affect student interest and enjoyment—and therefore student attitudes toward physical activity—so using a variety of teaching styles is necessary. You're sure to be the cure for insomnia if you rely solely on one style.

The Spectrum Approach

Mosston and Ashworth (2002) have defined a "spectrum of teaching styles" that move along a continuum from direct instruction (teacher initiated) to indirect instruction (student initiated).

In **The Spectrum Approach** each of these styles can enhance the health-related physical fitness education program. As you review this summary of the different styles, think about which styles will work with each lesson in your own teaching situation.

■ Command—The teacher makes all the decisions and gives step-by-step instructions that all students follow at the same time. This style is appropriate for teaching a new skill and for managing a class that needs a high degree of structure. It is also an appropriate style when task sequencing is essential and there can be no deviation from the sequence, as in teaching how to perform CPR. The command style is appropriate for lecture information that needs to be given to students before performing the task. Some other topics that might be taught using this style include how to calculate resting heart rate and how to record data on a graph to determine which exercise performed resulted in a higher heart rate.

■ Practice—The teacher decides what to teach, demonstrates or uses task sheets to introduce the skill, mandates the amount of time students will practice, and circulates among students, giving them feedback. Students determine the number of practice trials and the order in which they will practice skills (if more than one is part of the lesson). This is the most used style in a physical education setting, and although it is valuable, it should not be overused. This style is appropriate for teaching a new skill and for skill refinement; it affords students more latitude than in the command style as to how much practice they think they need. For example, you might ask high school students to bring their heart rates into their target heart rate zones but allow them to choose from four different activities to do so. Another example might be having the students rotate from station to station performing different exercises presented on a task card, but giving them an option of which modification they choose (e.g., Perform push-ups for one minute. You may choose from regular, modified, or wall.).

TEACHING TIP: Varying Your Teaching Style

Most effective teachers have a variety of teaching styles in their repertoires. Different classes, skills, and concepts will benefit from using different styles, and it is a challenge for teachers to find which styles produce the most learning in various situations. The better grasp you have of the different styles, the more likely you will be to try to use them. It can be compared to learning carpentry. If you only have a hammer and a saw in your tool belt, you will be limited in what kinds of work you will be able to produce. Likewise, if you as a teacher only have two teaching styles in your repertoire, you will be limiting the possibility of reaching all your students—and the opportunity for them to learn more.

Catherine Himberg, Professor of Physical Education
California State University
Chico, California

From *Teaching Secondary Physical Education: Preparing Adolescents to Be Active for Life* 2003.

■ Reciprocal—This style begins to lead a student to more independent, critical thinking. The teacher designs the tasks to be performed, and students work collaboratively (usually in pairs or groups of three) providing feedback about each other's performance. Each group of students is supplied with a task sheet that has the specific instructions and roles they are to perform. They are either the "observer" or the "performer." This style is used primarily for skill refinement and social interaction but may be used to teach new skills that are less complex. The teacher's role is not to correct performance but to monitor student interactions and to encourage the observers to give quality, positive feedback to the performers. This allows students to become more actively involved in their own learning, which can result in a greater depth of understanding. An example of this style is preparing students for taking the *FITNESSGRAM* tests by having them practice the tests in pairs and give each other feedback on technique.

■ Self-check—This style is similar to the reciprocal style, but instead of working with others, the students are involved in evaluating their own performance. The teacher still determines the tasks to be completed and designs the task or criteria sheet to be used. Then each student performs the tasks and provides his or her own feedback by completing the sheet. This style is appropriate for refining skills and for building self-reliance, but it limits interaction with the teacher and fellow students. This style must also be used with tasks that can be self-monitored. The self-check style works extremely well for homework assignments that encourage skill practice. For example, ask students to log aerobic fitness activity time performed outside of class. Allow students to select the appropriate activities for themselves and to monitor their own progress, giving themselves feedback through self-assessment of their aerobic fitness.

■ Inclusion—In this style, the teacher still designs the tasks to be completed, but students have options of "difficulty" levels they can choose to perform at. This puts the responsibility of learning back on the student, since the student takes responsibility for deciding when to move to a more difficult level of performance. This style helps the teacher both individualize lessons and empower students to move closer to independence in their health-related physical fitness activity. For example, give students the choice of jogging or walking briskly as a warm-up activity or let them choose between a variety of push-ups (e.g., with hands on a bench or on the floor) when working on muscular strength and endurance. Make

sure students know that they are expected to increase the difficulty when they judge they are ready.

■ Guided discovery—In this style, the teacher is not only working to enhance the physical abilities of the student but also to enhance critical thinking skills. The teacher determines the task and then designs a sequence of questions or problems that will lead students to one right answer. The teacher may also need to respond with an activity through which students may practice what they've learned. Student success depends on the teacher's ability to arrange questions or problems in a logical sequence posed at the right time in the learning experience. Although time consuming for both teacher and student, this style helps students remember the answer better than with less involved approaches, because students must take more responsibility for discovering the answer. An example of a guided discovery lesson might be assigning students to write a report answering the following questions:

■ What is one jogging or in-line skating route in your community that allows you to jog for 20 minutes starting from school or home? In this example, students might have to try several routes to find the one that meets the criteria.

■ What should you wear? How might this change with the time of day and weather?

■ What are the safety issues that you have to pay attention to? Do these change with the time of day or weather (figure 10.1)?

Another example might be for students to practice several ways of balancing and to determine which balance puts them in the best position to complete a certain skill.

■ Convergent discovery—This style extends the guided discovery style. The teacher poses a problem or question, but students go through the discovery process to converge on the one right answer without the teacher's guidance (while adhering to the principles of safety). In this style, students are encouraged to become more independent, critical thinkers. The teacher provides the setting in which students may discover the answer through a process of trial and error. This style is appropriate for students who have become proficient at finding answers through the guided discovery approach. For example, ask high school students to complete a report on what it would take to begin participating in a beneficial aerobic fitness activity in their community. Have them research

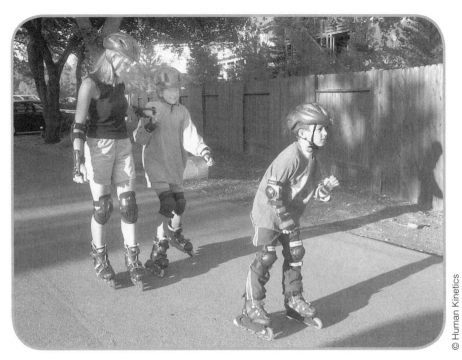

© Human Kinetics

■ **Figure 10.1** An example of a guided discovery assignment might be assigning students to write a report that answers questions such as, "What safety concerns should you address when in-line skating in your neighborhood?"

the aerobic fitness benefits of various activities, find ones that can be done in the community, find out the costs for equipment, where to do the activity, what prerequisite skills are necessary, and so on. Another example might be to pose the question, "What effect does gaining or losing weight (body fat) have on your heart rate?" Allow the students to perform several tasks adding or subtracting more weight that they have to carry around during the activity for each trial so they discover the answer. To increase or decrease the resistance, have students use hand weights, ankle weights, books, and so on, appropriate to the activity.

■ Divergent production—The teacher poses an open-ended problem for students to solve. Students learn that many physical activity situations have multiple solutions. This style is appropriate for students who are ready to work more independently of the teacher to meet health-related fitness challenges. For example, pose this situation to students: You have broken your ankle, but you want to maintain good aerobic fitness while wearing your cast. Devise an aerobic fitness plan to meet this challenge. Another example for younger students might be to have them perform three locomotor skills that will increase their heart rate.

NOTE: The following three styles are designed to allow the student the most independence and flexibility in their learning but are often the most

difficult to incorporate due to school restrictions or curriculum mandates. It also takes students time to understand the objectives of these styles, so there is some time involved in "teaching" the students how to be independent learners. These styles are most appropriate with older, highly motivated students or can be used quite effectively in "advanced" classes.

■ Individual program-learner's design—The teacher chooses the general subject area, but the student determines the task and possible solutions. This style encourages students to design their own learning programs based on their abilities, interests, and learning styles; therefore, this style more closely simulates real-world situations. It also allows the students to be independent learners and critical thinkers. An example might be for students to design their own personal health-related fitness plan.

■ Learner initiated—This style is similar to the previous style, but the students choose the general subject area and how they will go about completing the task on their own, not in response to teacher prompting. It is similar to contract learning. This style evolves in some older students who, for example, may have specific sport interests that compel them to seek teacher input.

■ Self-teaching—The extreme opposite of the command style, this style empowers students to make virtually all the learning decisions. This style is appropriate for high school students who have proven, through the learner-initiated style, that they can pursue their own interests independent of a teacher, and for adults engaging in physical activity on their own.

Work to incorporate several different teaching styles into your program to create variety and give students opportunities to practice greater independence. This will help you reach the goal of producing adults who independently pursue health-related fitness as a way of life. The styles that facilitate learner independence also, quite naturally, encourage students to use higher levels of thinking (e.g., synthesis, analysis, and evaluation). This, in turn, enhances the development of life skills, such as problem solving and making accurate judgments and wise decisions, that can be used both within and outside of the realm of health-related fitness. This is an important consideration when tying your curriculum into a school's overall mission of producing independent learners and doers.

One last thought to remember: Although the styles described form a continuum from teacher directed to independence, a student does not fully "graduate" from any one approach. For example, the command and practice styles will be appropriate at times all the way through high school, at least for part of a lesson. Even a highly motivated adult will benefit from a more directed style when learning a new physical activity or perfecting a familiar physical activity. However, give students more and more practice further along the continuum as they grow older and more experienced. This broader experience in self-directed approaches to physical activity will serve them well as adults.

Gardner's Theory of Multiple Intelligences

Just as students learn through different teaching styles, they also possess different learning styles. One way to examine this aspect is to look at **Gardner's theory of multiple intelligences.** Gardner (1983; 1993) asserts that different individuals are strong in different "intelligences." In other words, each person learns and produces best through various avenues. Each of your students needs to have opportunities to develop weak avenues and to excel through strong avenues. This section provides a brief summary of Gardner's intelligences and some examples of how they might be used.

Challenging yourself to address each type of intelligence when designing in-class activities is another way to create variety and spark interest in the class or lecture setting. Also, keep the various intelligences in mind when creating follow-up homework assignments (in both lecture and physical activity situations).

Bodily-Kinesthetic Intelligence

Moving to learn isn't just for the gymnasium! Individuals strong in bodily-kinesthetic intelligence solve problems or create with their bodies. Mime, crafts, hands-on science, dramatics, physical education, and other creative movement opportunities interest them. Skilled actors, dancers, athletes, surgeons, and craftspeople are likely to be high in bodily-kinesthetic intelligence.

To address this intelligence in health-related physical fitness education, be sure to have students actually apply health-related fitness concepts. For example, don't just talk about designing a personal fitness plan; have students actually design and use such plans. Find ways students can move in the class setting as well. Depending on age, students may enjoy miming actions (e.g., actions of a muscle), crafts that reinforce concepts (e.g., a valentine promising yourself to eat more heart healthy), a hands-on science lesson (e.g., capillary action shown by dropping colored water on a good brand of paper towel), drama (e.g., act out oxygen exchange in the lungs), and other creative movement opportunities. Middle or high school students might be asked to create a video for teaching elementary students about health-related fitness.

Spatial Intelligence

Understanding how objects orient in space is the strong suit of individuals with high spatial intelligence. A strong sense of direction and the ability to visualize end products accurately are evidence of this intelligence. Skilled architects, sculptors, and navigators are most likely strong in spatial intelligence. Sketching ideas; using charts, graphs, maps, diagrams, and graphics software; and building models are the preferred modes of learning. Assign these forms of conveying ideas as project options. In addition, incorporate teacher and student demonstrations into your teaching as much as possible. For example, have students show and analyze each other's running technique.

Use charts, graphs, diagrams, graphics software, and three-dimensional models to teach. Have students make their own similar items to reinforce their learning. This works well for charting heart rates, recording weight-training progress, logging physical activity, and so on.

Interpersonal Intelligence

The ability to understand and relate well to others, as in the case of psychologists and social workers, indicates strong interpersonal intelligence. Group brainstorming, cooperative activities, peer tutoring, simulations, and community-based activities interest these individuals. Incorporate cooperative learning approaches to foster interpersonal intelligence. A health-related physical fitness education example may be having students work in small groups to develop an aerobic fitness circuit. Brainstorm solutions to problems as a class or in small groups. Use simulations to teach real-world interpersonal skills. For instance, ask, "How would you spend 100 dollars in this community to participate in physical activity?" Have students collect data on the cost of facilities, equipment, and so on as homework, then work in small groups to help each other make wise and satisfying choices. Train students to participate as peer tutors or in the community on a health-related fitness service project (e.g., leading active games at a day care center).

Musical Intelligence

Fascination with sound and the ability to interpret, transform, and express musical forms indicates strength in musical intelligence. Skilled musicians and dancers are strong in musical intelligence. Use raps, chants, songs, rhythms, and musical concepts to reach these students.

Music and movement are almost impossible to separate. Consider allowing students to report on health-related fitness research through music. Use music to enliven and set the pace for physical activities as well. Allow students to give research reports in the form of raps, chants, and songs.

Logical-Mathematical Intelligence

A strong ability to reason and use numbers very effectively indicates high logical-mathematical intelligence. Scientists, mathematicians, and engineers are good examples of people high in logical-mathematical intelligence. Science demonstrations, math problems, sequential presentation of subject matter, critical thinking activities, and problem-solving exercises are preferable ways to learn for these individuals.

Challenge middle or high school students to solve health-related fitness problems, for example, calculating target heart rate zones or the percent of calories (kilocalories) of fat provided in a serving of a particular food, how much work is done climbing a flight of stairs, or how many kilocalories are expended walking versus running a mile. Elementary students can create movement sequences and patterns, such as a jump rope routine or counting reps of selected skills to repeat a pattern, while developing muscular strength and endurance or aerobic fitness.

Intrapersonal Intelligence

Those people who know both their strengths and weaknesses well can be said to be strong in intrapersonal intelligence. They are self-reliant and independent, preferring to learn through making personal connections, using interest centers and self-paced activities, reflecting, and goal setting. A health-related physical fitness education program should guide all students toward becoming more independent through, for example, self-testing and reflective journal writing opportunities. Help students make personal connections to the information you're providing. For example, encourage students to research and try out various physical activities they find interesting. Provide self-paced activities and learning centers, and give students time and guidance to select and set goals regarding physical activity and health-related fitness.

Naturalistic Intelligence

People who are adept at identifying flora and fauna are strong in naturalistic intelligence. Address this intelligence by using themes from nature as well as stories and poems about nature to encourage movement experiences that develop health-related physical fitness. For example, performing the crab walk, bear walk, and seal crawl helps young children study movement in nature while developing muscular strength and endurance (figure 10.2 *a* and *b*). At the middle or high school level, you could ask science teachers to create a study of how plants and animals live at high altitudes, and what the physiological implications of performing at high altitudes are for humans (i.e., What adaptations have plants and animals made at high altitude? What are the acute changes humans face when performing at high altitudes, and what are the chronic adaptations to high altitude?). Middle and high school students can also consider the value of physical activity in natural settings, such as hiking, canoeing, rafting, and so on.

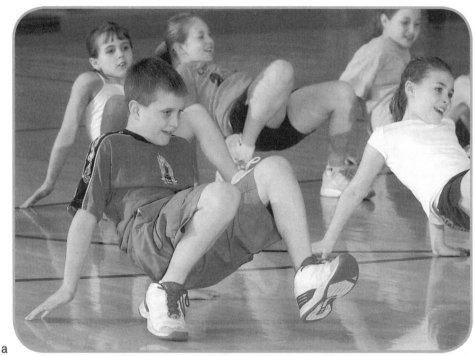

a

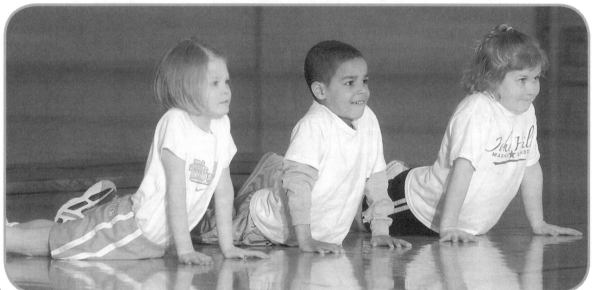

b

■ **Figure 10.2** Performing *(a)* the crab walk and *(b)* the seal crawl helps children study movement in nature while developing muscular strength and endurance.

Prepare students to get the most out of field trips to inspiring outdoor locations. For example, work with the science teacher to learn about the plants and animals you may see on a hike through a local park. Show students how fresh air, a change of scenery, and physical activity can work together to foster a sense of well-being.

Linguistic Intelligence

Linguistic intelligence involves using words very effectively. Skilled writers, poets, and public speak-

ers display linguistic intelligence. Opportunities to read, tell stories, listen to lectures, debate, perform writing activities, and participate in small- and large-group discussions interest these students. To speak to this intelligence, require students to keep a written log of their health-related physical fitness education activities.

Cooperative Learning

Cooperative learning is a style that has been around for a long time. As its name implies, students will be working together to complete a specified task or assignment. It is an extremely flexible style that has the potential to incorporate all three learning domains, to use several intelligences, and to provide for a more positive learning environment. One example of cooperative learning is a strategy known as "jigsaw."

In jigsawing, each member of a team is given a particular assignment to complete; each team member then brings back her product and places her piece of the "puzzle" with other team members' pieces to form a complete picture. Figure 10.3 provides two examples of how this might be accomplished in a physical education environment. The end result is smaller group instruction, and students are empowered to be responsible for their own learning. All

three domains are reinforced, and the teacher is able to serve as more of a facilitator and wander among the groups for individualized instruction and feedback.

The Classroom Approach

The most ideal teaching situation would be to have a gymnasium with an attached "smart" classroom and a two-hour block of time daily to teach health-related fitness education. But, of course, many physical educators are in less than an ideal situation. Imagine this situation: Your gymnasium has been overtaken by the annual science fair. What are you going to do for the next three days? You have three options available: (1) allow your students to sit and idly chat with their

---

Jigsawing Assignment

Unit: Tennis

- Divide your students into teams of six and assign each team member a stroke to teach.
- Give team members one or two drills that will reinforce his or her particular stroke. If time allows, have students design or locate the drills themselves.
- Allow time for practice and provide materials (videos, textbooks, and so forth) to help each member learn his or her stroke.
- After a set period of time (usually one class period), have each member teach his or her group the particular stroke and perform applicable "drills" to enhance the stroke.
- Upon completion, each group has been taught the basic tennis strokes.

Unit: Health-related fitness components

- Divide your students into groups of four and either assign each member a fitness component or allow them to assign themselves a fitness component.
- Give team members three to five activities that will enhance their components. If time allows, have students design or locate the activities themselves.
- All members regroup and design three or four warm-up routines that have all four components of fitness included.
- Once again, be certain to have the appropriate material on hand.
- Another approach is to have the first part of this assignment as homework and then devote one class to the group portion.
- Then you can have the group lead the class in the warm-up routines for the next couple of weeks.

Figure 10.3 Jigsawing assignment.

Adapted from J.E. Rink, 1998, *Teaching physical education for learning*, 3rd ed. (New York, NY: McGraw-Hill Companies), 89-94. Reproduced with permission of The McGraw-Hill Companies.

friends, (2) take your students to a corner of the gym or the top of the bleachers and attempt to keep their attention on some lesson you have prepared that involves you talking and them listening, or (3) locate an empty classroom and have a quality lesson prepared. The answer should be obvious. Teachers must make the most of their class time to prepare their students for lifetime physical activity, and choices one and two will not help reach that goal.

One of the primary principles taught in a teacher preparation program is "be prepared for the unexpected." If you live by this principle, when you find yourself without your gymnasium, you will be prepared with a group of activities that can be moved to another environment and still allow you to engage the students in active learning. One way to be prepared is to develop a core of health-related fitness classroom lesson plans for each course or grade that you teach. The number you develop should depend on the content you want to cover and the number of class periods you project you will be without physical activity facilities in the course of the school year or grading period. Then use the lessons as the need for alternative plans arises.

This method, however, is not intended to relegate health-related fitness teaching to a catch-as-catch-can status. It is simply a way to maximize your students' physical activity time when you have the facilities you need and to teach fitness concepts and skills when you don't—as long as this takes place within a well-organized and well-developed curriculum. If you make sure these lessons develop basic fitness concepts and skills in an age-appropriate, progressive manner, students will receive as complete a health-related fitness education as possible before leaving your program.

One efficient way to organize these lessons is to create a file folder or box for each one. Place any audiovisual materials (e.g., videotapes, prepared overhead transparencies, posters, and the like) along with handouts, written lesson plans, and any other supplies you'll need in the file. Marian Franck, a retired high school physical education teacher (Lancaster, Pennsylvania), calls this an "emergency kit." With one for each unit or lesson, you'll be prepared at a moment's notice.

Then, when you get to school and discover that the principal forgot to tell you the gymnasium would be used that day for the dress rehearsal for the eighth-grade class play, you'll be ready. All you need now is a portable kit with the general supplies you'll need (e.g., one pencil per student, art supplies, overhead marking pens, tape, and so on) and a room to meet

in with the audiovisual equipment you'll need. Some physical educators are fortunate enough to have such a room available full time, but most likely, you will have to find your own space. Plan for this possibility before school starts by seeking administrative support or by finding your own reliable solution.

In addition to having your "traveling lessons," you should plan these lessons to engage the students actively and provide them avenues for being responsible for their own learning. The concepts presented earlier in this chapter under the heading "The Spectrum Approach" work in an alternate environment as well. You need to advance the students from the direct instruction approach (command) to indirect teaching situations (student initiated).

Teaching Fitness Skills in the Classroom Setting

Certain fitness skills lend themselves to being covered in the in-depth time a classroom setting provides. Of course, all of these topics can be addressed in the physical activity setting as well if you divide the material into small enough pieces so that you don't take away from physical activity time.

Interpreting Heart Rate Data   A kindergartner can understand why his or her heart beats faster after moderate to vigorous physical activity. Third- or fourth-grade students can begin to understand the reasons for maintaining vigorous physical activity for a specified period of time. Middle school students can begin to draw correlations between types of exercise and how hard the heart works by monitoring various activities and charting either perceived exertion or actual heart rate. In high school, students can calculate their heart rates and target heart rate zones (see chapter 5), chart heart rates in graph form, log workout results, and calculate averages.

Treating Injuries   Naturally, preventing injuries is the way to go, but students need to understand that injuries do occur at times even when you're careful. Contact the American Red Cross or the National Safety Council for more information on basic first aid and cardiopulmonary resuscitation (CPR). Recommended injury treatment topics to be covered include the following: RICES (rest, ice, compression, elevation, support) principle; heat- and cold-related problems (heat stress, heat exhaustion, hypothermia, and hyperthermia); fluid intake (dehydration); sunburn and skin protection; differences between sprains and strains; assessment of injury situations (and when to see a physician); and basic life support. This list is by no means inclusive but designed as a starting point for developing classroom activities.

Becoming a Good Fitness Consumer   In this age of advertising blitzes and cable shopping networks, being a good fitness consumer is an essential skill. Students need to know how to comparison shop to get the most for their money when paying for legitimate equipment, supplies, and services, and how to discern when a product isn't worth the container it comes in. The following are suggestions for consumer education activities (you can adapt these activities to fit your students' ages and abilities):

- Ask students to compare vitamin supplement claims with the research and then make recommendations to their classmates based on their findings. (Have the class discuss whether they agree or not.)

- Direct students to bring in an advertisement for a fad diet or a piece of exercise equipment that promises miracle results. Have them report (orally or in writing) on whether or not the ad's claim is true and why or why not.

- Discuss what might make an advertisement effective (e.g., flashy, quick "bytes" of information, enthusiastic claims, and so on). Have students in small groups develop magazine ads or act out TV commercials that advertise the benefits of a health-related fitness activity or practice (e.g., drinking plenty of water before, during, and after exercise; playing an active game instead of watching TV; and the like).

- Take a field trip to a local sports equipment store. Have students prepare specific questions to ask about the equipment they're interested in. Ask the salespeople to help the students compare the features of similar products; then for homework, have each student choose one of the products and explain in writing why he felt it was the best buy for his needs.

Logging Physical Activity Data   The classroom provides an ideal setting for teaching students how to set up meaningful physical activity logs. Emphasize the importance of recording data accurately. Share with students ways to make helpful and thoughtful comments alongside their physical activity data. Then show students the connections between keeping these records and making future plans and setting future goals. For example, if a certain activity always

elicits negative comments, encourage the student to choose a different activity to meet the same goals. Finally, show students how to use technology to help them keep physical activity logs. Spreadsheet programs, computer-based calendars, and computerized logbooks for running and other aerobic activities are available for classroom use.

Setting Goals   Whereas you should be able to help each student set health-related fitness goals at a station on a circuit in the physical activity setting, the classroom setting provides opportunities to explain the purpose and mechanisms of goal setting. Sample class activities include the following (as always, tailor these suggestions to fit the ages and needs of your students):

- Use the information on goal setting in chapter 2 to help a fictional person set appropriate goals (e.g., How might Jack build upper body strength so he can climb up the beanstalk? or, Victor wants to improve his body composition. What are realistic ways he can approach this?).

- Have students work with a friend to help each other set realistic goals and plan activities to reach the goals in one health-related fitness area. Instruct them to help each other think of incentives they can offer each other (e.g., "If we both follow our plan, we'll buy matching workout outfits," or, "We'll walk to school together so we can have fun talking while we exercise").

- In small groups, brainstorm reasons people might not stick to their physical activity plans until they reach their goals. Then choose one problem and list ways to overcome it.

Designing a Personal Health-Related Fitness Plan   Students as young as the primary grades can begin to make choices about how they will reach their goals in each component of health-related fitness. As an instructor, it is your task to divide the material into small enough pieces so that students can understand and apply it. How small those pieces are depends on the ages and abilities of your students. *The Physical Best Activity Guides* provide examples of how to focus on one component of health-related fitness at a time in age-appropriate ways. Following such a program means that, over time, each student will have developed his or her own personal fitness plan. You can give an overview of this procedure in a lecture setting to "prime the pump" for personal planning activities to be done in the physical activity setting or as homework.

Students also need to know that effective personal health-related fitness plans are dynamic, or ever changing. Illustrate this point by sharing your own or a fictitious personal plan, and showing how the goals kept being reset and specific plans changed as old goals were achieved. In this way, students see the process of tailoring a program to fit individual needs, which they can apply as adults. (Refer to chapter 9 and the *Physical Best Activity Guide: Middle and High School Levels* for more information relating to this topic.)

The Homework Concept

Homework in physical education—how absurd! This is a statement often heard (and duly modified) from parents and students alike. Physical educators have not efficiently done *their* homework and have allowed this perception to become the norm rather than the exception. But today with many states revising their educational standards, school districts and teachers are taking another look at this concept and beginning to incorporate this into their programs. The advantages of this concept are numerous. Homework allows students to explore a topic more in depth; it allows for a greater variety of strategies to be incorporated; it allows for learning in all three domains; it allows for more "activity" time in the regular class; and it allows for another avenue of communication between the parents, the student, and the school. But where does a teacher begin when it comes to assigning homework?

First, remember that the homework assignment should not be something that is random or something you are assigning "just because." This serves no purpose and only creates another time-consuming task, without an educational benefit, for the student as well as yourself. (See "Sample Homework Assignment" section for examples.)

Second, make sure homework assignments are connected to the lessons you are currently teaching.

Sample Problem-Solving Activities

The following are sample problem-solving activities designed for applying appropriate knowledge in a personal lifetime health-related fitness course.

- Discuss how there are times when the heart rate increases, not in response to physical activity, but rather due to caffeine, stress, or other stimulants. Have students research this topic.
- Compare and contrast the health-related benefits of in-line skating with those of lap swimming.
- Case study: Read aloud to students a true personal story from a fitness magazine, sharing only the description of the person's fitness and health dilemma. Have students work together in small groups to design a realistic, beneficial, and interesting fitness plan for this person. Then have groups share and discuss their plans with the rest of the class. Read the rest of the true story aloud. Discuss the person's actual choices in light of the small groups' plans and the principles of safe and effective health-related fitness plans the students are learning to apply.

Through its core philosophy, Physical Best and the health-related physical fitness education that stems from it promote problem solving as a way of life. While other curriculum models espouse problem solving as an important component, most of these add it as just another ingredient in the recipe—not a basic philosophy. Physical Best believes, however, that problem solving must arise from the core of a program, not be tacked on almost as an afterthought. When students learn to design and implement personal fitness plans and leave physical education programs prepared and empowered to modify these plans to suit their individual needs over the course of their lifetime, they have truly learned problem-solving skills that will transfer to and apply in a variety of life's situations.

They should reinforce and be an extension of the topic. Homework assignments are also an excellent way to tie diverse components together, such as fitness and sports or attitudes and sports.

Third, explain to the students why they are doing this particular assignment. Initially, you are going to get groans and "ughs," but don't all teachers who give homework? If you make the assignment meaningful and relevant, and students understand the connectivity of the assignment, then it provides tremendous benefits down the road.

Possible homework assignments are numerous; they can be as simple as completing a worksheet or as comprehensive as developing a portfolio. Kindergartners as well as seniors in high school can do homework. It is just a matter of designing the appropriate assignment. Much of the information described in the preceding section (as good topics for the classroom setting) could be modified to present as homework for students, thus allowing more class time for actual activity.

Strategies for Successful Program Scheduling

Students might not remember the details of your program when they're in their 50s, but chances are they will remember how they felt about the program and about physical activity. Work to make good memories for tomorrow's adults, while providing a balanced health-related physical fitness education program.

The goals related to the development of self-esteem, self-direction, and a sense of responsibility for self and others, which we share with all educational programs in the school, may actually have more of an impact on maintaining an active lifestyle than our unique contribution in motor skills and fitness.

Judith E. Rink (2002)

Scheduling

Physical education should be scheduled in a way that provides the best opportunity for effective teaching to take place. Unfortunately, too often a physical education program schedule ends up being the result more of available facilities and other schoolwide priorities than of sound educational thinking.

Extending Physical Activity Time

The amount of time that physical educators have with their students varies widely from state to state, school to school, and level to level. But whether you see your students just once a week (as, unfortunately, some elementary physical education teachers do) or every day, you should take advantage of a number of proven strategies for extending physical activity time beyond your program. The goal is to get students into the habit of being physically active on their own; keeping activities personally enjoyable is important so students don't view these extra activities as drudgery. Adapt the following suggestions to fit your students' age range, your school's facilities, and other pertinent factors. Note that these ideas should all serve as extensions of physical education, not replacements. In other words, they serve in a sense as physical education homework and are meant to enhance what is taught during physical education class. Your administrators and colleagues must understand this so that they don't think it would be okay to cut back on physical education classes since students can participate in these activities outside of class.

■ Fitness breaks—The guidelines in the Surgeon General's report (USDHHS 1996) assert that physical activity can be accumulated throughout the day in short bouts, making this an increasingly popular and beneficial option in some districts. As you train classroom teachers to conduct these breaks, offer concrete reasons that are important to them, such as exercise increases blood flow to the brain, helping a person think better. The trained and certified physical educator must take responsibility for this information. Perhaps offer a five-minute summary of several possible activities at each staff meeting and help teachers solve any problems they're having.

■ Recess—Ensure that students have ample equipment and input for fun and beneficial

Sample Homework Assignments

These are examples of either a reflection/closure activity or a simple homework assignment for your students to complete.

Question for the Day

Design a question that will cause the students to reflect on the day's lesson. For example, when teaching a unit on golf, you might ask, "Which of the health-related fitness components will be maintained or improved through regular participation in golf?"

Research Paper

Students pick a successful athlete (either currently successful or in the recent past) and locate information about the workout regimen that the athlete uses to stay on top of his or her game physically and emotionally.

Active Andy and Suzy Slug

An example of an assignment for primary students might begin by having a discussion about what it means to be active and some activities they can do at home or after school to stay active. Reproduce pictures of children either being active or not active and send them home with the students. Have the students then draw a happy face beside the pictures that show kids being active and a sad face beside those being inactive.

Health Calendar

Have your students design a calendar that celebrates physical education, fitness, and being healthy. The calendar can cover a week, two weeks, or a month (teacher's choice). The students should plan activities to do during that time and log their success. Figure 10.4 is one such calendar that was designed to celebrate National Physical Education Week, which is always the first week of May.

MAY

Sunday	Monday	Tuesday	Wednesday	Thursday	Friday	Saturday
1	2	3	4	5	6	7
	No television or video games today. Go outside and do something physical.	Jump rope for a least 15 minutes today.	Take a 20-to 30-minute walk around the park or neighborhood today; go with a friend or walk the dog.	While watching your favorite television program, do sitting exercises such as crunches, push-ups, stretching, leg raises, biceps curls; and so on.	Ride your bike for 30 minutes. Tell a parent where you are going. Follow the laws of the road. Be safe!	

Figure 10.4 Keeping calendars is a motivating way to help students track and plan the frequency of their participation in physical activity.

physical activities during recess. Don't hesitate to teach activities during physical education that students can easily use during their free times—then point these out. After all, this can form the beginning of self-responsibility for physical fitness.

■ Lunchtime—Lunchtime free play is simply a longer recess in most schools, but you can make it so much more. Consider making yourself available as a personal fitness consultant to interested students, or train student volunteers to conduct fun fitness activities during free play times or to assist you with younger students in physical education class. You can even start a fitness club and offer incentives for participating.

■ Intramurals—These are physical activity programs conducted between teams of students or individual students from the same school. Adapt a program to augment your fitness curriculum in specific, stated ways, then work to ensure the program is fun and friendly, welcoming all who wish to participate. When creating teams, be sure to make them as even as possible. Then insist that participants focus primarily on skill, fitness, and social development, not cutthroat competition. Consider having students keep track of minutes of activity or calculate calories burned as a way of keeping activity and fitness as the focus. You might also consider allowing students to add points for using encouraging words to classmates in order to keep the focus on social development and fun. Think of other innovative ways to keep score that encourage student development toward program goals.

■ After-school programs—Consider creating a new program or working to enhance an existing after-school child care program. If you cannot commit the time to after-school activities, train others who can, such as parent or senior volunteers or child care workers.

■ Home-based activities—Send home assignments for the entire family to participate in such as "The Family Health Minute." Present a specific health topic to your students and have them go home and discuss the information with (or explain it to) their families. Try to get them to set aside a few minutes two or three times a week. It might be new information each time or one topic with different subtopics.

■ Encourage families to make physical activity a fun and regular family event. They can even create ways to work out while watching television (such as jumping rope, stretching, or doing sit-ups). Plan a calendar of events for students to do during a particular month. Figure 10.4 depicts one week of such a month. Designing the calendar is also a great homework assignment for students.

■ Community events—Family nights, health fairs, and Jump Rope/Hoops for Heart (American Heart Association and AAHPERD) events involve the wider community, from parents and siblings to senior citizens. Not only are such events ways to help students become more fit and healthy, they also provide good public relations for your program.

South Carolina has established a student performance standard for high school students that requires activity participation outside regular class. See the "South Carolina's Approach" section.

Block Scheduling

In the mid 1990s, the National Education Commission on Time and Learning disseminated a report concerning the lack of actual learning time versus the amount of time students spent in schools. It was critical of the rigidity of time schedules in both calendar and clock hours in American schools. Out of this report several recommendations were made regarding learning and the daily schedule of school. One of the recommendations was to encourage schools to redesign the school day to provide for greater learning time (quality over quantity), even if that meant extending the school day or decreasing the number of daily courses (U.S. Department of Education 1994; Hastie 2003). As a result, many schools (particularly at the high school level) began to move away from the traditional schedule in which classes meet each day for 45 to 50 minutes and students attend six to eight classes a day. The complaints about traditional scheduling include lack of time to explore a topic in depth, to use more involved teaching styles, or to apply higher-level thinking skills; too much time spent on transitions between classes and administrative chores; and difficulty getting to know each student personally.

Block scheduling attempts to resolve these problems by extending class periods to 80 or more minutes, reducing the number of courses a student takes in one day, and reducing the number of class

South Carolina's Approach

In 1995, South Carolina established a student performance standard for high school students that requires health-enhancing physical activity outside the physical education class. We have reproduced this standard here:

Criterion Three

Participate regularly in health-enhancing physical activity outside the physical education class.

Description of the Criterion

The intent of this standard is to help the student make a transition from physical education class to a physically active lifestyle and real-life opportunities. The high school student should participate regularly in physical activity outside the physical education setting if patterns of participation appropriate for a physically active lifestyle are to be established. Two dimensions of participation are critical. The first is the student should be exploring opportunities both in the school and in the community and surrounding areas for participation in a wide variety of physical activities. The second is the student should be developing the ability to make wise choices about how he or she spends time both in terms of the structured activities chosen to participate in as well as choosing more active alternatives in daily living (e.g., taking the stairs rather than the elevator). The student should independently seek opportunities for activity and design activity programs as a lifestyle issue. This criterion can be met through opportunities in the school and community as well as through independently designed programs of physical activity.

Definitions

- Regularly—Weekly over a nine-week period
- School activities—Sport teams, intramurals, club activities
- Community activities—Church sponsored, parks and recreation programs, YM(W)CA, commercial companies
- Health-enhancing physical activity—Moderate to vigorous exercise (consecutively and/or totally) for 20 minutes or more a day, three times per week
- Components of health-related fitness—Aerobic fitness, muscular strength, muscular endurance, body composition, and flexibility
- Independent programs—Family-designed structured programs and independently designed structured programs (The term *structured* here means designated time and place with planned regularity.)

Critical Aspect of Performance

The student provides evidence of regular participation for a minimum of nine weeks in an activity normally producing moderate levels of physical activity. The following are examples of student performance meeting the criteria:

- The student participates in a youth baseball league in the community.
- The student sets up a walking club with several other students during the lunch hour.
- The student sets up a personal fitness program consisting of weightlifting and aerobic exercise on a regular basis.
- The student participates in a folk dance or cycling club in the community.
- The student successfully participates as a member of a school athletic team. ☞

Assessment Example 1

The student keeps a daily journal of participation in his or her outside activity, recording each day of participation and what he or she does each day. The student evaluates his or her participation every three weeks, indicating the extent to which he or she is meeting the health-enhancing aspect of the criterion, the personal benefits of the participation, and the difficulties encountered in participating regularly in the activity. The journals are shared and discussed in the physical education class.

Assessment Criteria 1

- The student participates in the activity regularly for a period of at least nine weeks.
- The student evaluates the level of his or her participation appropriately.
- The student appropriately identifies both the advantages and disadvantages of participation.

Assessment Example 2

The student submits a signed form from a responsible adult describing the participation in an independent project.

Assessment Criterion 2

The student meets the criterion for type of activity and regularity of participation.

---

preps for each teacher. Another positive aspect of block scheduling, particularly in physical education, is that it allows for a stronger cognitive component to be added in the curriculum. There is now time to discuss the how and why of a particular topic, sport, or activity. For example, in an 80-minute class, students can spend 20 to 30 minutes discussing the benefits of aerobic fitness, then spend 30 minutes actually participating in an aerobic activity, and still have time for a quality closure activity.

If you were to look at schools offering block scheduling, you would find numerous variations from a "four × four semester block" to an "alternating block plan" (see figure 10.5) to a "trimester system" (Hastie 2003).

Another advantage of block scheduling, especially for physical education, is that it allows the students to get out of the gymnasium and into physical activity settings in the community. For example, it allows the time to take trips to the local health club, wall-climbing facility, mountain-biking course, ice-skating arena, dance club, hiking trails, and so on. It also allows for more in-depth instruction on how to get involved in these lifetime activities.

Minimal research has been done examining the long-term benefits of block scheduling versus traditional scheduling. The research that has been done speaks positively from a teacher's point of view about block scheduling. Haynes-Dusel (2001) and Bukowski and Stinson (2000) noted that some of the perceptions from teachers using block scheduling were, in addition to the above mentioned advantages, a less hectic pace (not having to rush through the material) and more time for planning quality instruction (prep periods were longer).

What about the other side of the coin? For every advantage of block scheduling, you can cite a distinct disadvantage, the most prominent being less frequent meetings (which may potentially negate the top priority of getting individuals active most days of the week). A second argument against block scheduling is that the classes are 80- to 100-minute periods. Few teachers have been trained to actively hold students' attention for that length of time; therefore, there is a good amount of unstructured class time, which is wasted. In addition, students have not been conditioned for the longer periods, and when this is combined with the teacher's lack of experience,

In this type of scheduling, students complete a total of six or seven classes a semester, but they only attend them two or three days a week. This mimics the traditional college semester schedule.

Student 1 is on schedule A, and student 2 is on schedule B.

■ Both students attend all six of their classes on Monday.

■ Student 1 attends 1st, 3rd, and 5th period classes on Tuesday and Thursday.

■ Student 1 attends 2nd, 4th, and 6th period classes on Wednesday and Friday.

■ Student 2 attends the opposite schedule on Tuesday through Friday (schedule B).

Student 1 - Schedule A

	Mon	Tues	Wed	Thur	Fri
1st period – English	X	X		X	
2nd period – History	X		X		X
3rd period – Spanish	X	X		X	
4th period – PE	X		X		X
5th period – Math	X	X		X	
6th period – Biology	X		X		X

Student 2 - Schedule B

	Mon	Tues	Wed	Thur	Fri
1st period – English	X		X		X
2nd period – History	X	X		X	
3rd period – Spanish	X		X		X
4th period – PE	X	X		X	
5th period – Math	X		X		X
6th period – Biology	X	X		X	

■ **Figure 10.5** Alternating block plan scheduling sample.

quality learning and student performance may decrease (Hastie 2003).

In any case, whether you are a proponent of block scheduling or not, you might not have the option, so you must make do with what you have. If it's 50 minutes, pick up the pace, cover material you think is absolutely essential, and provide students with a positive atmosphere. If you have block scheduling, then dig in, prepare quality, structured lessons using a variety of strategies, and once again provide a positive atmosphere.

Team Teaching

Team teaching is a great avenue to help solve space, equipment, and scheduling issues in the gymnasium as well as capitalize on an individual teacher's area of expertise. Team teaching allows one or more instructors greater interaction with individual students to assist in the learning process. Take the following scenario: There are two physical education classes scheduled in the gym at one time, and space is at a premium. It is difficult to conduct two different activities at one time without one interfering with the other; therefore, teacher A and B decide to team teach. Today's fitness lesson is on the proper form for performing push-ups at various levels (from the floor, from a bench, inverted, and so on). Teacher A is going through the technique with the entire combined class while teacher B is wandering among the classes correcting individual students' form (Rink 2002). In addition, team teaching allows each teacher to teach in his or her area of expertise more often, and the potential for developing strong units of instruction is enhanced. As the saying goes, two heads are better than one (in most cases).

There are drawbacks to team teaching. The main one is that, in most cases, one teacher tends to be the leader, and the others just go along with the program. If all teachers don't buy into the concepts, not only does the program suffer, but lesson quality decreases, the teachers themselves become resentful of the "slacker," and student motivation decreases. Therefore, before jumping into a team-teaching environment, have long and hard discussions about the benefits and disadvantages to determine if it is a potential solution for your program.

Environment

Regardless of whether you are in a gymnasium, outdoors, or in a classroom, the teaching environment sets the tone for your program. Your environment should be attractive and invite learning.

■ Create an attractive learning environment. Get rid of the torn, faded, and outdated posters, and take the time to create bright and interesting bulletin boards and other wall displays that teach. Integrate student work and pictures of your students in action whenever possible. Create kits of teaching aids (e.g., models of the human heart and lungs, oversized rubber band to represent a muscle stretching, and so on) to set up as attractive focal points during a lesson (figure 10.6). Such displays will enhance your students' chances of learning the material. Older stu-

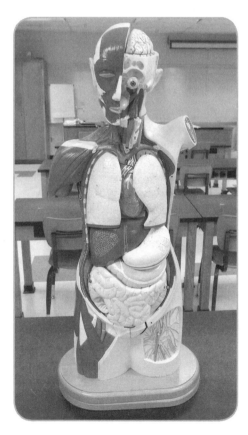

■ **Figure 10.6** Teaching aids can provide good focal points during a lesson in a lecture setting.

dents, parents, and other volunteers can help create these displays.

■ Ensure student safety. A safe learning environment is the foundation of learning and fun. After all, no one can learn about or enjoy physical activity if he or she is afraid of being injured. Be certain your environment is free of debris, and mark potential hazards clearly. Make sure your activity areas, locker rooms, and classroom are clean, freshly painted, and safe. Teach students specific safety information so that they can participate safely. Remind them often about safety concerns, and practice emergency procedures at least once a quarter.

■ Coordinate and schedule facilities. If you must share your gymnasium with the lunch staff because it doubles as a cafeteria, work with these personnel to make transitions smooth for both programs, minimizing lost instructional time. At the middle or high school level, you may need to work with coaches with whom you share facilities (gymnasium, track, and playing fields) to make sure everyone is able to use these facilities to their fullest. Try to look at these potential irritations as opportunities to network with other school staff—and as a stepping-stone to more significant interactions such as cross-curricular units. If you share facilities with other physical educators, strive to coordinate units so that each teacher can meet his or her objectives in a logical sequence. Finally, insist that facilities are kept in good repair so that instructional time is not lost due to hazards.

■ Play music. Music can welcome students, signal station changes, and provide a stimulating background. Within the bounds of good taste, allow students to bring tapes or CDs from home (screen before using in class).

Equipment

Certainly no one ever developed health-related fitness waiting for a turn; therefore, it is essential to have enough equipment to maximize student time on task. This ranges from having enough jump ropes in the gymnasium to having enough pencils in the classroom. While this may seem like common sense, for many schools and programs, obtaining and maintaining equipment are an ongoing headache.

■ Set up equipment before class. If this is not possible, have it ready to go in your storage area. Test audiovisual equipment and computer programs before trying to use them in class. Train students to help with setup and cleanup.

- Once you have a piece of equipment, take good care of it. The primary ways to extend the life of equipment are to provide regular maintenance, to teach students proper usage (and monitor how they are treating the equipment), and to store it properly when not in use. Consider providing official "certification" to students who have demonstrated they know how to use certain pieces of equipment (e.g., weight-training equipment, heart rate monitor) properly.

- Maintain your equipment by regularly inspecting it and repairing or replacing items as needed.

- Appropriate storage saves time, trouble, and needless wear and tear on equipment. See-through bins, baskets, and bags for small items; hanging bags; organized shelves; and labeled storage containers keep equipment safe and accessible. Secure exercise equipment, such as treadmills and stationary bikes, so that it cannot be used without adult supervision. If you share equipment with other teachers, install a sign-out procedure and carefully oversee timely and accurate returns.

- Assign squad leaders, specific students, or student assistants to pass out and return equipment.

- If you have equipment shortages and a small budget, contact community members to see if they will donate quality used equipment (as a tax deduction of course) for your program. You might also scour garage sales and classified ads. Parents may also be willing to donate used equipment. See *Creative Physical Activities & Equipment: Building a Quality Program on a Shoestring Budget* (1998) by Bev Davison for ideas about making some equipment.

- Consider fund-raising projects to help purchase equipment. Another way to gain equipment is by writing and applying for grants. There is a lot of money out there, so be on the lookout for state and federal grants that are available to support your program.

Technology

Although not essential to a good program, technology can help you teach health-related physical fitness. VCRs, computers, and video equipment can greatly enhance the teaching of health-related fitness

concepts. You can show videotapes or DVDs about health-related fitness topics, such as the functioning of the cardiorespiratory system, training principles, false advertising, and many other areas. Students can use computers to download, analyze, graph, and store heart rate monitor data. Have students use the Internet to research health-related fitness topics or to encourage "fitness pals" in other schools through e-mail. Divide students into small groups to develop health-related fitness reports, then videotape a "newscast" to share with peers or younger students. Some schools are equipped with in-house TV and radio stations that you may be able to use for the same purpose. HyperCard stacks for Macintosh computers are innovative tools available in some schools.

Other forms of technology are emerging for physical educators. One of the most popular items today is a heart rate monitor. Physical educators are investing in these to help students learn how to monitor their aerobic workout. There are simple two-function monitors that provide minimal feedback and sophisticated multifunction models capable of programming individual heart rate information, and upon completion of a workout, downloading information to a computer for analysis. Pedometers or Digi-Walkers are two other forms of technology physical educators are using to have students become more aware of their daily activity levels. If possible, tap into equipment that your non–physical education colleagues already have. You might consider scheduling time in the school's computer lab for students to learn to log physical activity time. *FITNESSGRAM* software not only provides teachers with functions, such as the ability to print out reports and keep information organized, it also provides a mode through which individual students (using passwords) can keep track of their own progress in health-related fitness. Another feature is the *ACTIVITYGRAM*, which allows teachers and students to monitor activity levels.

Technology can also provide an efficient and interesting medium for team teaching and cross-curricular learning. The science department may have items you can use, such as interactive CD-ROMs that teach about the human body.

Before deciding to purchase new technology, try to borrow it from a colleague or see a demonstration given by a salesperson to determine if the item is right for your program and student population. Then decide how many you need and can afford.

One final point to remember: Technology can help you teach, but it is no substitute for a solid program.

So don't turn technology into expensive toys. Make sure your reasons for using each item are sound and that your applications of the technology are relevant, both to your students and your program goals.

Summary

Bring your health-related physical fitness education program to life by creating an effective learning environment. By incorporating the principles described in this chapter, along with your own talents, you will encourage and assist students to pursue lifelong health-related fitness activities.

Yes, it's more work to provide a superior program that is health related, but the rewards are worth the effort. Create a fun and active learning environment, use appropriate teaching styles, and apply Gardner's theory of multiple intelligences to truly individualize your program to your students' needs, thereby generating interest in the class. Select a variety of developmentally appropriate learning experiences by ensuring that each is sequential, fun, safe, inclusive, serves a purpose, and can be connected to real life in meaningful ways. Then make sure your students not only understand basic skills (fitness and motor), but also understand how they can apply and monitor them in real-life situations.

Although Physical Best promotes the belief that it is usually ideal to integrate health-related fitness knowledge into actual physical activities, there are times when it is appropriate to share this information in greater depth in a classroom setting. But this doesn't mean you must give boring lectures! Don't be afraid to let students move in the classroom—interested and actively engaged students learn more.

CHAPTER

11

Chapter Contents

Including Everyone

Inclusion refers to the process of teaching students with disabilities together with their typically developing peers, using appropriate support systems that they otherwise would have received in a segregated setting. While this chapter explores that concept in greater depth, it also looks at how to meet the needs of each student, regardless of gender, cultural or ethnic background, or ability level (whether or not a student has been identified as having a disability).

In the Physical Best program, **inclusion** refers to the process of creating a learning environment that is open to and effective for all students whose needs and abilities fall outside of the general range of those for children of similar age or whose cultural or religious beliefs differ from that of the majority group. In short, inclusion means that *all* students are included in an appropriate manner, so that *all* students can reach their maximum potential.

Relevant Laws

Although inclusion is the general trend in education and society at large (and the ethical philosophy to adopt), it is not mandated by law. The law mandates only the least restrictive environment (LRE) and civil rights. Public Law 105-17, the Individuals with Disabilities Education Act Amendments (1997), mandates that students with disabilities are to be educated in the least restrictive environment. Least restrictive environment (LRE) mandates that students with disabilities are to be educated with their nondisabled peers to the maximum extent possible. Figure 11.1

shows a continuum of placement options available to students with disabilities. It is important to note that children with disabilities can move up and down the continuum based on their unique needs. Although some would advocate total inclusion at all times, physical educators should keep the intent of the law in mind and work to ensure that a quality program is provided for children with disabilities regardless of their particular placement option.

The Individuals with Disabilities Education Act (IDEA) sought to change the status quo and integrate students with special needs to the fullest extent possible, based on each individual's needs and abilities. This was the beginning of educators learning to focus first on what an individual *could* do, rather than on what he or she *could not* do. In a similar vein, Title IX of the Education Amendments of 1972 prohibited discrimination based on gender and spelled out how public institutions should ensure an individual's civil rights regardless of gender. The Americans with Disabilities Act (ADA) has broadened the scope of inclusion and integration by defining a disability as any individual characteristic that significantly impairs a "major life activity."

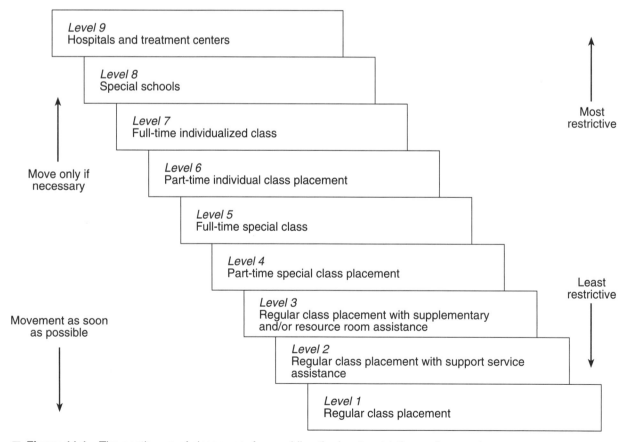

■ **Figure 11.1**   The continuum of placements for providing the least restrictive environment.

Reprinted, by permission, from J. Winnick, 2000, *Adapted physical education and sport*, 3rd ed. (Champaign, IL: Human Kinetics), 21.

Along with other civil rights legislation, this branch of law has created an acute awareness of the rights and needs of the individual. Aside from legal issues, however, offering a learning environment in which all students feel welcome and successful, achieve to the best of their abilities, and learn from diversity is simply the ethical action to take. Remember, diversity is part of our society, and it is important to simulate the society in which your students will function as adults as closely as possible—and to model appropriate behaviors toward those individuals who appear, at least on the surface, to be unlike oneself.

Benefits of Inclusion

All students can benefit from true inclusion—from experiencing the diversity of our society, from learning from those who appear to be unlike them, and from opportunities to find common ground despite differences. Inclusion allows students from other cultures to see a model of cultural inclusiveness that may positively influence their reactions to other cultures in the future, that validates their own culture, and that facilitates their own learning within the majority culture. Students with disabilities benefit from having peer models and from greater opportunity to participate in physical activity. Peer tutoring is an appropriate and effective strategy to provide meaningful practice and high levels of motor activity. It also assists in maximizing active learning time (Lieberman and Houston-Wilson 2002). All students benefit from being part of the problem solving that goes into being truly inclusive. Not only does inclusion benefit the child with a disability, but students without disabilities benefit from these interactions as well. The hope is that these interactions will break down barriers and lead to acceptance and friendships between the two groups. Ultimately, your program benefits because it is more effective for all students as you work together toward the goal of developing positive lifelong physical activity behaviors.

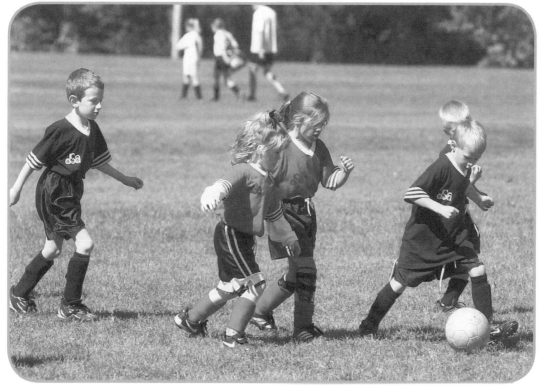

© Human Kinetics

Girls and boys should learn to participate together in physical activities. As adults, men and women participate side by side in coed volleyball and softball leagues, as well as in fitness clubs, biking and running clubs, and so on. Learning together at an early age prepares students for better cooperation later in life.

Including Students Who Don't Seem to Fit In

I was working with a group of teenagers, many of whom seldom dressed appropriately for physical activity and were considered by other instructors as "misfits." Instead of the prescribed activities, I introduced games analysis. We used leftover, abandoned, and broken equipment, such as broken bats and partially deflated balls. We also used as much other equipment as possible (e.g., more than four bases, lots of balls of different sizes and shapes, large discarded orange cones from a local construction site). Gradually, as they embraced the idea of changing games, they invented a baseball-like game. To this day I don't understand all aspects of their game—but they did!

The game involved eight bases; a player could run in any order he or she chose; more than one person could be on a single base at the same time; three teams competed simultaneously; and batters selected not only the type of pitch but also the type of ball to be pitched. It was a crazy game, but it wasn't long before every player was thoroughly engaged in the process of games modification, wearing appropriate attire, and creating and completing related homework assignments. Through games analysis, ownership of the program had shifted to the players.

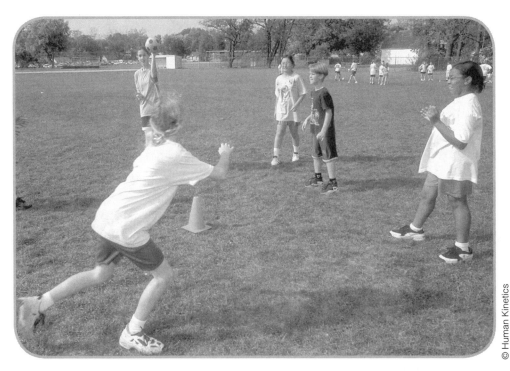

© Human Kinetics

Text is reprinted, by permission, from G.S.D. Morris and J. Steihl, 1998, *Changing kids' games*, 2nd ed. (Champaign, IL: Human Kinetics), 41-42.

Methods of Inclusion

What does all this mean for a health-related physical fitness education program? When your program includes students who fall below the expected range of skill and ability, the answers include further individualizing based on each student's needs, modifying the activity for all students, and collaborating with peer tutors, parents, other volunteers, and colleagues.

An example of modifying an activity for all students is to allow students to choose which test of aerobic fitness they prefer to practice and perform. That way a student with a disability can choose the test that allows him to use his abilities to their fullest, such as a blind student who chooses to perform the step test independently instead of the mile run, which would require the help of an assistant (AAALF/AAHPERD1995). A student with lower body paralysis may need the activity to be changed completely, because she may benefit more from testing for the upper body strength and endurance needed to power a wheelchair and get into and out of a wheelchair (AAALF/AAHPERD 1995).

Adaptations to Meet Unique Needs

You might find that changing an activity for everyone means that more students are actively engaged in the activity (both students who need special consideration and those who don't). There are several ways that

Disabilities Awareness Field Days

Teachers at Western Union Elementary School (Waxhaw, North Carolina) wanted to increase students' understanding and acceptance of children with disabilities. The children began learning about various disabilities at the beginning of the school year to prepare them to get the most out of a two-day field event. Just before the field days, students were briefed about the activities and their purpose, and they were reminded that they would be hosting special guests. This helped students understand that the events were for understanding what persons with disabilities *can* do, not to make fun of them. Students also raised money for the Special Olympics in a "Run for the Gold" event held the day before the main event began.

The first day of the main event, third through fifth graders participated in six indoor activities: An Easter Seals Society representative explained the proper etiquette and preferred language to use when speaking to or about persons with disabilities; a teacher with a hearing impairment shared her daily life experiences; students taped their fingers together, splinted their arms, and so on, to simulate physical impairment; students wore glasses covered to varying degrees to simulate visual impairments; students wore socks on their hands and tried to perform fine motor tasks to simulate learning difficulties of people with mental handicaps; and students tried to speak with a marshmallow in their mouth to simulate speech impairment. Students were also encouraged to process what they had learned through various art and writing activities. Meanwhile, preschool through second graders enjoyed six outdoor activities (what was simulated appears in parentheses): charades (nonverbal communication); sit-down basketball (wheelchair basketball); nondominant hand beanbag throw (physical impairments such as cerebral palsy); floor volleyball (physical impairments experienced by persons with amputations and paralysis); and silent 100-yard dash (hearing impairment). A member of the Tarwheels (a North Carolina wheelchair basketball team) also displayed his talents and spoke of never giving up. A parent of a child with a visual impairment shared the child's successes in judo and track and field. The second day, the two age groups followed the reverse schedule.

Reprinted, by permission, from M. Jobe, 1998, "Disabilities awareness field days," *Journal of Teaching Elementary Physical Education* 9(1): 10-11.

activities can be adapted to meet the needs of all students. Whenever a student with special needs is being evaluated regarding adaptations for physical activity programs, the following safety protocols should be implemented:

- Review of the student's records
- Conference with parents
- Possible contraindications (e.g., for scoliosis, repeated bending; or for autism, large noisy areas for instruction)
- Appropriate class size and instructional support
- Instructional environment
- Instructional strategies

After collecting the necessary information from the safety protocol, this information should be organized onto a student profile sheet (see figure 11.2).

Once you have the necessary information to support the individual's needs, you then need to give consideration to four areas that cover different attributes of the teaching and learning environment (Lieberman and Houston-Wilson 2002). See table 11.1 for a list of questions to ask yourself.

The sidebar "Including Pablo" shows creative ways to adapt a high school weight-training class to be more inclusive. You can use questioning strategies and opportunities in class to have students modify the games, drills, and activities to meet the needs of everyone in your class. These extensions and refinements of lessons will develop a positive environment in your classroom, school, and community. In the *Physical Best Activity Guides*, an inclusion tip is provided for each activity. The tips represent a variety of needs that physical educators encounter in their students, and many ideas can be easily transferred from one activity to another.

Student Profile Sheet

Student: _____ Date of birth: _____

Classroom teacher: _____ Physical education teacher: _____

Occupational therapist: _____ Physical therapist: _____

Speech and language therapist: _____

1. Medical information/precautions:

2. Speech/language programs used (devices):

3. Behavior program and/or protocol:

4. Positioning/adaptive equipment/braces:

5. Nursing plan:

6. Dressing:

7. Other:

■ **Figure 11.2** Teachers should organize and store information about students in a record such as the student profile sheet. A reproducible version of the student profile sheet is available in appendix A.

TABLE 11.1 Teaching Considerations for Developing Activities

Teaching areas	Question	Answer
Instruction	1. What modality is optimum to maximize comprehension of instruction?	1. Students often benefit from a visual demonstration while receiving verbal directions.
	2. What supports need to be in place to assist with instruction (e.g., communication system, staff, and so on)?	2. It is important to consider the need for supports such as adapted equipment, technology, communication systems (e.g., Mayer-Johnson symbols), or staff.
Rules	1. Do the rules allow for everyone to participate and maintain the integrity of the game?	1. During a basketball game, a student with special needs may take three steps without dribbling before a violation.
	2. Can everyone understand the rules?	2. Complicated rules such as offsides are omitted or simplified to assist with comprehension.
	3. Do the rules provide a safe environment for everyone?	3. A student in a wheelchair is provided a "buddy" to assist with the throwing and catching as well as creating a "safety circle" around the wheelchair.
Environment	1. Is the size of the area appropriate to the students and the activity?	1. A large multipurpose gymnasium has a line of cones down midcourt to create a smaller area to work. This is done when instructing a small first-grade class who has a child with autism included for physical education.
	2. Are areas of instruction clearly delineated?	2. An inclusive second-grade class is taught in a fenced area because a child who has a tendency to run off is in the class.
	3. Are the noise, temperature, air quality, and lighting in the area appropriate to the needs of the students?	3. The custodian at the school has the grass cut at night so that students with allergies and asthma can participate in the outdoor physical education classes.
Equipment	1. Is the equipment such that all students can participate or are there modifications that will assist with ensuring total participation?	1. Jump ropes are modified; the ropes are cut in half for those who aren't able to get their feet off the ground. Beeper balls or Velcro balls and mitts are used.
	2. Is the equipment developmentally appropriate?	2. Students who are included in high school programs are participating in developmentally appropriate activities and are not throwing beanbags at a target.
	3. Is the equipment safe for all students (e.g., latex)?	3. Nonlatex equipment is provided.

Including Pablo

The 10th-grade weight-training class at Centerville High School had several students who had been identified as having a disability. One student's name was Pablo; he was nonambulatory and moved in a manual wheelchair. Pablo had been in school with many of the students in the class, but it had been a long time since they had seen him out of his wheelchair. Most of the time Pablo had participated in physical education by being the referee, keeping score, being an extra person on the team, or participating in an alternative activity on the side of the gymnasium. All of the students liked Pablo and interacted with him, but they were unsure of what he was really capable of doing physically.

During the first week of school, an adapted physical education teacher came to the class to work with Pablo. She created a weight-training sheet similar to the one used by the class, but with Pablo's activities and the weight and number of repetitions he was to complete specifically marked. The adapted physical education teacher asked for volunteers to be Pablo's weight-training buddy. She explained that the buddy would be working at the same machine as Pablo in order to help him if he needed it, but that the buddy would have time to complete his own workout. The buddies would rotate so that Pablo and the buddies would have a chance to work with other people. The adapted physical education teacher talked to the buddies and Pablo. She asked Pablo to demonstrate how he could transfer to the various weight room equipment independently but would need help to set the pins for the weight amount. Everyone in the class was excited that Pablo was able to transfer out of his chair; it had been a long time since they saw him out of his wheelchair while participating in physical activity. They also realized how important weight training was for Pablo. This class would help him develop strength so he could continue to get out of his wheelchair independently.

The buddies soon became unnecessary for Pablo because everyone in the class would help with anything Pablo needed, and he needed very little. The students were happy to have Pablo as part of their class and included in activities. The adapted physical education teacher would stop by the weight-training class periodically to see how Pablo was doing in weight training. Everyone in the class would tell her how great Pablo was doing and if he was improving.

This story was taken from an Adapted Physical Education Teacher who provided consultative adapted physical education in Maryland.

Teaching Strategies

Several different teaching strategies can be effectively utilized to teach students physical and motor activities in physical education. These strategies include the multilevel approach and task analysis. In the multilevel approach, all students work on the same targeted areas (e.g., flexibility), but each student works toward different goals appropriate for his or her abilities. For example, fourth graders without disabilities might explore stretches specific to an area of physical activity interest. At the same time, students with mild disabilities might focus on learning a new stretch, while students with severe disabilities might work on mastering one stretch without bouncing. Plan an activity for each level and decide which level is appropriate for which students, so that the entire class is actively involved in learning. Figure 11.3 shows a sample form that may be used to assess the level of assistance an individual with a disability needs to perform a curl-up. Note that the task has been broken down into its component parts in a process known as **task analysis.** An individual may need a task to be broken down more or less, depending on his or her disability. A score reflecting percentage of independence can then be calculated, giving you valuable information about

Curl-Up

Name: _____ Date: _____

Directions:

Circle the level of assistance the individual requires in order to perform the task. Total each level of assistance column and place the subtotals in the sum of scores row. Total the sum of scores row and place the score in the individual's total score achieved row. Determine percent independence score based on the chart below. Place number of repetitions in the product score row.

Key to levels of assistance:

IND = Independent—the individual is able to perform the task without assistance

PPA = Partial Physical Assistance—the individual needs some assistance to perform the task

TPA = Total Physical Assistance—the individual needs assistance to perform the entire task

Curl-Up	IND	PPA	TPA
1. Lie on back with knees bent	3	2	1
2. Place feet flat on the floor with legs slightly apart	3	2	1
3. Place arms straight, parallel to the trunk	3	2	1
4. Rest palms of hands on the mat with fingers stretched out	3	2	1
5. Rest head on partner's hands	3	2	1
6. Curl body in a forward position	3	2	1
7. Curl back down until head touches partner's hand	3	2	1
Sum of scores:			
Total score achieved:			
Total possible points:	21		
% Independence score:			
Product score:			

Percentage of independence

7/21 = 33%	12/21 = 57%	17/21 = 80%
8/21 = 38%	13/21 = 61%	18/21 = 85%
9/21 = 42%	14/21 = 66%	19/21 = 90%
10/21 = 47%	15/21 = 71%	20/21 = 95%
11/21 = 52%	16/21 = 76%	21/21 = 100%

■ **Figure 11.3**   A sample form to assess the level of assistance needed by an individual with a disability. This sample focuses on the assistance necessary to perform a curl-up. A reproducible of this form is available in appendix A.

Reprinted, by permission, from AAHPERD, 1995, *Physical best and individuals with disabilities: A handbook for inclusion in fitness programs* (Champaign, IL: Human Kinetics), 100.

the level and type of support that you must provide for the student. You should then develop a plan to increase independence, because this enhances the "development of the fitness abilities of the participants" (Houston-Wilson 1995).

Collaboration

To successfully include students with disabilities in physical education, a network of support systems must be in place. The ideas presented below can be used in the regular class setting or in expanded opportunities, such as before- and after-school programs. These can be optional opportunities or chances to help students experiencing difficulties catch up.

You can collaborate with many different people, including peer tutors, parent and community service volunteers, paraprofessionals, and consultants. Choose the type of collaborator based on the student's needs, available resources, and the individualized education plan (IEP) or 504 plan (discussed later in this chapter).

To determine the type of help a student may benefit from, first consult with the student's direct service providers, including classroom teachers and adapted physical education specialists as well as the occupational therapist, physical therapist, speech and language therapist, or other related service providers. You should have all the relevant information you can for each student prior to implementing that student's program. The medical and behavioral

needs of some students can be overwhelming. The information you receive through collaborating with other professionals involved in a student's plan will have a direct impact on the quality of instruction and physical activity for that student. After consulting with other professionals who are working with these students, you can organize the collected information into the student profile sheets. For many students, this profile sheet can be very important in the process of ensuring safety and success (see figure 11.2).

You must properly train any teaching assistants or volunteers you may use. They need to know how to help a student, how not to do any harm (physical or emotional), and when to call on you for assistance. Take the time to develop a specific training program for these helpers before using them in the physical activity setting. Discussing the student's basic needs and abilities (while ensuring privacy) and simulating learning situations are good ways to provide training. Include these professionals in your collaborative team meetings. Students with severe disabilities need assistants who are professionally trained by those qualified to do so.

Major Areas in Which to Ensure Inclusion

To ensure an inclusive learning environment, the following must be addressed: students with special needs, gender, culture, and ability levels outside the "norm."

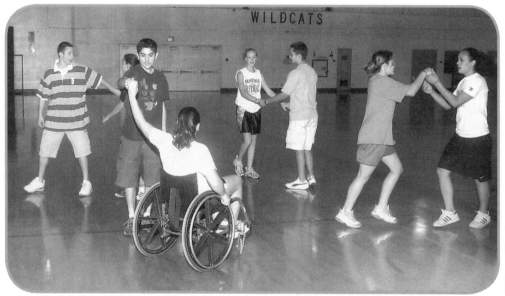

Individuals with disabilities generally display the same physiological responses to exercise found in nondisabled persons, though some factors such as heat dissipation and heart rate responses may be different.

Students With Special Needs

Each student with special needs should come to your class with either a 504 plan or an individualized education plan (IEP). An IEP will list a student's present level of performance; identify attainable annual goals and objectives; include clear instructions on how much time the child will spend in regular physical education class and with what support services; and identify the level and purpose of support services. Although being part of an IEP team is a time-consuming part of teaching, this process is vital to the student's learning and must receive proper attention.

Based on the IEP or 504 plan, adapt your curriculum and teaching methods to meet the child's interests. You should make direct and repeated contact with involved special services staff, parents, and medical personnel. If available and appropriate, work with an adapted physical education teacher to ensure that the student receives the instruction he or she needs. When designing health-related fitness plans for students with disabilities, keep the following in mind (adapted from DePauw 1996):

- Individuals with disabilities generally display the same physiological responses to exercise found in nondisabled persons. (Be careful, though, because some people with disabilities do not respond the same as those without disabilities; for example, heat dissipation and heart rate response may be different for a person with a spinal cord injury. Ask the family to consult with their physician.)

- Although specific disabilities may affect the intensity, duration, and frequency of exercise, individuals with disabilities can benefit from training, including improving their performances.

- Wheelchairs can be adjusted or modified (by those qualified to do so) to improve physical activity performance.

- Athletes in wheelchairs play basketball, tennis, and many other sports.

Use this information to ensure that students with disabilities are included in class activities to the greatest extent possible.

When deciding how best to teach an individual with a disability, focus on the individual, rather than the disability. In other words, refrain from making automatic judgments about an individual's condition. Look at what each child *can* do, instead of assuming he or she cannot do an activity.

Developing a Respectful Environment

Craft (1994) suggests the following for teaching children without disabilities appropriate inclusive behavior:

- Do not allow students to show disrespectful behavior toward anyone.

- Let students know it's okay for everyone to make mistakes—including you.

- Help students understand that often people tease or put down others because they feel insecure, scared of others' differences, or unsure of their own abilities.

- Teach students to ask questions about differences in a positive manner; this helps combat ignorance.

- Have positive role models with disabilities share how they enjoy physical activity.

This list of suggestions can help encourage children to be more inclusive in regard to culture, gender, and race as well.

Gender Inclusion

If you separate genders for activities, ensure that the activities are reasonably equivalent and not stereotypical. Physical Best recommends that you do *not* separate genders at the elementary level and try to avoid doing so at the middle and high school levels as well. After all, there are many activities that both genders can do together to reach the physical education standards. Remember, you should choose activities for a purpose (e.g., meet-ing the national standards), not simply because they have traditionally been used. Some professionals say that there may be rare cases where privacy, size and strength differences, and safety require some temporary gender separation at the middle and high school levels. But keep in mind that goal-based curriculums have a plethora of choice. Therefore, focus on the idea that activity choices are not an end in themselves. View activities as *strategies* for reaching program goals.

Coeducation Classes and Physical Education

One of the most widely debated areas of equity in physical education is coeducational classes. In today's society, most teachers would never think of segregating students by different ethnic groups, but some still have a hard time accepting students from different gender groups in the same classes. Segregated classes prevent boys and girls from interacting with one another and learning how to work and play together. Segregation by gender limits opportunities for boys and girls to reconsider their stereotypical assumptions in the physical domain.

Placing boys and girls in the same physical education class is only the first step toward providing students with the opportunity to examine their preconceived ideas about the opposite gender. The figure that follows shows six steps to equity. Not every teacher needs to pass through all six steps; however, you should be able to identify the step you currently occupy. Step six is complete equity, including opportunities for both genders to demonstrate skills, answer questions, receive feedback, and feel respect from the teacher and other students. It also includes an environment in which the teacher uses inclusive language (referring to the class as "students" instead of "you guys") and omits stereotypical phrases (e.g., "You throw like a girl").

As you progress through steps two through five, continually reflect on your own teaching behaviors. When boys and girls appear to not be working well together, examine the learning environment and determine what might be causing the problem. Often I hear physical educators state that the boys won't let the girls touch the ball. Sometimes, the physical educator states that a girl must touch the ball before the team can score. When I question the teacher as to whether or not all the boys in her class refuse to share, she typically responds, "No, it is a few aggressive boys." This tells me that the situation has little to do with coeducational physical education, since these same boys are also preventing the other boys from touching the ball. The remedy is either to make a rule that everyone must touch the ball, or better yet, reduce the size of the teams, so that everyone on the team must be involved for the team to be successful. Requiring that a girl must touch the ball before scoring sends the message that girls need special treatment, which only serves to reinforce the stereotype that the girls are not as competent as the boys (Mohnsen 1997).

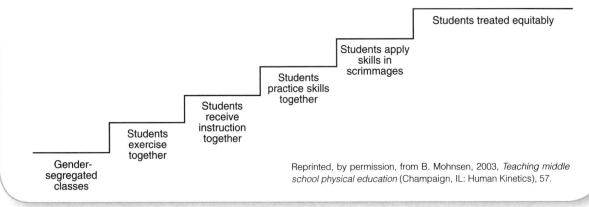

Gender-segregated classes → Students exercise together → Students receive instruction together → Students practice skills together → Students apply skills in scrimmages → Students treated equitably

Reprinted, by permission, from B. Mohnsen, 2003, *Teaching middle school physical education* (Champaign, IL: Human Kinetics), 57.

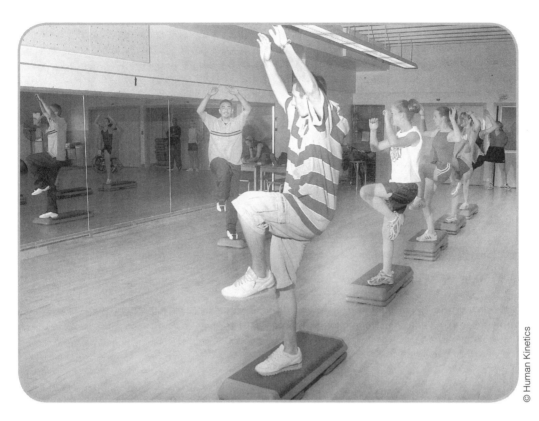

Both male and female students can enjoy the benefits of a steps aerobics class.

Remember, as adults, the majority of physical activity opportunities are not gender segregated. Men and women participate side by side in health clubs, biking and running clubs, dancing (a great activity to build aerobic fitness), wall climbing, in-line skating, and most other physical activities. In many communities, the most popular adult sports are coed softball and coed volleyball.

Students need to experience equal opportunity within each lesson as well. Unfortunately, however, educators in general tend to inadvertently favor boys. In physical education, for example, boys are more likely to give and receive positive specific feedback or specific corrective feedback (e.g., "I noticed how evenly you paced your mile run," or, "Push off with your toes more"). Girls are more likely to be passive observers and to receive general feedback (e.g., "Good job," or, "Try again"). Boys are also more likely to be pushed to complete a task, whereas girls may be allowed to quit (Cohen 1993; Hutchinson 1995; Sadker and Sadker 1995).

TEACHING TIP:
The Educational Value of Gender Inclusion

I have found coeducational physical education to be highly successful, both for girls and boys. Certainly the skill levels of girls have improved. . . . The boys, too, have benefited from exposure to a greater diversity of activities, experienced more opportunities to be successful, and learned more social skills—with no decline in their learning of movement skills.

Jean Flemion

1990 NASPE Secondary PE Teacher of the Year
Arthur E. Wright Middle School Calabasas, California

One way to monitor your instruction for gender bias is to videotape yourself. Then watch the tape and keep score of the type of feedback you give boys and girls. If you do not have access to videotaping equipment, a colleague or other trained observer could keep score for you. Figure 11.4 shows a sample tally sheet.

Another way to fight gender bias is to ensure that the visual aids you use show both genders partici-pating on equal terms and in nonstereotypical ways. Invite guest speakers who have crossed gender lines to play sports that are nontraditional for their gender. Finally, expose all students to a variety of activities that develop health-related fitness, regardless of gender. For example, a boy's lungs don't know that society says that dance is a "girl's thing," while a girl's muscles don't know that society says that tree climbing is a "boy's thing."

Equity Checklist for Physical Education

- Is your curriculum gender inclusive?
- Do students participate in gender-integrated classes?
- Are teaching styles varied to accommodate different learning styles and preferences?
- Is gender-inclusive language used?
- Do instructional materials portray both genders as active participants in a variety of activities?
- [Do you give] equal attention to boys and girls during classroom practices such as questioning, demonstration, and feedback?
- Are local community resources used to help erode gender barriers to sport participation?
- Is time consistently reserved for gender dialogue?
- Do you hold high expectations for both boys and girls?
- Is gender equity a pervasive schoolwide goal?

Reprinted, by permission, from L. Nilges, 1996, "Ingredients for a Gender Equitable Physical Education Program," *Teaching Elementary Physical Education* 7(5):28-29.

Girls			Boys		
Positive general feedback	Positive specific feedback	Corrective feedback	Positive general feedback	Positive specific feedback	Corrective feedback
⁊⁊⁊ II	II	I	⁊⁊⁊	⁊⁊⁊ IIII	IIII

Figure 11.4 Sample tally sheet.

Reprinted, by permission, from L. Nilges, 1996, "Ingredients for a gender equitable physical education program," *Journal of Teaching Elementary Physical Education* 7(5):28-29.

Cultural Inclusion

Cultural influences can greatly affect what an individual is interested in learning and doing. Since helping students find out what physical activity is enjoyable for them is an important part of health-related physical fitness education, it is essential to be sensitive in this area. Develop a survey to help you determine student interests, then incorporate the survey results into program plans. Your obvious desire to respect other cultures will go a long way toward bridging cultural gaps. Indeed, Lowry (1995) writes, "If your students believe that their opinions and perspectives are valued and used, then you have taken the first step in setting up a culturally sensitive environment." You can take these basic steps in tandem with teachers of other subjects to help make your health-related physical fitness education curriculum more culturally inclusive (and for that matter, more cross-curricular). Try to incorporate the physical activities, games, holidays and traditions, and music of other cultures.

Banks (1988) suggests that teachers consider three areas when they plan their lessons and overall programs:

- Integrate content—Use activities from other cultures to achieve your program goals. For example, an active game from another country is just as good for developing aerobic fitness as a familiar game.
- Plan how to reduce prejudice—Plan awareness activities that facilitate understanding among cultures, such as discussing different ways of dressing for exercise, based on cultural differences.
- Employ culturally responsive pedagogy—Respect differences and learn the history and meaning behind traditions and values.

Ask students and parents from various cultural backgrounds to share their beliefs and any individual requests with you. This process will further sensitize you to the philosophies and sociological issues that

Teaching the Limited English or Non-English-Speaking Student in Physical Education

A student who doesn't speak English as his first language can succeed in and enjoy physical education. The following may help such a student:

- Assign an English-speaking buddy to help the student in physical education class. If possible, choose someone who speaks the same language as the non-English-speaking student (Mohnsen 2003).
- Physically move a student through a skill to help her comprehend what you want.
- Use gestures and other visual aids, such as toy people and small balls (Mohnsen 2003).
- Use facial expressions and voice inflections to emphasize your points.
- Remember to speak slowly and enunciate clearly, as you would in the regular classroom (Mohnsen 2003).
- Emphasize the target skill's key word or phrase as you work with the student, and have the student's buddy do so as well.
- Encourage the student to repeat the **cue words** or phrases as she executes the skill so she will learn the vocabulary that goes with the actions.
- Learn some of the important words and phrases from the child's native language.

Reprinted, by permission, from B. Pettifor, 1999, *Physical education methods for classroom teachers* (Champaign, IL: Human Kinetics), 259.

may affect physical education learning and fitness attitudes. Finally, respect diversity in cultural values. For example, gender equity may be an offensive concept in certain cultures, so respect the different expectations for girls and boys within each culture you encounter. Provide equal opportunity for all, but if a student and her parents, for example, elect not to take advantage of the equal opportunity you provide for girls because of religious beliefs, you might discuss other options with the student and her parents. You might involve a school counselor or administrator in such a discussion as well, depending on the circumstances. If religious beliefs mandate that girls not wear shorts, you can discuss appropriate alternatives with the family and determine some other appropriate dress for participating in physical activity (e.g., culottes, which look like a skirt, but function like shorts; Mohnsen 1997). Keep in mind that not everyone in a class has to dress alike to be able to benefit from physical activity. As another example, Hispanic girls in one class would not perform any type of straddle stretch, so their teacher offered all students a choice from a group of stretch pictures (Lowry 1995). Building in choices helps build on cultural diversity, rather than trying to eliminate it.

Ability Inclusion

Some students are either extremely talented or extremely challenged (but not classified as having a disability); these students deserve inclusion, too.

Physically Elite Children

Although Sara, who can run a mile in under six minutes, or Jimmy, who can do 150 curl-ups, may not need much of your attention, don't neglect these students. You may find that the physically elite make good peer tutors. This will help keep them interested in your program, and it may also help them build social skills. However, do not have them tutor so much that their own needs go unmet or that other students sense favoritism. In addition, challenge the physically gifted students in your classes to explore advanced participation in physical activity. A student who might otherwise be bored (and, as a result, disrupt class) is instead challenged and is an asset to the class. For example, you might have a physically elite high school student read a book on becoming a personal trainer and then let the student serve as an assistant during class helping other students. You might also make arrangements for this student to interview a personal trainer at the local health club (and have the student write a report). Show interest in such students' extracurricular sport activities, and have them share their experiences with the rest of the class. Encourage independence and fitness gains in middle and high school students by encouraging them to use health-related fitness training principles to continually challenge themselves.

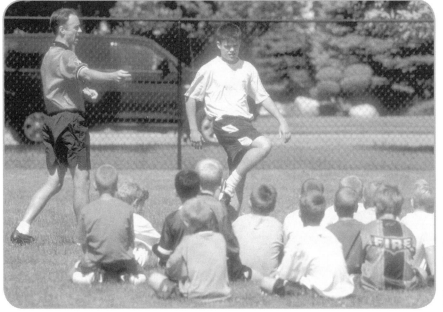

© Human Kinetics

Physically elite students can build social skills by serving as peer tutors.

TEACHING TIP: Reaching Students Who Are Afraid to Try

Ben came up to me after the first class and quietly, but in a serious tone, said, "Mr. Hichwa, that was a good talk, but, you know, I don't do gym." Ben informed me that he was cut from his fourth-grade travel soccer team, his physical educational experience in the elementary school was far from positive, and he did not intend to expose himself to further failure or ridicule in the sixth grade. . . . I thanked Ben for being so forthright and suggested that he come to our next class as an observer, which he agreed to do. At the end of that class, I asked him if he thought he could feel comfortable taking part in future class activities. Because I took the time to listen to Ben, showed respect for his concerns, and gave him time to feel comfortable in his new environment, Ben agreed to give it a try! Throughout the year, Ben tried his best, participated fully, and eventually learned to enjoy the many challenges.

At the beginning of sixth grade, Clare was very tall for her age, fairly heavy, and extremely clumsy. She would go through the motions, but even encouragement from her peers was construed as a personal affront and caused her great anguish. But by making developmentally appropriate changes, the activities became less threatening. Clare started to experience a little success, and her self-concept began to rise. She excelled at the problem-solving initiatives and slowly gained respect from the other students. Her running times improved as she participated more enthusiastically; she didn't feel inadequate when competing with herself and enjoyed monitoring her progress. By eighth grade, Clare felt confident enough to demonstrate the layup shot in basketball!

John Hichwa, Educational Consultant

1993 NASPE Middle School Physical Education Teacher of the Year
Redding, Connecticut

From J. Hichwa, 1998, *Right fielders are people, too.* (Champaign, IL: Human Kinetics).

Physically Awkward Children

Wall (1982) defines the physically awkward child as one "without known neuromuscular problems who [fails] to perform . . . motor skills with proficiency." Don't assume a physically awkward child will outgrow the problem on his own; many do not (Schincariol 1994). Such children tend to get discouraged and, consequently, drop out of physical activity never to return, compounding their problems.

You should first screen such a student for motor skill delays by administering a test of motor proficiency (Schincariol 1994). For example, the Test of Gross Motor Development (Ulrich 2000) may give you useful information. Then consult with an adapted physical education specialist and the child's parents to individualize the child's physical education program (Schincariol 1994).

The physically awkward child needs remedial help in the form of extra practice time, instruction, and encouragement (Schincariol 1994). This student may need one-on-one help, the same as a student with special needs; if so, arrange for a trained volunteer, teacher's aide, or peer tutor.

Create learning situations in which the child who is physically awkward can learn, succeed, and have fun, making it more likely that the child will learn the value and benefits of physical activity. Offering choices and variety is especially critical to enticing the physically awkward child to persist in physical activity. For example, in conducting a fitness circuit with a jump rope station, you can also offer the choice of doing step aerobics (step up and step down) to those physically awkward children who are unable to jump rope. This allows those children to participate in an activity when their lack of motor skills might otherwise prevent them from getting a good workout.

Low-Fit or Obese Children

There are many causes of poor fitness and obesity: lack of physical activity, poor diet, cultural beliefs, family situation, and too much time watching TV and playing video games, to name a few. Your job as a physical educator is to motivate all students to strive for greater levels of fitness (no matter their weight). Do not, however, assume these conditions arise from laziness. More likely, the younger obese or low-fit child tries harder in your classes, even though the results are poor. The older obese or low-fit student may avoid physical activity—by failing to dress for class or by simply refusing to participate—due to embarrassment and fear of failure.

For these children, your first step should be to have percent body fat measurements taken to determine the severity of the problem (see the *FITNESSGRAM/ACTIVITYGRAM Test Administration Manual*). Then ensure that the child's problems are not caused by disease, health disorders, or hereditary problems. This is best done through the family doctor at your request. Keep in mind that a little diplomacy can go a long way, so always maintain the student's privacy and respect the family's wishes. Consider holding a parent–teacher–student conference in which you express your concern and desire to help. If medical conditions are involved, work with the family doctor and parents to establish parameters for the student's participation in class. Middle and high school students may benefit from sharing their negative experiences and personal concerns regarding physical activity and body composition. A private conference with you or a journal-writing opportunity that allows the student to air his or her feelings may lead to improved attitudes toward appropriate physical activity and nutritional practices.

Once medical concerns have been ruled out, work with the student and family to set appropriate goals and design an individualized fitness plan, emphasizing fun and variety. An obese student also needs extra nutritional guidance. Stress the benefits of even mild exercise, because being expected to do too much too soon often discourages obese students. Let the student set an individual pace within each activity and in regard to the principle of progression. Encourage the entire family to become more active to increase the student's total physical activity time and sense of support. Reinforce achievements by having the student chart progress and by offering other rewards, such as the right to choose the game the class will play or the music the class will listen to.

You must deal sensitively with overweight or obese children when exercising to ensure that activity sessions are positive experiences for everyone. Some guidelines include the following. (The following list is reprinted, by permission, from J.P. Harris and J.P. Elbourn, 1997, *Teaching health-related exercise at key stages 1 and 2* (Champaign, IL: Human Kinetics), 27):

- Treat pupils as individuals, not comparing and contrasting them.

- Encourage a range of physical activities, including non-weight-bearing exercises, such as swimming, exercise in water, and cycling.

- Encourage low-impact activities, such as walking, and provide low-impact alternatives (such as marching) to high-impact exercises (such as jogging).

- Schedule rest periods to allow recovery from activity.

- Ensure correct exercise technique to minimize the risk of injury.

- Permit a choice of exercise clothing that reduces embarrassment.

- Ensure the wearing of supportive footwear during weight-bearing activities, and use soft surfaces, rather than hard surfaces (such as concrete), where possible.

- Provide differentiated tasks to cater to a wide range of abilities, including low-level, easier tasks.

- Be aware of potential problems, such as breathing difficulties, movement restriction, edema (fluid retention resulting in swelling), chafing, excessive sweating, and discomfort during exercise.

- Encourage routine activity around the home and school.

- Where possible, provide opportunities for overweight and obese children to be active in a private, rather than a public, context.

- Enable obese children to follow an individually designed exercise program, based on their particular needs and capabilities.

- Encourage guidance and support from school, family, and friends.

- Always provide positive feedback and constant encouragement.

Other Health Concerns—Asthma

Other health concerns may also affect a student's ability or willingness to fully participate in the classroom. Asthma is one relatively common example. People who have asthma are susceptible to narrowing of the airways, which makes breathing difficult. This narrowing can be brought on by a number of factors (such as irritants, allergens, weather changes, viral infections, emotions, and exercise). The factors differ among individuals and may vary over time.

Exercise-induced asthma may occur during or after exercise. The usual symptoms are wheezing, coughing, tightness of the chest, and breathlessness. However, regular physical activity has specific benefits for children with asthma (such as decreased frequency and severity of attacks and reduction in medication), over and above the benefits it has for children in general; therefore, children with asthma should be encouraged to be active and should be integrated as fully as possible into physical education lessons and sporting activities. Children with asthma should be able to participate in activities alongside their peers with minimal adaptation. A child is most likely to experience exercise-induced asthma when performing continuous aerobic exercise at a relatively moderate intensity for more than six minutes in cold, dry air (for example, cross country running). Appendix G contains a "Student Asthma Action Card" that can be used to document your students' information.

Although it is important to treat each child individually, here are some general recommendations that should be followed during exercise. (Reprinted, by permission, from J.P. Harris and J.P. Elbourn, 1997, *Teaching health-related exercise at key stages 1 and 2* (Champaign, IL: Human Kinetics), 25-27):

- Encourage the use of an inhaler 5 to 10 minutes before exercise.
- Encourage children to have a spare inhaler readily available for use.
- A child arriving for activity with airway constriction should be excused from participation for that session.
- Allow a gradual warm-up of at least 10 minutes.
- Permit and encourage intermittent bursts of activity interspersed with reduced intensity exercise.
- Permit lower intensity (easier) activity.
- Encourage swimming—the environmental temperature and humidity of an indoor pool is well tolerated by people with asthma.
- In cold, dry weather conditions, encourage the wearing of a scarf or exercise face mask over the mouth and nose in the open air.
- Encourage breathing through the nose during light exercise—this warms and humidifies the air.
- Do not permit children with asthma to exercise when they have a cold or viral infection.
- Where possible, advise children with severe asthma to avoid exercise during the coldest parts of the day (usually early morning and evening) and in times of high pollution.
- If symptoms occur, ask the child to stop exercising, and encourage him or her to use an inhaler and to rest until recovery is complete.
- In the case of an asthma attack, send for medical help, contact the child's parents, give medicine promptly and correctly, remain calm, encourage slow breathing, and ensure that the child is comfortable.

A Word About Inhalers

Although you should encourage children with asthma to participate in physical education as fully as possible, you must be aware of possible limitations. Children should have free and easy access to their inhalers. It is not wise for schools to keep asthma medication in a central store. Teachers who are better informed are more able to help children with asthma lead a normal life.

Adapted, by permission, from J. Harris and J. Elbourn, 1997, *Teaching health-related exercises at key stages 1 and 2.* (Champaign, IL; Human Kinetics), 27.

Nothing prevents the vast majority of children with mild to moderate asthma from participating in a range of physical activities with minimal difficulty, providing that they take appropriate precautions before and during exercise.

Summary

Inclusion in health-related physical fitness education means making it possible for all students to succeed in *and enjoy* physical activity. Thus, inclusion helps students meet the ultimate goal of becoming adults who value and pursue physical activity as a way of life. At the same time, inclusion teaches other valuable life lessons: social skills, cultural respect, and the feeling that you do not have to accept limitations unfairly assigned by those with limited visions of what people can be. To be truly inclusive in your program (as opposed to simply going through the motions), make a commitment to the planning and effort it takes. But you don't have to do so alone: Collaborate with both school and nonschool personnel to make the task of inclusion easier. Collaboration will also ensure that you have the input you need to tailor your program to your students' needs.

PART IV

Foundations of Assessment in Health-Related Fitness and Physical Activity

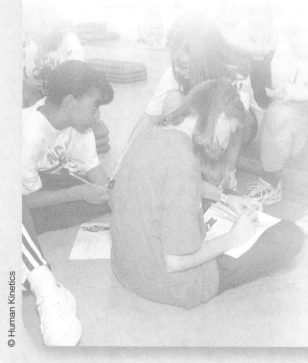

© Human Kinetics

Part IV provides an overview of assessment issues related to health-related fitness and physical activity. It covers basic assessment principles, how they relate to health-related physical fitness, and how to assess fitness knowledge, self-responsibility, and attitudes. Chapter 12 relates the foundation for assessment—the National Standards for Physical Education, Health Education, and Dance Education—to health-related fitness and physical activity. In addition, it outlines recommended assessment tools, how to apply assessment tools, and how to use assessments to shape program planning. The tools and concepts

☞

are applied as appropriate in the next two chapters. Chapter 13 explores appropriate methods for fitness testing and physical activity assessment. For each of these two major areas, it offers guidelines for assessing as well as for then sharing results in effective and helpful ways. Chapter 14 concludes this section on assessment with concrete suggestions for using the appropriate assessment tools to assess cognitive, personal responsibility, and affective realms. Applying the concepts and suggestions found in this part will challenge each student to develop positive lifelong physical fitness habits.

Principles of Assessment

If you hired a health fitness instructor or personal trainer, you would not expect to receive a letter grade as a result of working with this expert. You would expect the expert to assess your fitness level and then prescribe or advise a course of action so that you could work efficiently and safely toward a higher fitness level. The same needs to be true for today's physical education teacher: Students should expect to have their health-related fitness levels assessed, and then be advised on the best course of action based on those assessments. After all, a grade does not tell a student what he or she needs to know to become more fit.

In an ideal world, you would not have to assign a grade. Each grading period, you would have plenty of prep time to write detailed reports of each student's current fitness status. Then you would sit down for an hour or two with each parent and student to communicate this information in full, set goals, and help develop plans to meet those goals—in a private, quiet, and comfortable office. Although this is not possible in most physical education class settings, you can provide private, detailed feedback and adequate input into goal setting and physical activity planning, based on appropriate assessment data.

You must understand that grading and assessment are not one and the same: They have very different purposes. **Assessment** is continuous collection and interpretation of information on student behaviors, and it informs you and your students how they are improving in specific components. **Grading** attempts to communicate all that the individual has done in your physical education program. A grade is summative and often comparative between students. In this chapter, we first explore the issues and tools of assessment, then we outline alternative and appropriate ways to use this information, especially if you must assign physical education grades.

Assessment

There are many approaches to evaluation (grading) and assessment. In **traditional assessment,** results of tests are the main data used to assess student learning. In physical education, this has often taken the form of rules tests (e.g., for specific games and sports), skill test results, and teacher observation, all used for determining course grades.

Today, the term *alternative assessment* is often used interchangeably with *authentic assessment*, although they are not quite the same. **Alternative assessment** involves using tools other than traditional standardized testing—including tools such as portfolios, journals, and role playing—to collect evidence about student learning and achievement of program objectives. Alternative assessment becomes authentic when the assessment takes place in a real-world type of setting, such as analyzing a child's running stride during natural play on the playground, or having a student set up a personal fitness plan that will actually be used and altered over time. **Authentic assess-**

ment takes into consideration the many factors or the context of the activity, and it is more likely to assess a student's ability to perform or demonstrate knowledge in a game or real-life setting (Lacy and Hastad 2003). Applied specifically to physical education, developmentally appropriate authentic assessment will include individual assessments of children as they move and participate in a variety of activities. Comparisons should be made by examining the child's progress since the previous assessment and by examining benchmarks of growth and maturation, not on the basis of a single test score (summative evaluation) or the performance of other students in the class.

To avoid being artificial or contrived, authentic assessment in health-related physical fitness education must teach and motivate each student to apply fitness knowledge in the real world. In this section, we outline how. Specifically, we discuss the national standards in relation to assessment, explain the importance of assessment, and describe effective assessment tools.

National Standards and Assessment

As mentioned in chapter 9, the Physical Best program is aligned with the national standards for physical, health, and dance education. In standards-based instruction, such as the Physical Best program, students are assessed based on achievement of the standards as defined for each grade level. In addition to assessing students' health-related fitness knowledge and performance levels as outcomes measures, effort and improvement can be used as process measures. When student assessments are used to evaluate effectiveness of a program, the circle of instruction is complete.

Importance of Assessment

Given the time and energy commitment that assessment takes, you may be wondering, *Why bother?* But assessment provides

- opportunities to focus on each individual,
- specific feedback to guide each student's personal goal setting,
- feedback on the effectiveness of your teaching,
- feedback on the effectiveness of the overall program,

- important feedback about student instructional needs,
- information to guide future planning, and
- credibility in the minds of administrators and parents.

To assess and provide feedback that is helpful for each individual, you should assess students and monitor for progress in all learning domains (categories): psychomotor, health-related fitness, affective, and cognitive. The **psychomotor domain** refers to skills and motor or movement patterns. It is commonly assessed during drills, skill tests, and gamelike activities. The **health-related fitness domain** refers to developing health-related fitness and most often is assessed through fitness testing. The **affective domain** refers to the attitudes and values a student has toward and during physical activity. Although more difficult to measure, affective behaviors can be assessed through journals, rubrics, questionnaires, and systematic observance of student behaviors, including effort and compliance with directions. The **cognitive domain** refers to knowledge about rules, procedures, safety, and critical elements, as well as fitness knowledge that will contribute to the ability to make healthy lifetime activity choices and to participate in a variety of physical activities throughout the lifetime.

Both formal and informal assessments are important to a quality physical education program, and they can be used for assessing learning in different domains. Formal assessment lets you know more precisely how individual students are progressing and provides data for assessing your overall program. Informal assessment conducted by you is less time-consuming yet helpful for making decisions about teaching strategies, moving on, or changing the lesson to spend more time practicing a newly presented skill. Informal self-assessment conducted by students allows them to practice strategies they can use on their own outside your program—this is an important instructional strategy. Many of the same assessment tools can be used either informally or formally. An informal assessment of journal entries may simply involve the instructor scanning to see if the student completed the work assigned (affective domain—assessing personal responsibility), while a formal assessment may involve applying a rubric to assess the thoughtfulness and thoroughness of the entries (cognitive domain—assessing depth of knowledge).

Choosing What to Assess

We'll use the example of stretching to help illustrate assessment possibilities in each of the learning domains: cognitive, health-related fitness, affective, and psychomotor.

Cognitive assessment measures students' fitness and skill knowledge. Assessing cognitive knowledge of stretching, for example, would involve assessing students' knowledge of why it is important to stretch and knowledge of how to stretch safely—including questions such as, do they know that they should warm up? and, do they know why a warm-up is important before stretching?

Cognitive assessment does not have to involve giving a written test. Continuing the stretching example, it could be as simple as asking a question about how far to stretch, or about the muscles and joints affected by the stretch. However, we recommend many other methods of assessing the cognitive domain (see chapter 14), and we recognize that the cognitive domain involves more than knowing safety concepts or rules of games and sports. For instance, do your students know how much and how often to drink water when exercising or what makes their heart beat faster? Do they know the guidelines for safe stretching or the principle of specificity? Cognitive assessment includes gathering information about students' abilities to perform such tasks as taking their heart rates and using a pedometer. In the case of stretching, assessing fitness knowledge would involve assessing whether the student can identify the appropriate flexibility exercises for a specified activity. Knowledge can help students choose appropriate, safe, and enjoyable activities and prepare them to sort fact from fiction when viewing advertisements for new "miracle" exercise equipment. This knowledge is imperative if students are to be active for a lifetime. Assessing their progress toward fitness and their understanding of these concepts helps them assume personal responsibility for their own health and well-being.

Assessment in the health-related fitness domain means assessing components of fitness that contribute to good health and prevention of disease. Obviously, this area is the major focus of Physical Best and is addressed throughout the text. In chapter 13, we'll describe how to assess health-related fitness. Assessing the health-related fitness domain related to stretching involves measuring how far students can stretch, or more specifically, the range of motion of each joint of the body. One example would be using the back-saver sit-and-reach test.

The affective domain is perhaps the most difficult and abstract area to assess, and yet it can be done well and can be a powerful tool for motivating students to develop a lifelong desire to be physically active. Affective assessment measures a student's attitude and motivation level toward physical activity. Assessing the affective domain related to stretching could involve finding out how stretching makes a student feel. Does the student feel more competent because her flexibility is improved or empowered because she knows how to stretch correctly? Or does she not really care about stretching and not desire to increase her flexibility? In chapter 14, we'll explain ways to assess the affective domain without penalizing students who express a dislike for certain types of activities. Assessment of effort or participation involves assessing how much, how often, and to what degree students participate in physical activity. To complete our stretching example, assessing the area of effort would involve discovering whether and how often a student is stretching in and out of class. However, the effort or participation is actually a reflection of their attitudes about and values toward the importance of the activity. Participation is actually the behavior reflecting the affect or feelings, and it should not be graded separately or without an examination of the factors that lead to participation levels.

The psychomotor domain is usually the most common area associated with physical education. Assessment in this domain involves examining ability and skill, which are authentically assessed during game situations and sports contests. This area is well known to teachers and will not be discussed within this context.

Most important, regularly using assessment in authentic activity settings allows you to teach more effectively and motivate students. Assessment must be viewed as an integral part of teaching, not as an add-on or as a summative grade report.

Teaching Through Assessment

Assessment does not need to be time-consuming when it is planned as part of your instructional strategy. Indeed, assessment is critical for defining essential information about performance for your students. By emphasizing self- and peer assessment, personal responsibility, and goal setting, you can make assessment a learning tool in itself. In these ways, you teach your students how to learn, not just

why. This, in turn, empowers students to reach the Physical Best goal of becoming adults who know how to be physically active for life in safe, effective, and enjoyable ways. (We might add that this goal is shared by *FITNESSGRAM/ACTIVITYGRAM* and the CDC's Healthy People 2010 plan.) Your job is to facilitate this process while each student is in your program. We discuss self- and peer assessment in the section titled "Recommended Assessment Tools."

Recommended Assessment Tools

To assess authentically, you must apply a variety of tools to gather accurate information about a student's progress. A student might find one form of assessment easier to perform in and interpret than the others due to his or her individual strengths. By balancing the types of tools that you use, you give each student a chance to excel in one way or another, and you give students the opportunity to develop avenues of learning and learning intelligences that they are weaker in. Naturally, you must adjust each tool to fit the age and ability of each student as well. Finally, when selecting an assessment tool and designing

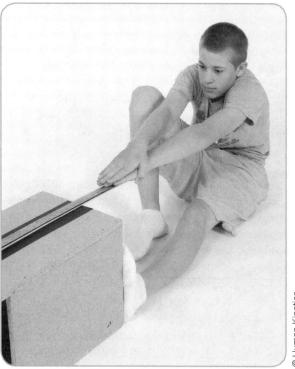

The back-saver sit-and-reach test is one method available for assessing a student's health-related fitness.

an assessment assignment, be sure the results will help you answer the question, Is the student moving toward the ultimate goal of health-related physical fitness education—that of becoming an adult who values, enjoys, and participates in physical activity?

Rubrics

A **rubric** is a scoring tool that identifies the criteria used for judging student performance (Lund and Kirk 2002). Rubrics range in complexity from checklists to holistic in nature and can be used to assess skills, attitudes, and knowledge. A checklist rubric might list certain skills—for example, "Runs tall, leans slightly forward" or "Offers encouragement and support to teammates"—and include a blank where a check mark or smiley face is placed if the skill is performed correctly. A rubric might also be analytic, where the skills are assigned point levels, perhaps from 1 to 5 for "Never" to "Always" or for more qualitative descriptions of levels of play. Finally, rubrics may be holistic, containing paragraphs written to describe various levels of performance. Each paragraph includes several different dimensions and traits (psycho-motor, health-related

fitness, affective, and cognitive) and is aligned with a point value or level number.

Well-designed rubrics inform students about expectations for the quality of work necessary to reach the standard or achieve a specific grade. Rubrics can be used by teachers, students, and peers to score or evaluate the information gathered by most of the assessment tools we describe in this chapter. A rubric can also double as a task sheet to keep students focused on critical elements or knowledge concepts during class, or as an observation checklist to guide feedback given by teachers and peers. Thus, being able to create and use effective rubrics is a vital teaching and assessment skill (see figure 12.1).

More information on using and creating rubrics for fitness evaluation is presented in chapter 14. There are also Web sites with examples of rubrics available to assist teachers in the design of their own rubrics. Some teachers have found the following sites helpful in creating rubrics for their classes: www.editor@ 4teachers.org; www.pecentral.org; www.pelinks4u.org.

Teacher Observations

In every lesson, as you circulate among students who are applying the concepts and practicing the skills

Assessing Knowledge of Calculating and Using Heart Rate

Student's name _____   Date _____   Score _____

Class _____

Target component	Score 1 point	Score 2 points
Can demonstrate sites at which to count the pulse	Knows one site	Knows two sites
Understands how heart rate information indicates intensity	Some understanding	Clearly understands
Can accurately count the pulse for a fraction of a minute, then accurately calculate heartbeats per minute with a calculator	Sometimes	Most of the time
Can describe ways and reasons to increase or decrease heart rate	Some understanding	Clearly understands

■ Figure 12.1   Example of a rubric to assess knowledge of calculating and using heart rate. A reproducible version of this rubric is available in appendix A.

Easier Said Than Done

In group projects, assessment of both the group's and each individual's performance to ensure everyone has done his fair share is very difficult (a big assessment issue in itself). For one thing, it is difficult to design the rubrics for these. At the beginning of each project, you should make students aware of the criteria by which you will be judging them. Simply sharing the rubrics you will use is very helpful. Then consider allowing groups and individuals to assess themselves and each other, alongside your professional assessments. For example, if three group members each privately rate the fourth group member poorly, this may support your conclusions regarding this student as well. But be careful! These can be touchy issues. The skillful teacher will work to ensure that the student is not embarrassed but is instead helped and encouraged to practice on the targeted activity. Developing a supportive and open teaching environment is the key to getting the best work out of everyone. Discussing any large discrepancies with those involved can be a valuable teaching technique. Using an individual accountability tool, such as a journal entry or quiz, can also help.

you have introduced, you should also be continuously observing and assessing both the overall performance of the class and each individual's performance. This informal process is an important part of "thinking on your feet," that is, adjusting lessons as they progress based on the needs you see arise. For example, you observe that many students are having trouble finding a site at which they may count their heart rates, so you regain their attention and review the two main sites.

If you have the equipment available to you, videotaping student performance is one observation technique that can help you assess students as well. Consider requiring each student to bring in a blank videotape at the beginning of the school year. Then you can periodically videotape each student performing a skill for closer scrutiny and analysis. Parents or older students can help with videotaping.

You can assess (using a rubric) as you replay the video; this frees you to concentrate on management and positive feedback during class. You can also have students self- or peer assess via videotape, perhaps at one station on a circuit. Using the videotapes and reviewing with a rubric allow you to systematically observe specific critical elements, behaviors, or events, and to record and analyze them with greater accuracy (Lacy and Hastad 2003).

Journal and Log Entries

Journal and log entries provide a way to integrate writing into the health-related physical fitness education curriculum, and they can be used to assess affect and knowledge simultaneously. **Logs** provide a baseline record of behaviors and help form the basis to set personal goals related to exercise frequency, intensity, or duration. Although logs can contain reflections on performance, strictly speaking, they are mainly for recording performance and participation data. Students can log the dates and times of each aerobic fitness activity they engage in outside of physical education, record heart rates before, during, and after each activity, and analyze whether their total aerobic fitness time each week has been sufficient to maintain or improve aerobic fitness.

A **journal** or reflection entry may include log data, but the student often adds a written record of how she felt emotionally and physically before, during, and after each activity. Journals are usually designed not only as records, but also as reflections. Logging and reflective journaling give students multiple opportunities to review their progress, which often motivates them to continue being physically active.

Teach students how to set up well-organized logs and journals, such as those shown in figures 12.2 and 12.3. Students often use logs without much difficulty but have trouble when they are asked to reflect in

Family Steps

Name	Steps Day 1	Steps Day 2	Steps Day 3	Steps Day 4	Individual total
Mom					
Dad					
_____					
_____					
_____					
_____					
_____					
Daily total					
				Grand total	

■ Figure 12.2   This sample log sheet shows how a family can track their steps using a pedometer. A reproducible version of Family Steps is available in appendix A.

Adapted, by permission, from R. Pangrazi, A. Beighle, and C. Sidman, 2003, *Pedometer power: 67 lessons for K-12* (Champaign, IL: Human Kinetics), 110.

a journal—yet reflection can offer the most useful insights for teachers and students alike. Reflection develops with maturity and practice. Students should be encouraged to reflect on likes and dislikes and on positive and negative feelings about participation. Reflection is a type of journal entry that involves thinking about the learning process itself to help improve performance and attitude (Melograno 1998).

Teachers should not expect young students to reflect competently without guidance and feedback on the process. With younger students, begin by having them log their activities. Older students should be encouraged from the outset to react or reflect on the activities, but they will still need guidance. Start by reviewing their logs and asking them specific questions to stimulate reactions. To progress from reaction to reflection, you might let them choose which questions to answer or let them write their own questions.

One way to transition from logs to journals is to give each student a small booklet and have students write data or log entries on the right-hand pages, leaving the left-hand pages blank for comments. Teachers use the left-hand pages to not only make comments or provide feedback, but also to ask more probing questions that stimulate student reflection. See the "Logs and Journals" section in chapter 14 for an example of using this technique with the PACER.

In assessing reflective journal entries, focus mainly on the student's understanding of the assignment, not spelling and grammar. Although you should reinforce learning in other curricular areas, don't spend too much time on these issues. You might encourage other teachers to assess them as part of a cross-curricular, team-teaching approach. If neatness and spelling count with you, let students know ahead of time; otherwise, settle for legibility and being able to understand what they mean. You can also have students complete journal assignments on a computer (if appropriate and available).

Finally, if you ask for opinions or for students to share their feelings, keep in mind that there are no

Turn a log into a reflective journal. Examine the "Family Steps" log. Reflect on the log with respect to the concepts of FITT. Your reflection should consider these questions:

1. During the course of the day, which family member had the most steps? Which family member had the least?
2. Explain why you believe the person with the most steps was more active.
3. Do you believe that the person who had the most steps is active enough to stay healthy? Why or why not?
4. In comparison to _____(family member), why do you think you had fewer steps?
5. Can you think of ways to increase the number of steps you had on any of the days you were lower? Describe the strategies you would choose.
6. Which days were you most active? What did you do differently on the active days than you did on the less active days?
7. Did you meet your daily goals for time?
8. Did you meet your weekly goals for frequency?

Figure 12.3 Sample reflective journal entries.

right or wrong answers, only degrees of thoroughness and thoughtfulness. In figure 12.4, NASPE offers sample criteria and scoring guidelines for journal entries made during an adventure education experience (e.g., ropes course, wall climbing, and the like).

See chapter 13 for more about using logs and journals to assess affect. See chapter 14 for more about using logs and journals to assess cognitive knowledge, skills, and affective development. *Moving Into the Future: National Standards for Physical Education* (NASPE 2004) also offers good examples and guidelines.

Student Projects

Student projects are multitask assignments that encourage individuals, partners, or small groups to apply basic fitness knowledge in real-life settings. Under teacher guidance, a student or group of students explores an area of interest, sets goals, plans how to achieve those goals, and then strives for those goals (Melograno 1998). For example, a student investigates how muscular strength and endurance may enhance performance in a favorite sport, then formulates, tests, and reports (verbally or in a journal) theories on exactly what helps performance. Projects tend to be cross-curricular in nature, bringing to bear skills developed in several

subject areas. Use a rubric to assess each part of such a project having teachers in other subject areas assess parts related to their areas, if possible.

NASPE (1995) offers the following guidelines for developing and using projects effectively. (The following list is reprinted from Moving Into the Future: National Standards for Physical Education [1995] with permission from the National Association for Sport and Physical Education [NASPE], 1900 Association Drive, Reston, VA 20191-1599):

- Use a variety of teaching styles.
- Start with small projects in the early grades to prepare them for more complex projects later.
- Explain criteria for assessment and scoring procedures at the beginning of the project.
- Have others also score the project, for example, community experts or colleagues in other disciplines.
- Pilot test any major project before using the results as a basis for promotion or graduation.
- Use this opportunity to individualize your program to meet each student's needs.
- Design a scoring rubric for each part of the project.

Criteria for assessing journal entries

- Analyzes and expresses feelings about physical activity
- Identifies evidence of success, challenge, and enjoyment present in the activity
- Explains challenge that adventure activities provide
- Describes the positive effects friends and companions bring to this experience

Scoring guidelines for journal entries

Exemplary: Expresses feelings of personal participation and about sharing it with friends

Acceptable: Identifies feelings of personal participation

Needs improvement: Has difficulty expressing feelings about participation

Unacceptable: Does not make journal entries

Figure 12.4 Criteria and scoring for reflective journal entries during an adventure education experience.
Reprinted, by permission, from NASPE 1995.

In addition, be sure to design group projects so that cooperation with peers is essential for success. This interdependence builds social as well as health-related fitness skills. For example, a group works together to design a training circuit to enhance health-related fitness components. Then they oversee the circuit while another group performs the activities.

Evaluate group projects on both overall group product and individual performance. In other words, make both the group and each individual accountable. In this way, you will be able to identify the "slackers" (those who are just along for the ride) and the "workers" (those who put a lot of effort into the project). You might, for example, use a rubric to assess the group's efforts, then have each individual turn in a journal entry or take a quiz to determine individual learning.

The *Physical Best Activity Guides* provide many suggestions for both individual and group projects in health-related physical fitness education.

Role Plays

Role playing is an informal way to assess students. Use it mainly to assess the affective domain, but keep in mind that it may also reveal clues about the degree of cognitive understanding. To create an effective role play, have students assume roles in a simulated social situation or psychological dilemma related to health-related fitness. For example, have small groups act out how they might convince a friend not to smoke, or how they might encourage an obese friend to join a physical activity.

When assessing a role-playing performance, you should listen for students to incorporate specific information in the dialogue and actions they develop. For example, in the case of convincing a friend not to smoke, you should hear several specific points, such as the increased risks of heart attack and cancer.

An event task is a more open-ended role-playing situation through which you encourage students to problem solve. For example, you could challenge students to design and demonstrate a flexibility training circuit for helping a student in a wheelchair increase flexibility. The possible correct solutions are perhaps endless, as long as they follow the principles of training and the FITT guidelines. Not surprisingly, event tasks are often the basis of effective group and individual projects.

To effectively manage role-playing activities, allow groups time to develop and practice their ideas. Then have them take turns performing in front of the class, at a station, or in small groups while you circulate from one to the next.

Health-Related Fitness Tests

Fitness tests, such as *FITNESSGRAM/ACTIVITY-GRAM* (developed by the Cooper Institute and endorsed by AAHPERD), provide standardized methods for assessing each area of health-related fitness (figure 12.5). As part of an authentic assessment approach, use the test results to help students plan how to maintain or improve each component. Teach students to perform fitness tests independently and informally. These self-testing opportunities are vital to preparing students for designing their own health-related fitness programs throughout their lives. Then, perhaps test students more formally each semester or quarter. Have the purpose of such testing firmly in mind, however. Know if you are using test results for individual goal setting or overall program evaluation. Teach realistic goal setting as described in chapter 2 to teach students how to safely apply the principles of overload and progression. We explore fitness testing using *FITNESSGRAM/ACTIVITYGRAM* in more detail in chapter 13.

Written Tests

Written tests are a traditional form of assessment in physical education and most other subject areas. They are, however, often maligned in physical education theory, probably because they have been overemphasized and overvalued in the past. But written tests still have their place as a valid assessment tool. Whereas less formal assessments, such as role plays and discussions, can reveal important general information about who understands the concepts you're teaching and who doesn't, written tests can provide more specific and accurate data on what each individual knows and doesn't know. Just beware of the potential problems: Written tests don't always assess what has been taught or learned. Often, a teacher writes a test based on what is important to him or her, regardless of what was actually taught. In addition, teachers tend to focus on only one form of written test, instead of using a variety of formats to draw important information from students.

Objective tests, such as multiple-choice or true-false, take little time to administer and are easier to score. Subjective tests, such as short-answer or essay tests, provide deeper insights into student understanding and are occasionally worth the teacher follow-up time they require. Figure 12.6 shows three examples of written tests appropriate for health-related physical fitness education. Choose the format that best fits the content you're teaching and the ages and abilities of the students you're testing.

Manage the workload by only giving written tests to one or a few classes at a time and by keeping the tests brief—no more than 10 quick questions (multiple-choice, true-false, short-answer) or 1 to 3 essay questions. Save class time further by asking a

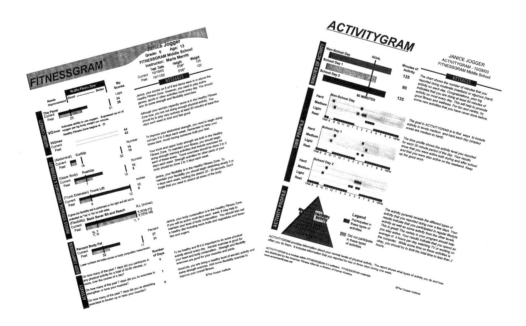

■ **Figure 12.5** *FITNESSGRAM* and *ACTIVITYGRAM* provide students with individualized reports based on their fitness test scores.

Reprinted, by permission, from The Cooper Institute, 2004, *FITNESSGRAM/ACTIVITYGRAM test administration manual*, 3rd ed. (Champaign, IL: Human Kinetics), 64 and 78.

Name ____________________

Grade: ____4____

1. When I run for a long time my heart
   (a) beats slower
   (b) stays the same
   (c) beats faster
   (d) almost stops
2. Which of the following is an example of muscular strength?
   (a) playing soccer
   (b) lifting a 50-pound bag of dog food
   (c) doing the sit-and-reach test
   (d) jumping rope
3. Being physically active is
   (a) fun
   (b) good for my heart
   (c) a way to stay well
   (d) all of the above

a

Name ____________________

Grade: ____7____

1. Target heart rate means
   (a) the rate you always want your heart to beat
   (b) the maximum heart rate you can achieve
   (c) the ideal heart rate at which to work out to improve aerobic endurance
   (d) the lowest rate your heart can go
2. Which of the following is an example of muscular strength?
   (a) running a mile
   (b) bench-pressing 150 pounds one time
   (c) doing 35 push-ups
   (d) riding an exercise bike for 30 minutes
3. To gain basic health benefits from physical activity you must participate in
   (a) three or more sessions per week
   (b) activities lasting 20 minutes or more
   (c) moderate to vigorous activity
   (d) all of the above

b

Name ____________________

Grade: ____10____

1. Determine the target heart rate for a person who is 17 years old (please show your work):

2. Define muscular strength and provide an example:

3. List five benefits of regular participation in physical activity:

c

■ **Figure 12.6** Examples of written tests appropriate for assessing the health-related fitness knowledge of students in *(a)* 4th grade, *(b)* 7th grade, and *(c)* 10th grade.

classroom teacher to administer quick written tests. This approach probably works best at the elementary level or at other levels that have self-contained classrooms.

Discussions

Discussions can provide the teacher with a wealth of information, but they can be time-consuming. Interview students at one station on a circuit, briefly pause mid-activity throughout a lesson, or lead a whole-class discussion to provide closure to a lesson. For a good discussion, set a clear objective, plan the questions that will guide students through the topic, keep students focused on the desired content of the discussion, and summarize the discussion at its end to provide effective closure.

To increase participation in a discussion and therefore its effectiveness, you might try the following (adapted from Woods 1997):

■ Make sure you wait at least three seconds before calling on anyone, so all students have time and motivation to ponder the question.

■ Ask one individual or group to provide an answer, but have the rest of the students in class raise their hands if they agree with the answer.

■ Have everyone respond verbally at the same time at a signal. You can also do this nonverbally by having students signal thumbs-up or thumbs-down for true or false and yes or no.

■ Direct partners to share their answers with each other, then raise their hands when they believe you have stated the correct answer (verbal multiple-choice).

■ Keep the questioning quick and to the point; don't take too much total time or unnecessarily disrupt the momentum of the class activities.

Discussions are quick, paperwork free, and especially helpful in assessing those students who find written communication difficult (Woods 1997). However, large-group discussions are not appropriate forums in which to assess individuals.

Polls

Polls can give you some of the same information as discussions, but more quickly. You can pose the same questions and have students "vote" in response. Older students can secretly mark a ballot, whereas younger students might enjoy participating in a "poker chip survey" (Graham 1992), in which they place one of two colors of poker chips to indicate yes or no, true or false, disagree or agree, and so on. Students can cast their votes on the way out of class. Use the results of a poll as a group assessment to help you plan reteaching lessons and to revise and improve lessons for future use. One effective use of polling is to ask the students, at the conclusion of a lesson, to raise their hands if they enjoyed the activity, or to give a "thumbs-up" if they would like to play the game again in class. Polling is a quick and efficient way to assess general group enjoyment, and it avoids singling out students by requiring them to provide individual responses.

Applying Assessment Tools

Some assessment tools lend themselves well only to certain situations. Other assessment tools work well in a variety of situations. In this section, we discuss which assessment tools work well for self- and peer assessment. We also discuss how teachers can use portfolios for student assessment. In addition, as you will see in chapters 13 and 14, different tools work best for assessing different areas—cognitive, affective, health-related fitness, and psychomotor.

Self-Assessment

Teaching students how to monitor their own progress, or **self-assess,** is an important key to reaching the ultimate goal of producing adults who know how to design appropriate physical activity programs for themselves. It also helps students focus on performance "progress," rather than "product," because students understand the critical elements (process components) better, which, in turn, improves performance standards and achievement. You can have students use rubrics, journals, or logs to monitor their progress and assess their performances in fitness testing, role playing, and group and individual projects. Journals and logs also help you make students accountable for staying on task during class. The following sample journal assignments provide opportunities for students to reflect on their learning and check for understanding:

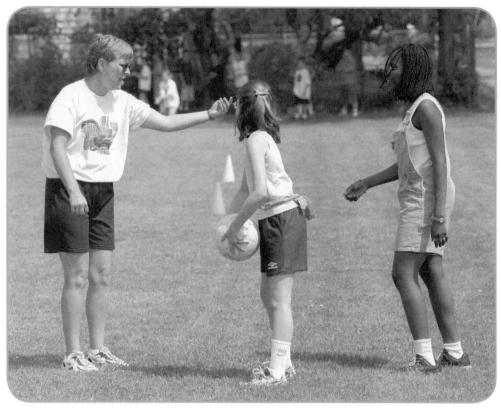

© Human Kinetics

A brief discussion with a student at a circuit station can provide a quick assessment.

- "Help your friend . . . " Have students describe in writing how to do a particular health-related fitness activity safely (or have younger students make appropriate selections from a pair or series of pictures that show right and wrong ways to perform).
- Record feelings. Occasionally or regularly have students record how they feel physically and emotionally after physical education class and other physical activity.
- Record performance. Have students record the number of times they performed a health-related activity, such as each stretch, by making check marks. Young children might enjoy recording a smiley or frowny face next to each check mark to indicate how they felt about each performance.
- Analyze performance. Have students record how well they feel they did on different fitness activities, and what exactly they will work on to improve their performances.

Peer Assessment

Peer assessment is an assessment method where students analyze the performance of other students and is an important part of developing physical, cognitive, and social skills. Analyzing others' performances helps a student focus on the key parts of a skill, reinforcing his or her own learning. Most students, however, need repeated instruction to learn to assess peers effectively. Make sure they have rubrics or other clearly listed criteria available, so that they can evaluate and make judgments accurately.

To organize peer assessment, have students work together in pairs or small groups to analyze each other's performances. Students should use the same rubrics as used for self-assessment. Teach students specific strategies for giving helpful feedback. Role playing acceptable peer assessment behaviors can be helpful.

When daily peer and self-assessment occurs, students learn more, retain more of what they learn, perform more accurately, and are more account-able. Thus, using multiple peer and self-assessments improves student understanding, retention, and accuracy of data collection and recording.

Using Portfolios for Student Assessment

Although most of your ongoing assessment should be informal, as in day-to-day observations and peer and self-assessment, you should periodically perform more formal assessments. For example, you should select certain self- and peer assessments, rubrics, and class assignments for closer scrutiny. These formal assessments can be combined to create a more complete, and therefore more authentic, picture of each student's progress in a portfolio (figure 12.7). A portfolio gives you a ready reference for assessment, grading, and parent–teacher conferences.

Sometimes described as an assessment tool in itself, the well-designed **portfolio** is a "tool kit" of sorts—a collection of tools that help you do a thorough job of assessing each individual. This "collection" might be contained within a three-hole folder, a hanging file, or any other type of container you deem appropriate. Because portfolios showcase student progress so well, they are a powerful way to build feelings of self-efficacy in students, those feelings that make students believe they have the ability to learn and the competence to participate.

What should you put into each portfolio? Select a wide variety of assignments and assessments to form a more complete picture of each student's progress and achievements. Include both informal and formal assessments: periodic fitness testing results; rubrics that reflect affective, cognitive, and physical development; journal entries; and projects. The older the students, the more you should strive to teach them to select their own portfolio pieces (based on criteria you set). This is part of making each student an independent learner.

Portfolios can go with students from grade to grade and school to school, making it possible to monitor long-term progress and persistent problems. Portfolios are also a tool for monitoring a program's effectiveness in terms of delivering a sequentially designed curriculum.

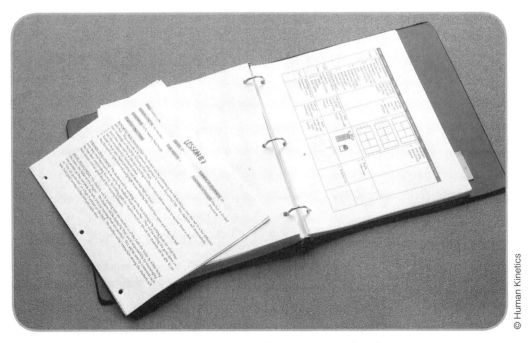

© Human Kinetics

■ **Figure 12.7** A portfolio system can provide an authentic assessment of student progress.

Portfolio Management

Assessing student portfolios is very time-consuming. Be careful what you choose to spend your time on, and think through a manageable plan for dealing with portfolios. Follow these tips to help turn portfolios into the teaching, learning, and assessing tool they are meant to be, without giving up your family life:

- First, determine the purpose for using the portfolio.
- Obtain or have students or volunteers make sturdy portfolios. Use a traditional three-hole folder, a folded piece of 12-by-18-inch construction paper with pockets added, a flat box, a hanging file, or another appropriate container.
- Store portfolios by class in milk crates, portable hanging file boxes, or larger bins. At the elementary level, try to get the classroom teacher to store the container and bring it to each physical education class.
- Train students to file their own papers or to file papers for younger students (but maintain confidentiality). Color coding by class or grade level can help. Establishing class management procedures for filing papers helps, too.
- Establish protocols for passing out and collecting portfolios.
- Periodically, select or have students select representative pieces from their assessment activities to retain in their portfolios. This leaves fewer bits and pieces for you to sort through. Designate how many pieces to select, taking the time to discuss what creates a good cross section of items. Send the rest home, after stamping each one with a message such as "COMPLETED ON TIME" to indicate you do care, but that you're not using it as part of your assessment of a student. This will eliminate a lot of paperwork in a professional manner. If you designate pieces to select after the work is completed, students will be motivated to try their best on each assignment.
- Staple or glue certain ongoing assessments, such as a fitness testing record sheet, onto the front or back cover of each portfolio.
- Decide whether you want to staple in several sheets of paper to form journals inside each portfolio, use a separate notebook for journals, or add individual sheets to portfolios with journal entries as they are written.

Grading and Reporting Student Progress

As mentioned at the beginning of this chapter, assessing and grading have very different purposes. Assessment tells you and your students how they are improving or what they need to work on with respect to specific program objectives or standards. A grade is a single summative or composite symbol or score that becomes a permanent record of student achievement, and it must be representative of

achievement of all program objectives (Lacy and Hastad 2003). If you must give a single letter grade, it needs to represent a compilation of many assessments and measurements of improvement—not a limited or single test of student status. Lacy and Hastad (2003) also caution that teachers must be sensitive to the impact of grades on youth, and that the grades must be tied to the school's procedures for issuing grades (p. 337). You can create an acceptable relationship between assessing and grading, but you must plan to do so even before the course begins.

Determining a fair and balanced single grade is without a doubt one of the most difficult aspects of the assessment process. Although fitness maintenance is a prominent program objective (i.e., NASPE Standard #4: Achieves and maintains a health-enhancing level of physical fitness), the criterion used to evaluate fitness involves assessing a variety of components and crosses over several standards. For our purposes, the best criterion for measuring student achievement is the "healthy fitness zone," which is age, gender, and component specific. A student who is in or above his or her healthy fitness zones in each fitness area should achieve a high mark related to Standard #4, but the teacher also needs to address other standards and program goals in the grading process. With respect to grading and fitness assessment, it seems more appropriate to focus on providing clear and accurate feedback regarding individual goals and student achievement of those goals, and then to encourage the student to self-assess. If a composite or single grade is required by the school district, teachers are encouraged to provide alternative and helpful fitness feedback, such as individual *FITNESSGRAM* reports attached to the composite grade. This approach will help students understand the process of achieving and maintaining healthful levels. Grades based primarily on achievement of specific fitness scores can discourage students from continuing to be physically active after they leave your program.

Including Fitness Scores

For teachers who are looking for ways to include fitness scores in a composite grade, some possible solutions are provided on the following pages.

Performance feedback on fitness test scores should do the following:

- Help the students understand where they can improve
- Help you recognize if students are meeting program objectives and content standards
- Show you where you should change your program (e.g., grades plotted on a graph to summarize trends)
- Promote your health-related physical fitness education program to the school and community
- Justify the ongoing need for health-related physical fitness education in the curriculum

Weighty Matters

What weight should you give each area you plan to rate in the final grade? This will vary according to district mandates, personal preferences, and program goals. We recommend that, in a health-related physical fitness education program, you strive for balance of program aspects—cognitive, affective, and physical assessment data—because each of these areas affects how students will be empowered to make lifestyle decisions regarding physical activity and health-related fitness.

Fitness Education Sample Grading Criteria Form

_____ Knowledge of fitness concepts (25 percent)
_____ Fitness testing—ability to self-test and interpret results (20 percent)
_____ Physical activity effort—in and outside of class (25 percent)
_____ Fitness skill application—for example, ability to take pulse or ability to pace while running (20 percent)
_____ Attitude toward physical activity (10 percent)

Sharing Information With Students and Parents Beyond Grades

Share assessment feedback with students and parents within the context of your entire assessment program. In other words, reinforce that you are using a balance of assessment tools across all domains to assess each student. You can do this by presenting knowledge assessment alongside affective and physical assessments. This will help both students and parents see how knowledge enhances development in other areas and vice versa. See figure 12.8 for a sample grading form.

Physical Education Progress Report: Grades 3-4

Student: _____ Date: _____

Teacher: _____

___ 1st qtr (Nov)   ___ 2nd qtr (Feb)   ___ 3rd qtr (Apr)   ___ 4th qtr (June)

	Working to achieve	Needs improvement	Achieved
Intellectual			
1. Knows rules and procedures governing movement activities and games	❏	❏	❏
2. Recognizes the effects of space, time, force, and flow on the quality of movement	❏	❏	❏
3. Applies basic mechanical principles that affect and control human movement	❏	❏	❏

Comments: _____

	Working to achieve	Needs improvement	Achieved
Social			
1. Respects rights, opinions, and abilities of others	❏	❏	❏
2. Shares, takes turns, and provides mutual assistance	❏	❏	❏
3. Participates cooperatively in student-led activities	❏	❏	❏

Comments: _____

	Working to achieve	Needs improvement	Achieved
Emotional			
1. Assumes responsibility for giving and following directions	❏	❏	❏
2. Makes decisions on an individual basis	❏	❏	❏
3. Responds freely and confidently through expressive bodily movement	❏	❏	❏

Comments: _____

	Working to achieve	Needs improvement	Achieved
Values			
1. Carries out tasks to completion	❏	❏	❏
2. Displays preferences for various forms of movement	❏	❏	❏
3. Engages in movement activities voluntarily	❏	❏	❏

Comments: _____

	Working to achieve	Needs improvement	Achieved
Physical			
1. Executes all locomotor movements in response to rhythmic accompaniments	❏	❏	❏
2. Controls body while balancing, rolling, climbing, and hanging	❏	❏	❏
3. Shows body control in manipulating playground ball, while stationary and moving	❏	❏	❏

Comments: _____

■ **Figure 12.8** Sample grading form. This form has been tailored to a specific school district's curriculum. A reproducible version of this form is available in appendix A.

Reprinted, by permission, from V.J. Melograno, 1998, *Professional and sport portfolios for physical education* (Champaign, IL: Human Kinetics), 109.

For assessment to be accurate, you must ensure that it is safe for your students to share their feelings about physical activity. You must also emphasize intrinsic over extrinsic motivators. What, then, do you do with the affective information you collect? Handle with care all affective assessment data you gather so that students will be honest with you, helping you make your program the best it can be.

Parent–teacher conferences are an excellent way to share this information. This personal contact makes it easier to convey information in a positive and genuinely caring manner. If you cannot meet systematically with every parent, try to at least meet with the parents of students who seem especially reluctant to participate in physical activity. Invite the student as well. At the conference, brainstorm ways to help the student enjoy physical activity more. Express any specific health concerns you may have, and explain your physical education program philosophy. Remember to be diplomatic and to ask for honest feedback on your program. Find out about lifestyle activities the family enjoys, such as fishing, and suggest they expand this outdoor activity to include hiking and canoeing. At the end of the conference, thank the parents for their time, and invite them to contact you whenever they have concerns, comments, or questions.

If you cannot hold conferences, send parents a detailed attitude and motivation report. Provide space for parent feedback, and leave the door open for further communication. Finally, involve parents in fun family events to help families learn to enjoy physical activity together.

Be sure to inform everyone—both students and parents—ahead of time what you're looking for in terms of development and participation and effort levels. This approach can prevent many misunderstandings. Communicate regularly through newsletters. If you focus, as we believe you should, on self-assessment, students will know their results already, but teacher–student conferences will cement these understandings. Consider setting up teacher–student conferences as part of an activity circuit, so that you can help each individual set goals based on your feedback and the student's personal objectives. Finally, ensure student and family privacy when interpreting and sharing assessment results. Remember, the idea is, over the course of a K-12 program, to guide each student up the Stairway to Lifetime Fitness (Corbin and Lindsey 2004), empowering each to take individual responsibility for health-related fitness.

Using Assessments for Program Planning

A central reason for using your valuable time to assess regularly should be to learn how to tailor your program to meet individual student needs. In response to poor cognitive assessment results, the temptation to overdo lecture lessons may be great, but resist this urge. Certainly, lecture settings have their place in the health-related physical fitness education program; however, a greater goal is to keep students as physically active as possible. In short, help students learn while they do. For example, if students are having trouble learning how to pace themselves while running the mile, design an active game that teaches this concept—or have groups of students do so.

Adapt activities that turn kids off; they'll be glad to suggest how. The process of working together not only improves your program, but it also helps model problem-solving skills. Remember, if students do not enjoy the physical activity in your program, they are much less likely to pursue it as a lifestyle choice. Naturally, this defeats your attempts to produce adults who love physical activity and seek it as a way of life. Be sure to include a variety of movement forms in addition to health-related fitness and sport activities; for example, dance, outdoor pursuits, and adventure programming can spark interest in physical activity in otherwise reluctant students.

Motivating Through Assessment

Of course, knowing how to be physically active for life isn't enough: Students must want to pursue such a lifestyle. Giving students the responsibility for tracking their own progress is highly motivating (Hichwa 1998; Hellison 2003). Avoid comparisons among students. Instead, focus on helping students set goals for personal improvement, so that they are more likely to feel successful each time they participate in physical activity. Even a very young child can set a simple goal, such as playing physically active games after school three times a week instead of watching television.

Goals should be set based on current personal health-related fitness levels, feelings of self-efficacy, knowledge of the FITT guidelines and training principles, access to various types of programs and activities, and the purposes you have established for setting goals.

To guide self-assessment and goal setting, set benchmarks (i.e., the healthy fitness zones) by which students can monitor their own progress (see chapter 2). This process makes students more accountable for their own learning and progress. This is in keeping with the philosophy of helping students move from depending on your guidance to independently pursuing health-related fitness as a way of life.

Specifically, students may be motivated by carefully monitoring self-recorded progress toward goals that they set with their teacher. For this to occur, sufficient time must be given to allow for progress. Focus on small steps toward improvement or toward the goal. It is the small steps that can actually be seen in the student's own writing that are the most motivating. These become fuel for developing a sense of competence. (Refer to chapter 2 for goal-setting strategies and guidelines.)

Summary

To be truly authentic, assessment in health-related physical fitness education must allow students to demonstrate, in real-life settings, that they are moving toward the goal of becoming physically active adults. Thus, your program should motivate students to apply fitness knowledge in the real world as they make progress in the physical, affective, and cognitive domains. Within the context of "motivation," teachers should separate health-related fitness assessment from the grading system in physical education, and they should provide specific feedback using alternative methods that inform students about progress toward personal goals and about strategies to achieve them. In chapters 13 and 14, we show you how to apply the tools discussed in this chapter in specific ways to assess progress toward health-related fitness, knowledge, and affect.

CHAPTER

13

Chapter Contents

Assessing Health-Related Physical Fitness

If your ultimate goal is to help students become physically active for a lifetime, students in your classes must not only be developing health-related physical fitness, but they should also be developing physical activity habits. Students should participate daily in physical activities outside of physical education, and they need to develop the skills and knowledge to help them remain physically active throughout their lives. In this chapter, we explain how to assess health-related fitness levels and physical activity levels both within physical education and outside of the regular physical education class. Many of today's physical education teachers have already updated their fitness testing and curricular programs to reflect the emphasis on the components of health-related fitness as recommended in state and national standards. Others are still in the process of making the change from skill-based to health-related fitness testing. Quality programs use pretest assessments to establish a starting point for students to plan individualized programs; these scores are used for goal setting and to regularly check progress toward goals. Records are individualized and include physical activity participation data, not merely one time scores. Teachers look for improvement in every student, and the focus is on how a student's personal choices can affect each health-related physical fitness component.

Fitness testing has had a somewhat controversial history. In the past, many teachers placed more emphasis on skill- or sport-related fitness. (An example of sport-related fitness is assessment of speed, as measured by an individual's 100-yard dash time.) Many tests compared students to other students (using normative scoring), leading many children who were actually healthy individuals to perceive themselves as unfit. Conversely, some students who were practicing unhealthy behaviors were still able to achieve good scores, giving them a false picture of their present and future health and fitness. For example, these students may have matured physically earlier than most students of similar age, or may have inherited good upper body strength, thus scoring higher on some tests, even though they were not regularly physically active (something that would catch up to them later in life).

Today, there is greater awareness that comparing students does more harm than good. Therefore, current guidelines for teachers include recommendations to

- use fitness assessment as only one of several criteria for assigning grades, and avoid using fitness scores in the composite grade;
- use fitness test results as only one of several indicators of program effectiveness;
- avoid posting test results in public places or where other students can see them; and
- base awards on personal achievement of or progress toward goals rather than on student test scores (see figure 13.1).

Furthermore, in the past, sometimes test results were inconsistent: A student would pass one test and fail when taking another similar test in a different battery. This problem had to do with assessment design, not teacher practice, and it created problems even for teachers who used fitness testing appropriately.

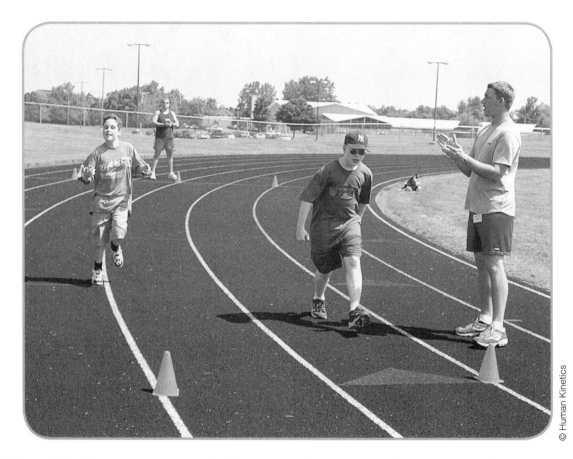

© Human Kinetics

■ **Figure 13.1** Many students are turned off to physical activity when awards are based on outperforming or being compared to others rather than on personal improvement, achievement, or progress toward realistic goals.

Norm-Referenced Versus Criterion-Referenced Testing

Norm-referenced tests—no matter the subject area—are tests for which an individual's score is compared to the average **(norm)** and standard deviation (average difference) of all the students who took the test. In fitness testing, norm-referenced tests were initially developed using a large sampling of student performances on fitness test battery items to establish the average (norm) and to figure out the scores achieved by the most fit or the top-level students. Norm-referenced testing is not necessarily a bad thing. However, the purpose of the norms was often misinterpreted, and they were often used to set up a reward system for the top-level students. For example, the early versions of the President's Challenge test battery only awarded the "President's Physical Fitness Award" to students who scored at the 85th percentile on all test items, meaning, to earn this award, a student had to perform in every test item as well as or better than 85 out of 100 of the students for whom data was collected; however, criterion-referenced standards are now available for this test battery. Another example of norm-referenced tests using recognition awards based on competitive scoring is the AAU Physical Fitness Program. This program gives its top award to those who score in the "Outstanding" (as compared to others) range in all five test items (Craft 1994).

In contrast, *FITNESSGRAM* is a **criterion-referenced test;** student scores are compared to preset standard score ranges that indicate levels of health-related fitness necessary for good health and reduced risk of diseases associated with sedentary lifestyles. The goal is to score in the healthy fitness zones (HFZs) in each component of health-related fitness: aerobic fitness, muscular strength and endurance, flexibility, and body composition. It is important to understand that criterion-referenced tests are initially developed using a normative procedure—testing a wide sample of individuals over a range of ages and from diverse populations. However, once the scores are averaged (normed), the scores are also analyzed with respect to the individuals' risk factors for or their development over time of chronic diseases such as heart disease, or for impairments affecting long-term quality of life. Thus, criterion-referenced scores are actually normative scores in comparison to risk factors. The healthy fitness zones are the range of scores achieved by students considered to be at minimal risk for development of chronic diseases or impairments. Students at the low end of the **criterion zone**—the healthy fitness zone (HFZ)—are considered to be at a minimum level of health to lead active and healthy lives, but they can be encouraged to maintain or increase their fitness to further enhance their health. Students at the high end of the HFZ are considered to be healthy and fit enough to participate in lifestyle activities and are least likely to develop the diseases associated with sedentary lifestyles. In most cases, exceeding the zone will not be harmful (with the exception of being too lean or of hyperextending joints), and further development in fitness may contribute to better performance in sports or motor activities.

In some situations, teachers may elect to have students stop the test when they have achieved a score equal to the upper limit of the healthy fitness zone. Stopping the test performance in this manner can reduce required testing time. It may also reduce embarrassment and create a less threatening and less competitive environment for students who are less capable. If this approach is used, parents should be informed about the process, so that they understand that the performance reported on *FITNESSGRAM* does not necessarily represent a maximal effort. Also, if performance during class time does not allow a maximal effort, it is good to give those more highly motivated students the opportunity to do a maximal test at some other time. An after-school fitness challenge may prove to be very popular with students who are high-level performers.

FITNESSGRAM acknowledges performances above the HFZ but does not recommend this level of performance as an appropriate goal for all students. (Note, too, that scoring above the

(continued)

HFZ in body composition is undesirable at all times.) However, students who want to achieve a high level of athletic performance may need to consider setting goals beyond the HFZ (for example, a gymnast who needs exceptional flexibility for a variety of reasons, or a basketball player who can use additional flexibility to improve shooting accuracy). Students, especially younger students, will need teacher assistance in setting realistic goals. But with practice, over time students will be able to set goals with less help and will become more self-reliant.

Using HFZ scores allows students to achieve a level of fitness associated with good health. More students can be successful and score in the HFZ than can meet the levels listed in the tables of earlier norm-referenced tests. This method of scoring removes more of the competitive emphasis previously associated with fitness testing and puts the focus on the achievement of health-related fitness. This provides greater opportunities for students to experience feelings of success through the testing experience.

Guidelines for Appropriate Fitness Testing

To make fitness testing a viable component of authentic assessment, it must do the following:

- Give students the opportunity to demonstrate the desired behavior—Teaching students to self-test gives them opportunities to demonstrate the behaviors they'll need to create their own effective physical activity programs throughout life.

- Link directly to the curriculum—Self-testing as a self-teaching activity helps make health-related fitness concepts "essential content" of the curriculum.

- Occur on an ongoing basis—Self-testing makes it easy to test on an ongoing basis, because it saves teacher time. More important, it individualizes the instruction and sequence of learning.

- Give students the practical experience they need to feel confident in their abilities to apply the tests and seek improvement in real life.

- Be tied to the goal-setting process—Teachers must help students understand how assessment and goal setting are integrated into lifestyle changes.

Some children will need more supervision and help than other children. Teach all students proper procedures and periodically conduct more formal tests, regardless of your students' levels of inde-

pendence. Figure 13.2 shows a continuum from just beginning to learn how to self-test to formal, but independent, self-testing (along with the goals at each stage in the continuum). The more experienced the student, the more independent he should be of teacher supervision, because the ultimate goal is to produce adults who can conduct their own tests in the context of self-designed physical activity programs. Some students may, however, stay at one stage on the continuum longer than others, depending on their needs and abilities. For example, most elementary students will require a high degree of direct teacher supervision. Students in middle school will likely be capable of cycling through the first three steps (teacher-directed self-testing practice; formal, teacher-administered testing; and informal self-testing, checked by peer) repeatedly, but they may not progress to informal self-testing (without being checked) until they are older. High school students should be able to progress to formal self-testing (not checked by peer or teacher). Note that goal setting and physical activity are important steps after the initial self-testing practice (teacher directed) and will perpetuate a continuous cycle of testing, goal setting, and participating in physical activity as illustrated in figure 13.3.

Administering FITNESSGRAM

When administered correctly, **FITNESSGRAM** overcomes many of the problems fitness testing has experienced in the past. *FITNESSGRAM* sets

	Format	Goal
1	Teacher-directed self-testing practice	To familiarize students with testing procedures
2	Formal, teacher-administered testing	To provide accurate baseline data
	Goal setting	To focus training efforts
	Physical activity	To reach goals
3	Informal self-testing, checked by peer	To compare to baseline data, to provide more testing practice, and to ensure accuracy
	Reset goals (if necessary)	To focus future efforts
	Physical activity	To reach goals
4	Informal self-testing	To self-monitor progress, to provide more testing practice
	Reset goals (if necessary)	To focus future efforts
	Physical activity	To reach goals
5	Formal self-testing, checked by teacher	To ensure accurate current data
	Reset goals (if necessary)	To focus future efforts
	Physical activity	To reach goals
6	Formal self-testing, not checked	To monitor progress independently

■ **Figure 13.2** An example of a continuum for moving students from teacher-directed testing to self-testing.

performance standards—called healthy fitness zones, or HFZs—that reflect the basic health-related fitness levels required for good health, instead of comparing children's performances (figure 13.4). Thus, the likelihood that each child will feel successful in fitness testing is greater, increasing the probability that he or she will view physical activity and health-related fitness in a positive light.

Furthermore, as part of the *FITNESSGRAM* reports, students not only receive scores, but they also receive interpretations of the scores and recommendations that are individualized to help them improve in the aspects of fitness where scores fell below the HFZ. This immediate educational feedback teaches students how the specific test relates to the achievement of a healthy lifestyle. All students are also provided reinforcing statements regarding their healthy behaviors and are encouraged to continue these behaviors.

The *ACTIVITYGRAM* portion of the program helps students understand how activity behaviors outside of school contribute to health and well-being. Students are encouraged to think of the assessments as lifestyle assessments, rather than school-based tests. (See figure 13.5 and the *"ACTIVITYGRAM"* sidebar.)

Some argue that health-related fitness testing, even when conducted properly and with sensitivity, is too artificial and contrived to be part of authentic assessment. Physical Best asserts, however, that developmentally appropriate health-related fitness testing, conducted in a sound physical education program, helps teach students how to be fit for life. Moreover, it provides a "snapshot" of each student's current fitness level, allowing both teachers and students to plan for improvement.

Prepare for testing

— Precede with regular enjoyable exercise

— Explain reasons for testing

— Precede with knowledge of how to take tests

— Precede with knowledge of exercise warm-up

— Explain recognition opportunities

Testing

— Follow basic exercise principles

— Test properly

— Consider student feelings

— Consider student confidentiality

— Teach while you test

— Consider self-testing opportunities

After testing

— Report results

— Interpret results

— Recommend program of exercise

— Carry out program

Implement recognition programs

— Explain recognition philosophy

— Use recognition to foster competence and confidence

— Use recognition to stimulate intrinsic motivation

— Use recognition to foster parent interest

— Implement recognition for everyone

Quality physical education program

— Learn about fitness and exercise

— Learn to self-test

— Learn to interpret test results

— Learn to plan personal program

— Do regular vigorous exercise

— Learn to enjoy exercise

■ **Figure 13.3** Testing is part of the overall educational process leading to a physically active, healthy lifestyle.

This material is reprinted with permission of R. Pangrazi and C. Corbin, 1994, Teaching Strategies for Improving Youth Fitness, page 5, a publication of the American Alliance for Health, Physical Education, Recreation and Dance, 1900 Association Drive, Reston, VA 20191.

ACTIVITYGRAM

A new feature of *FITNESSGRAM*, revision 6.0, is the inclusion of physical activity assessments. These assessments were added because of the need to reinforce to students the importance of developing lifetime habits of regular physical activity. While students' fitness is important, it cannot be maintained unless they remain physically active as adults.

The *ACTIVITYGRAM* assessment is a recall of the student's previous day's physical activity, based on a validated physical activity instrument known as the Previous Day Physical Activity Recall (PDPAR) (Weston et al. 1997). In the assessment, the student reports his or her activity levels for each 30-minute block of time during the day. The format is designed to accommodate both school and nonschool days.

The assessment, provided through the available software, includes detailed information about the student's activity habits and prescriptive feedback about how active he or she should be. It is very similar to the *FITNESSGRAM* assessment.

Because of the cognitive demands of recalling physical activity, it may be difficult for young children to get accurate results. Thus, it is recommended that the *ACTIVITYGRAM* program be used with students in fifth grade and higher.

FITNESSGRAM®

Janice Jogger
Grade: 6   Age: 13
FITNESSGRAM Middle School
Instructor: Marie Merritt

	Test Date	Height	Weight
Current	10/15/03	5'06"	125
Past	10/11/02	5'05"	122

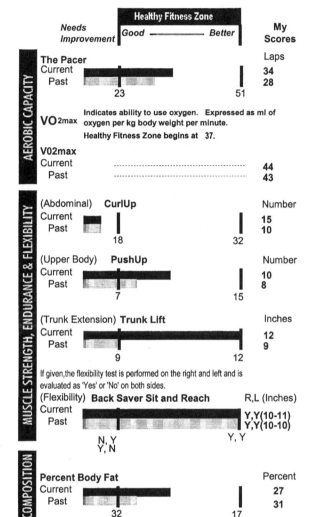

Healthy Fitness Zone

Needs Improvement	Good ——— Better	My Scores

AEROBIC CAPACITY

The Pacer — Laps
Current 34
Past 28
23   51

VO2max Indicates ability to use oxygen. Expressed as ml of oxygen per kg body weight per minute.
Healthy Fitness Zone begins at **37**.

VO2max
Current 44
Past 43

MUSCLE STRENGTH, ENDURANCE & FLEXIBILITY

(Abdominal) CurlUp — Number
Current 15
Past 10
18   32

(Upper Body) PushUp — Number
Current 10
Past 8
7   15

(Trunk Extension) Trunk Lift — Inches
Current 12
Past 9
9   12

If given, the flexibility test is performed on the right and left and is evaluated as 'Yes' or 'No' on both sides.

(Flexibility) Back Saver Sit and Reach — R,L (Inches)
Current Y,Y(10-11)
Past Y,Y(10-10)
N, Y   Y, Y
Y, N

BODY COMPOSITION

Percent Body Fat — Percent
Current 27
Past 31
32   17

Lower numbers are better scores on body composition measurement.

ACTIVITY

Number of Days

On how many of the past 7 days did you participate in any physical activity for a total of 30-60 minutes, or more, over the course of a day? **4**

On how many of the past 7 days did you do exercises to strengthen or tone your muscles? **1**

On how many of the past 7 days did you do stretching exercises to loosen up or relax your muscles? **0**

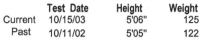

MESSAGES

Janice, your scores on 5 of 6 test items were in or above the Healthy Fitness Zone. However, you need to play active games, sports or other activities most every day. You should also do some strength and flexibility exercises.

Although your aerobic capacity score is in the Healthy Fitness Zone now, you are not doing enough physical activity. You should try to play very actively at least 60 minutes at least five days each week to look and feel good.

To improve your abdominal strength, you need to begin doing curl-ups 3 to 5 days each week. Remember to keep your knees bent. Avoid having someone hold your feet.

Your trunk and upper body strength are both in the Healthy Fitness Zone. To maintain your fitness, you should begin doing strength training activities that include exercises for each of these areas. Trunk exercises should be done 3 to 5 days each week. Strength activities for other parts of your body should be done 2 to 3 days each week.

Janice, your flexibility is in the Healthy Fitness Zone. To maintain your flexibility you should begin stretching slowly 3 or 4 days each week, holding the stretch 20 - 30 seconds. Don't forget that you need to stretch all areas of the body.

Janice, your body composition is in the Healthy Fitness Zone. If you will be active most days each week, it may help to maintain your level of body composition. You should also eat a healthy diet including more fruits and vegetables and fewer fats and sugars.

To be healthy and fit it is important to do some physical activity almost every day. Aerobic exercise is good for your heart and body composition. Strength and flexibilty exercises are good for your muscles and joints.

Good job, you are doing a healthy level of aerobic activity and some strength exercise. Add some flexibility exercise to improve your overall fitness.

©The Cooper Institute

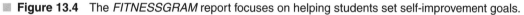

Figure 13.4 The *FITNESSGRAM* report focuses on helping students set self-improvement goals.

Reprinted, by permission, from The Cooper Institute, 2004, *FITNESSGRAM/ACTIVITYGRAM test administration manual,* 3rd ed. (Champaign, IL: Human Kinetics), 64.

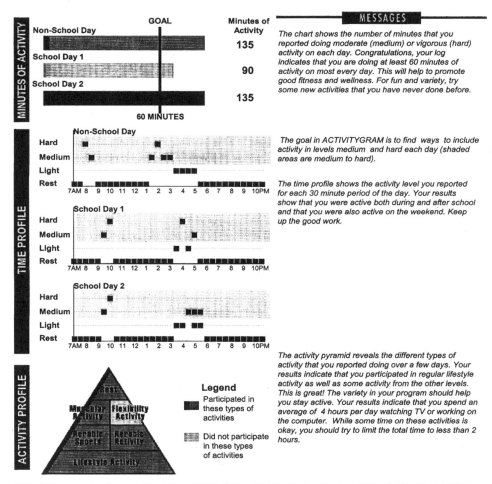

ACTIVITYGRAM

JANICE JOGGER
ACTIVITYGRAM - 10/28/03
FITNESSGRAM Middle School

MESSAGES

The chart shows the number of minutes that you reported doing moderate (medium) or vigorous (hard) activity on each day. Congratulations, your log indicates that you are doing at least 60 minutes of activity on most every day. This will help to promote good fitness and wellness. For fun and variety, try some new activities that you have never done before.

The goal in ACTIVITYGRAM is to find ways to include activity in levels medium and hard each day (shaded areas are medium to hard).

The time profile shows the activity level you reported for each 30 minute period of the day. Your results show that you were active both during and after school and that you were also active on the weekend. Keep up the good work.

The activity pyramid reveals the different types of activity that you reported doing over a few days. Your results indicate that you participated in regular lifestyle activity as well as some activity from the other levels. This is great! The variety in your program should help you stay active. Your results indicate that you spend an average of 4 hours per day watching TV or working on the computer. While some time on these activities is okay, you should try to limit the total time to less than 2 hours.

ACTIVITYGRAM provides information about your normal levels of physical activity. The report shows what types of activity you do and how often you do them. It includes information that you reported for two or three days during one week.

ACTIVITYGRAM is a module within FITNESSGRAM 6.0 software. FITNESSGRAM materials are distributed by the American Fitness Alliance, a division of Human Kinetics. www.americanfitness.net

©The Cooper Institute

■ **Figure 13.5** Sample printout of an *ACTIVITYGRAM* report.

Reprinted, by permission, from The Cooper Institute, 2004, *FITNESSGRAM/ACTIVITYGRAM test administration manual,* 3rd ed. (Champaign, IL: Human Kinetics), 78.

Preparing for Testing

Fitness testing doesn't have to be an administrative nightmare. By following some simple guidelines, your *FITNESSGRAM* experience should be a positive one. Simply being ready to administer fitness testing makes the entire process flow more smoothly. The following suggestions will help streamline the process of administering *FITNESSGRAM*. (The following list is adapted, by permission, from The Cooper Institute, *FITNESSGRAM/ACTIVITYGRAM Test Administration Manual,* 3rd ed. Gregory J. Welk and Marilu D. Meredith (Champaign, IL: Human Kinetics, 2004).

1. Prepare students for the test—Allow two to six weeks for students to practice test items and increase their fitness levels. Administering the tests at the very beginning of the school year may lead to muscle soreness and discouragement. It may also cause misleading follow-up test results because students improve more rapidly once they get used to the testing procedures. (See "Involving Students" later in this chapter.)

2. Read all test instructions carefully— These are located in the *FITNESSGRAM/ ACTIVITYGRAM Test Administration Manual,* 3rd ed.

3. Collect the necessary testing equipment—Obtain the testing equipment you need, and ensure that it is working properly. Sources of equipment are listed in the *FITNESSGRAM/ACTIVITYGRAM Test Administration Manual.*

4. Prepare record-keeping forms—Reproduce necessary forms (see the *FITNESSGRAM/ACTIVITYGRAM Test Administration Manual*). Record student names as appropriate, depending on the form you use.

5. Organize testing stations—Create a kind of circuit, such as that shown in figure 13.6. Be sure your setup allows both you and your students to flow easily from one station to the next. In addition, locate the stations so that you can see the entire activity area, making adequate supervision easier. Make sure forms, pencils, and clipboards are available at each station to allow students to record their test results.

6. Organize students—Decide in advance how to group students and which group will begin at which station.

7. Maximize instruction—Plan testing with other activities to continue the learning process and keep all students active.

In addition, if you are new to fitness testing or unsure of a procedure, practice administering the test to a small group of students or colleagues prior to testing on a larger scale.

Involving Students

All people learn best by doing, so if your goal is to produce students who can self-direct their own physically active lifestyles, you must involve them as fully as possible in each part of your program—including fitness testing. At the heart of this approach is teaching students to self-test. You should give students feedback to help them establish appropriate goals, such as to improve the number of laps they are able to complete on the PACER test, or to improve their sit-and-reach score. Beyond this, have students record their own test results. Even second graders can record numbers if you take the

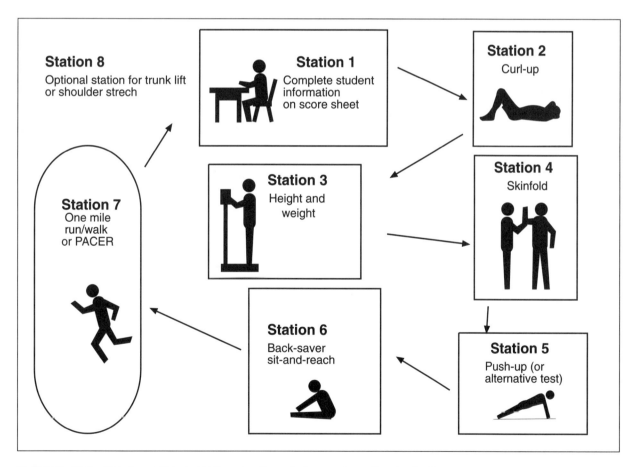

■ **Figure 13.6** Creating a fitness testing circuit can help you streamline the testing process.

Effective Test Item Practice

For optimal test performance, students need to practice each item ahead of time, repeatedly. The practice helps to ensure that the results are based more on true differences in fitness, rather than on knowledge about how to perform the test items. The following are simple suggestions for making this practice worthwhile:

- Discuss and demonstrate the correct techniques (critical elements) involved in each test item. Deliver this information in multiple forms: posters, listed critical steps in word or picture form, or checklists of test steps for self and peer checking.
- Have students practice the test items with a friend. Provide rubrics for students to use during this practice, so that their partner can provide feedback on technique as well as emotional support. Then have them practice and practice some more.
- Make testing stations available during class so that students can self-test regularly. Use posters to guide the students.
- Assign fitness homework that involves parents.
- Send weekly workout reports home.

Encourage students to make their best efforts when they practice the test.

time to show them the appropriate place on the form. The *FITNESSGRAM/ACTIVITYGRAM* software is simple enough for almost all students to be able to enter their own scores. For any of these administrative tasks, you can also train older students and parents to assist you (as long as you ensure the privacy of tested students).

Test Protocols

As mentioned, you should prepare the test setting in advance so that you're ready to supervise, troubleshoot, and discuss results with students during the actual testing. Adequate preparation also makes it easier to record results efficiently. (See "Preparing for Testing" earlier in this chapter.)

FITNESSGRAM test protocols are specifically addressed in the test manual, and most teachers are adept at giving the tests. However, when teachers want to move from a teacher-centered model to a more student-centered model (which helps create students who take personal responsibility for their fitness), the following strategies can increase student adherence to proper test protocols, help students become more skillful at self and peer assessment,

and help make fitness testing a positive experience for both teacher and students:

- Explain the testing procedures and purposes to students over several preceding lessons. Have them practice, practice, practice. Review this information on test days.
- At the stations, use the same posters, rubrics, or task cards (listing the critical elements or common errors) as were used during practice sessions.
- Use drawings or diagrams depicting correct form, and also some depicting common errors.
- Always announce test days in advance. "Pop quiz" fitness testing can lead to negative attitudes toward both fitness testing and physical activity. Remember that if preparation and practice are sufficient, anxiety will be reduced, and with encouragement to do their best, motivation will be maximized.
- Conduct the test under good environmental conditions. Postpone fitness testing if the testing environment is too hot or too cold. Encourage students to dress appropriately. Provide water before, during, and after strenuous tests, such as the PACER or one-mile run.

Set the tone for student-friendly testing by always focusing on personal improvement and by carefully guarding student privacy. Do not allow fitness testing to become a competitive sport. Never compare one student's performance to another's. Refrain from judging student effort. For example, telling a student, "You're not even trying," discourages rather than motivates.

Teach through testing by explaining the concepts behind each test and discussing results with students.

Train and use parent, community, and student volunteers to make test day proceed more smoothly. Be sure to brief them on your testing philosophy.

TEACHING TIP:
Spreading Out Fitness Testing

Instead of administering an entire fitness test battery all at once, you can incorporate fitness testing with other units and activities throughout the school year. Specifically, you can test various health-related fitness components at various times as the assessments match the concepts the students are studying. Students will be more motivated to self-test as they see the connections between concepts, class activities, and testing. This saves time and "kills several birds with one stone," because you are teaching concepts, relating assessment to each concept, and having students practice self-assessment all at once. This can be more beneficial than conducting a formal testing time.

Laura Borsdorf, Professor
Exercise and Sport Science Department
Ursinus College,
Collegeville, Pennsylvania

Tailoring Health-Related Fitness Testing for Your Students

FITNESSGRAM is designed to meet the needs of students within a wide range of abilities. As a general rule, teach and use alternative test items if they fit your program and your students' needs better. For example, in using the one-mile run, if your students represent a wide range of aerobic fitness, you will have many less-fit students running long after the more aerobically fit students have completed the run. This scenario could result in the less-fit youth feeling very self-conscious. In such a case, you might choose the PACER test instead, in which students who are more aerobically fit finish last. Thus, the students with lower fitness levels are far less likely to be "exposed." You can also stagger the start in the one-mile run, so that it is more difficult for others to discern who is running slower. Another idea is to have students of similar ability run in small groups together, at different times or on different days. Ideally, the students would choose which aerobic test they prefer, increasing not only their autonomy, but also their motivation to do their best.

Elementary or Inexperienced Students

Elementary and less experienced students need to practice individual test items more, and they also need more supervision, during both formal and informal testing. Pair younger or inexperienced students with older or more experienced students or adult volunteers for both the test item practice sessions and actual test days. Be sure to thoroughly train your helpers. Consider introducing, teaching, practicing, and then testing each test item in a given time period, perhaps integrating one test item into a three-week skills unit, and then introducing another test item during the next skills unit. For example, focus on flexibility (e.g., back-saver sit-and-reach test item) while teaching an educational gymnastics unit. This approach helps younger and inexperienced students get used to one test item at a time, while teaching them the health-related fitness component in the context of a real life activity. A test circuit may consist of alternating warm-up and test stations, all related to a single health-related fitness component and its corresponding test item.

Middle and High School Students

Be sure to offer older students increasing independence within the context of adequate supervision. Overdirecting students sends the unwelcome and counterproductive message that you consider the students to be incapable of functioning fully in the test situation. Carefully gauge the maturity and understanding levels of each student and strive to provide the right level of independence and self-direction. Viewing yourself as more of a fitness consultant than teacher can help you assume a more low-key role in the testing environment. You can also train older students to help younger or less experienced students learn to be more self-directed. This may motivate the tutor to learn the material to be taught more thoroughly, in order to do a good job teaching another student. Furthermore, it reinforces the main concept that students need to take personal responsibility for assessing and maintaining their personal health and fitness.

Reluctant or Overanxious Students

Some students may have had poor fitness testing experiences in the past or may be more reserved and private than others. Reluctance and anxiety are common emotions in every assessment situation. Create the most positive fitness testing environment you can to help these students and to prevent such problems from developing in other students. As described earlier, one of the best actions you can take is to have students practice the test items frequently, over an extended period of time, before conducting more formal testing. You can also offer a choice of test items that test the same component, such as the PACER, the one-mile run, and the walk test for testing aerobic fitness (for middle or high school students). Work hard to ensure student privacy regarding test scores, and students will learn to trust you. Treat student feelings in a sensitive manner and reassure students that personal achievement is the focus of your program. Finally, allow extremely anxious students to exempt themselves from formal testing, regardless of their reasons. They will still gain a lot from self-test practice, but students gain nothing from being forced to perform in more formal tests. In fact, forcing the issue can reinforce negative feelings toward physical activity—the opposite of the ultimate goal.

Students With Disabilities

In general, where appropriate and possible, you should use the same definitions, components, test items, and standards of health-related fitness for individuals with disabilities as you do for those without disabilities (Lacy and Hastad 2003). You can, however, modify *FITNESSGRAM* to meet the needs of many students with disabilities. You may need, for example, to provide assistance to varying degrees to help the student with a disability perform a test. Or, if the tests do not measure the abilities an individual needs to lead an active and independent life, you may need to select alternative tests. For example, a person who does not have use of the legs may benefit more from testing and developing flexibility in the upper body, rather than of the back and hamstring muscles (CI 2004; Lacy and Hastad 2003).

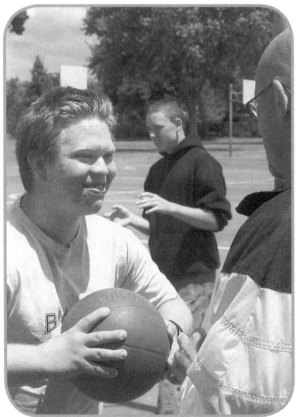

© Human Kinetics

Fitness testing for students with disabilities should measure the individuals' ability to function in everyday activities and should take into account the students' interests.

Health-Related Fitness Tests for Persons With Disabilities

FITNESSGRAM tests can be modified for students with disabilities. Information on how to do this is found in chapter 4 in a section entitled "Considerations for Testing Special Populations" of the *FITNESSGRAM/ACTIVITYGRAM Test Administration Manual,* 3rd edition. As a complement to *FITNESSGRAM,* the Brockport Physical Fitness Test also tests the health-related fitness of individuals with disabilities (Winnick and Short 1999). The Brockport tests are specifically designed to accurately assess the physical fitness of individuals with a wide range of physical and mental disabilities and were developed through Project Target, a research study funded by the U.S. Department of Education.

The Brockport Physical Fitness Test resources include the following:

- The *Brockport Physical Fitness Test Manual*
- The *Brockport Physical Fitness Training Guide*
- The *Brockport Physical Fitness Test Administration Video*
- The Fitness Challenge software

For more information or to order the Brockport Physical Fitness Test Kit or materials, contact Human Kinetics at 800-747-4457 or on the Web at www.HumanKinetics.com.

As you design an individualized fitness program for a person with disabilities, keep in mind that a major reason for fitness testing should be to measure an individual's ability to function in everyday activities. Thus, it's important to look at each individual, assess needs and limitations, and design alternatives to bypass those limitations. An individual's interests should be taken into account as well. For example, if an individual in a wheelchair would like to be able to play wheelchair basketball more proficiently and with greater stamina, the fitness program should work to enhance the person's abilities in this area. Fitness testing should then discern whether or not the person is making progress in areas relevant to enjoying this interest. Whenever possible, the individual should be part of this design process: "A personalized program should be planned with, rather than for, individuals with disabilities" (Winnick 1995).

Using Health-Related Fitness Testing Results Appropriately

Much of the "bad press" related to fitness testing, both in the past and the present, can be attributed to improper use of test results. To help rectify this, you should explain the reasons for the tests to students and parents, use fitness test results to help students

plan for future gains, and use fitness test processes or goal achievement as only one of several means to arrive at a letter grade.

Sharing Results With Students and Parents

Keep in mind, from the first lesson in which you introduce a test item and throughout all formal tests with respect to that item, that you should discuss and explain the reasons for the tests and the meanings behind the results. With students, you can do this as part of your set induction at the beginning of a lesson. Prior to testing, remember to contact parents with a letter that explains your testing philosophy and approach and how you plan to use the results. It is especially important to reassure both students and parents that you will do your utmost to guard student privacy. Share the actual forms you will use to record and interpret the test results, so that all involved can clearly see what you plan to focus on (the relevant forms are provided in the *FITNESSGRAM/ ACTIVITYGRAM Test Administration Manual* and software). You may want to set up the tests during parent nights and take the parents through each of the items as a group. These actions set the stage for clear and productive communication when test results become available.

When sharing test results, use blank *FITNESS-GRAM* forms to review the purpose of the test items and the meaning of the test results. Distribute individual report forms in a private manner, such as in a sealed envelope or during a student–teacher or parent–teacher conference. You may find it helpful to set up a station on a physical activity circuit at which you privately discuss test results, while the rest of the student's group participates in an activity.

Along with test results and interpretations, you should share information and offer guidance on how each student can improve health. Help the student set realistic goals and subgoals at this time as well (see chapter 2 for more on goal setting).

Grading

Despite the difficulty of assigning grades to students, it is a reality that most teachers have to deal with. However, we cannot emphasize enough that *fitness test results should not be used as a basis for grades*.

Lund and Kirk (2002) summarize the appropriate use of health-related fitness assessment as follows:

> Unless results of fitness testing are used to improve student learning, testing should not be done. Additionally, the Physical Education Content Standards call for students to use this information to develop personal fitness improvement programs (NASPE 1995). Performance-based assessment might call for students to create such a plan based on the analysis of personal fitness test results and knowledge of what optimal levels of fitness should be, causing students to use fitness results in a manner that would be helpful to them as adults (p. 15.)

Expanding on this concept, grades can be based on age-appropriate abilities to self-test and interpret test results, as well as on written tests of knowledge of fitness concepts and principles. Assignments relating to the process of how to set goals and plan personal programs are also excellent to grade and include in the summative grade report. Such emphases help students become adults who are physically active for life in self-designed, enjoyable fitness programs. In contrast, grades based solely on test results are likely to discourage students from continuing to be physically active after they leave your program. If you choose to give credit for showing improvement in fitness test scores, remember that improvements will come in smaller increments for students who have already achieved a high level of fitness than for those who have not, and your grad-

ing system should not penalize high-fit students for this reason. Consider reporting the accomplishment of fitness goals as the measure of success and the achievement of a health-enhancing level of physical activity as the basis for feedback to parents. Many teachers send home a grade for physical education and attach a separate *FITNESSGRAM* report as the feedback related to health-related fitness. This method requires no extra work—and is a more authentic and appropriate means to report student test results and health.

Planning

Testing just to test is a waste of both teacher and student time. To be part of authentic assessment, fitness testing must provide feedback to shape your health-related physical fitness education program into the best it can be. So use test results to help both you and your students plan for future learning and fitness gains. For example, if you find that students are making little or no progress in muscular strength and endurance, design and use more activities that enhance these areas. Involve older students in this problem-solving process. Encourage students to set specific process-oriented goals related to the targeted areas, such as "I will do push-ups four times a week, and each week, I will increase the number of push-ups I do by at least one repetition, until I reach my healthy fitness zone. I will then continue to do push-ups four times a week to maintain upper body strength in the healthy fitness zone. If I'm able, I will attempt to continue to increase the number I can do." This helps students learn to tailor their personal fitness programs to their own specific needs. By following up on results, you continue the planning-teaching-assessing-planning cycle.

The misuse of results, inappropriate test selection, and use of insensitive testing protocols have created controversy with respect to the use of fitness testing and the reporting of results. Appropriately applied, however, *FITNESSGRAM* is an excellent health-related fitness test battery that provides an up-to-date and sensitive health-related assessment program that is easy to implement. Use the information in this chapter to plan, conduct, and follow up on fitness testing that teaches students what they need to know to participate throughout their lives in effective, personally designed fitness programs and physical activities.

Guidelines for Appropriate Physical Activity Assessment

Many teachers report that they grade students on effort and participation. This practice is unfair and lacks reliability and consistency because students may have widely varying physical fitness test results and yet be applying similar levels of effort. In fact, students who are obese or less fit actually require greater effort to accomplish even simple movement (such as walking) than students who are already fit or who possess greater muscular strength. **Effort** infers how hard a student tries. Although putting forth effort or trying hard is a highly valued characteristic in a competitive society, the appropriate benchmark for assessment is the authentic assessment and quantification of physical activity frequency, intensity, and time levels that contribute to attainment of the HFZ in each test or component area. Furthermore, effort is directly related to motivational level, and motivation is best enhanced in children by creating a safe learning environment and success experiences. Finally, assessment of effort is laden with bias toward student affect—a student who grumbles may be exhibiting poor affect, yet working hard. Another may grimace, feigning effort, yet actually be expending little or no intense energy. Hence, teachers who rely on the assessment of student effort are more likely measuring their own teaching effectiveness and their ability to motivate students, not actual student achievement. Therefore, the ensuing sections of this chapter will focus on accurate assessment of levels of physical activity—quantifiable through reliable assessment of physiological indicators of progression toward healthy fitness outcomes.

Why Reward Physical Activity Instead of Effort or Results?

The goal of a quality physical education program is to develop a lifelong pattern of physical activity among our total population. This focus is different from other subjects, such as math or driver education, where there is a need to be able to do primary tasks before moving forward. The difference is the desired outcome. Presumably, once you learn to add, subtract, multiply, and divide or learn to drive a car, you'll be able to do it correctly for the rest of your life. However, when it comes to health-related fitness, scores today do not necessarily indicate long-term results. The fifth grader born with the "right" genes might score well on the one-mile run without much effort, whereas a classmate might make a great effort but still record a poor time. However, in the long run, if the student with the good time becomes a "couch potato," and the student with the poor time continues to spend time being active in a variety of different activities, it is likely that the latter student will live a healthier life.

Ultimately, physical educators want a nation of physically active, healthy citizens, not a nation of ex-athletes who follow a couple of years of excellent fitness levels with 50 years of TV watching that results in declining health, high medical bills, and poor productivity. Reward time or persistence in physical activity, because that is what will, in the long run, result in lifelong health and fitness.

It is fine to encourage results, as well as activity time, but this needs to be individualized. The *FITNESSGRAM* criteria help teachers obtain appropriate results for a broad range of individuals, set individual goals for improvement, and provide encouragement for reaching higher levels. For example, did the student with the best one-mile run time in class spend as much time in a target heart rate zone as the individual who took longer to complete the same distance? You might challenge the high achieving student to do even better—to set increased time and distance goals; maybe he or she will end up running cross country and really enjoy it. Encourage excellence! However, don't let that discourage students who don't have the genetic potential to be star athletes but who will benefit just as much from physical activity. Remember, challenge each student individually to be his or her individual physical best, and reward that physical activity time.

Strategies for Assessing Physical Activity

The best strategies for assessing physical activity link fitness concepts such as intensity, frequency, and time to the type of activity. Students may appear to be fairly active when you are casually observing them, but closer assessment of activity data is necessary to determine whether students are truly applying the fitness principles of overload, intensity, and specificity to progress toward lifetime health-related fitness goals.

Logs and Journals

As discussed in chapter 12, logging physical activity information in a table, chart, or journal provides you with evidence of actual total time spent in physical activity. Time alone, however, does not necessarily demonstrate appropriate activity levels. Use these strategies to gain more robust information on activity from logs:

- Teach students to use the perceived exertion scale as shown in figure 13.7 so that they can record these data in their logs as well.

- Look for and graph intensity levels with duration of activities in the logs. Students who do not demonstrate changes over time should be encouraged to examine their goals and revise strategies in their personal plans.

- Incorporate technology effectively by having students use heart rate monitors and pedometers. Recording indicators of intensity such as heart rate or steps over time, in addition to the duration of activity time, increases the efficacy of assessment.

- Depending on your students, you may want to have parents or guardians verify student participation time by signing their child's log or journal periodically.

Heart Rate Monitors

According to Kirkpatrick and Birnbaum (1997), **heart rate monitors** make it possible to fairly and more accurately assess each student's intensity level. Heart rate monitor data provide individualized feedback. Students can use the monitors as a self-assessment tool in the aerobic fitness component of health-related fitness. For example, a high school

6	No exertion at all
7	
8	Extremely light
9	Very light
10	
11	Light
12	
13	Somewhat hard
14	
15	Hard (heavy)
16	
17	Very hard
18	
19	Extremely hard
20	Maximal exertion

Borg RPE scale
© Gunnar Borg, 1970, 1985, 1994, 1998

Figure 13.7 If you teach your students to use the Borg rating of perceived exertion scale, they can record these data in their activity logs.
Reprinted, by permission, from G. Borg, 1998, *Borg's perceived exertion and pain scales* (Champaign, IL: Human Kinetics), 47.

student may find it is no longer possible to elevate the heart rate into the target heart rate zone by walking fast. The student can determine the need to choose to perform a more vigorous aerobic fitness activity, such as jogging or playing one-on-one basketball, to increase aerobic fitness. This process enhances physical activity independence.

As previously detailed in chapter 5, target heart rate zones are not effectively used for younger children (elementary through middle school). However, heart rate monitors can still provide an avenue to motivate young students. You may teach younger students to examine resting heart rate prior to an activity and then compare the difference between exercise heart rate and resting heart rate, thereby incorporating math into the lesson.

You may also want to play a version of heart rate bingo (Kirkpatrick and Birnbaum 1997). Plan your bingo card with a wide range of anticipated resting and exercise heart rates. Provide a card for each child or use a class card. Include a free space on the card where the child may record his or her resting heart rate. At the end of an activity, have the children find their final exercise heart rate or their average heart rate (if using heart rate monitors that track heart rate over the period of activity and provide an average heart rate). Mark this heart rate on either the class bingo card or the child's personal bingo card.

Children keep track of their exercise heart rate each day and begin to fill their card. When a child gets a typical bingo such as a row, column, or diagonal, he or she brings the card to you. You may choose a reward such as being an exercise leader or getting to choose the class activity from a list that you provide. If using a class bingo card, when the class scores a bingo, they get to choose the next class activity from a list you provide (or other incentives you may have developed). This allows the use of heart rate monitors in the classroom to motivate younger students, without using target heart rate zones.

Pedometers

Another good way to quantify physical activity is to count the steps taken daily. **Pedometers** can be used as a motivational tool to provide feedback on the duration (distance) or intensity (distance over time) of the physical activity. Between 9,000 and 10,000 steps has been recommended as the daily number of steps for maintaining a health-enhancing level of activity. However, step counts vary greatly from day to day. Monitoring weekly, rather than daily, steps can help avoid feelings of failure. To begin, have students keep track of their daily steps in a journal and average the first three days. This is the baseline from which they will begin their walking program and set personal goals. Work up to the long-range goals—established by the President's Challenge—of 11,000 steps per day for girls (ages 6-17) and 13,000 steps per day for boys (ages 6-17). Children can also encourage parents to target daily step goals (adults should get 10,000 steps per day, or 12,000 steps if weight loss is a personal goal); this may increase family activity outside of school time. Refer to table 13.1 to assist students in setting step goals.

A free exercise logging tool is available from the President's Challenge Web site at www.presidents challenge.org.

Pedometers may report steps, distance, calories burned, time spent exercising, or heart rate averaged over time. The simplest ones count steps only. Some have the capacity to adjust the stride length. For an average adult, 10,000 steps is approximately 3 miles, and this will be different for children. Teachers can instruct students on how to determine the number of steps per mile. Mark off 100 feet and have students count the number of steps they take in that amount of space. Figuring out the distance between two heelstrikes, or **stride length,** (dividing the number of steps/100 feet), and then dividing 5280 feet by the stride length estimates the student's steps per mile. Providing the formula and task to the math teacher is an excellent strategy to share content across the curriculum—and to inform other teachers about quality physical education at the same time.

Combining the recording of steps with heart rate is an ideal format for combining the concepts of time (distance traveled) with intensity. Increasing either the number of steps or the heart rate provides the overload needed for appropriate progressions to enhance cardiorespiratory endurance—aerobic fitness.

Chapter 2 contains information about the Presidential Active Lifestyle Award (PALA). The PALA is an embroidered blue presidential emblem accompanied by a certificate signed by the president of the United States. Students who are active for 60 minutes per day, five days a week, for six weeks are eligible to receive this award. The award can also be earned by keeping track of steps per day using a pedometer (see page 24).

TABLE 13.1　Setting Step Goals

Start point	Goal	How to reach goal	Time needed
Less than 2,500 steps	5,000 steps/day	Increase 250 steps/day	10-20 days
2,501-5,000 steps	7,500 steps/day	Increase 300 steps/day	8-16 days
5,001-7,500 steps	10,000 steps/day	Increase 400 steps/day	6-12 days
7,501-10,000 steps	12,500 steps/day	Increase 500 steps/day	5-10 days
10,001-12,501 steps	15,000 steps/day	Increase 500 steps/day	5-10 days

*From Sportline's Guide to Walking (Sportline, Inc, Campbell, CA)

Using Physical Activity Assessment Results Appropriately

Many questions arise when deciding how to use participation or physical activity data appropriately. Should you set a minimum out-of-school physical activity participation level for a grade (e.g., three hours per week is an A)? What if the child's family or day care situation makes engaging in physical activity outside of school difficult? Should you fault the student who cannot yet run properly but who is trying hard to learn? What about the child who participates in many extracurricular activities but does not keep a journal up-to-date and is unable to quantify the activity levels accurately? Use the following information to deal with these common dilemmas in ways that encourage, rather than discourage, physical activity participation and, therefore, improve health-related fitness.

Sharing Information With Students and Parents

Keeping parents informed in these areas helps you gain their support. As suggested in chapter 12, communicate through conferences, detailed report cards, and newsletters. Be sure to inform everyone—both students and parents—ahead of time what you're looking for in terms of physical activity level. By sending home current *FITNESS-GRAM* and *ACTIVITYGRAM* printouts that provide information that links assessment to strategies and goals for each child, parents will also learn what they need to know to be able to help students accomplish goals. Make clear your view on the child who does not possess outstanding motor skills but who persists and progresses toward goals. Make accommodations for students whose family situations make it difficult for them to participate in physical activity outside of school. These tactics help individualize your approach and prevent many misunderstandings, especially when assessing the fairly subjective idea of effort.

Follow up further by making yourself available for parent and student consultation. Help each individual set goals based on your feedback and the student's personal objectives (see chapters 2 and 12). Brainstorm with the family who finds it difficult to fit in physical activity because of work, day care, and neighborhood situations. Teachers using *FITNESS-GRAM* reports and goal setting in this manner have found that parents become the best advocates for quality physical education, and the added bonus is that they have fought hard to keep or increase the physical education time and requirements for these programs.

Grading

Once again, it is important to be up front with students and parents regarding what weight, if any, you will give physical activity level in the final grade. Be sure to reward and praise the achievement of physical activity goals—and progress toward goals. Remember, the gifted athlete who does not try to do his or her personal best is not getting nearly as many benefits from physical activity as the less gifted child who participates fully. Possessing fitness skill knowledge does not do any good for an individual who does not know how to apply it to the greatest benefit. It can be difficult to be the judge and jury deciding how much effort a child puts forth. Be sure to use a variety of assessment tools as described in this chapter (and other chapters in part IV) to support the grades you assign.

Teachers who include activity in the grades of students owe it to the students to provide an accurate and authentic accounting of scores when assigning grades. Frequency, intensity, and time can be quantified and evaluated effectively through the review of student reflection in journal entries, achievement of goals, records of intensity and duration of activity, and portfolios that demonstrate participation regularly in a variety of outside activities.

Planning

As with other areas we have examined, all worthwhile assessment feeds back into the planning process. If students are not making adequate progress toward personal goals, consider the program and its motivational components. Remember that enjoyment and fun are the primary motivational components for children. Of critical importance, too, are the feelings of emotional safety and comfort when participating with others. While it is easy to assign blame to students for not trying, the physical educator's job involves creating a climate where students can learn, feel safe, and develop competence.

Summary

By sensitively and authentically assessing physical fitness and physical activity, you will help students see that the two go hand in hand and can be used to monitor their health-related physical fitness and to reduce their risk factors across their lifetime. When students are involved in self-testing and logging of time, duration, or intensity of activity, they become further empowered to self-assess, to make decisions to change unhealthy behaviors, and to use effective strategies for adopting more healthy habits. If your students improve in these areas while under your supervision, you will have made great progress toward reaching the Physical Best goal of helping students become physically active for a lifetime.

CHAPTER

14

Chapter Contents

Assessing Fitness Knowledge, Self-Responsibility, and Attitudes

For all the time and energy assessment takes, it's important to use the information you collect to the greatest advantage. Whenever you're not sure how to use assessment data, simply ask yourself if your use of it furthers a student's chances of reaching the ultimate goal—that of increasing and maintaining physical activity, and carrying that activity into adulthood. In this chapter, we discuss tools and strategies for assessing fitness knowledge (the cognitive domain), personal responsibility, and attitudes (the affective domain).

Assessing Fitness Knowledge: The Cognitive Domain

Helping students gain health-related **fitness knowledge** is a crucial component of a quality physical fitness education program for many reasons:

■ Knowledge of physical fitness and personal exercise behavior are related. People tend to make a personal investment in activities that have meaning (Carron, Hausenblas, and Estabrooks 2003).

■ Understanding the science behind health-related physical fitness exercises prepares students to sort fact from fiction when reading advertisements for quick weight loss plans or new "miracle" exercise equipment.

■ Knowing how to exercise, such as appropriate stretching, correct strength-training techniques, and proper hydration, prepares students to safely benefit from physical activity.

■ Knowledgeable students are better prepared to make informed decisions in starting and maintaining physical activity programs.

To find out what your students have learned about fitness and what they still need to learn, you need to periodically assess their knowledge. As teachers consider the limited time available for physical activity each day and week, a dilemma arises about the trade-off between time spent assessing knowledge and the resulting time taken away from physical activity. On the one hand, the goal of Physical Best and the Healthy People 2010 plan (USDHHS 2000aa) is to increase daily activity. On the other hand, teachers are asked to integrate more assessment. How can you accomplish this?

The key to meeting both objectives is to assess students' fitness knowledge through alternative assessment tools and strategies, to reduce reliance on traditional written tests, and to move toward more authentic and direct methods such as brief questions, interviews, and after-class projects. Asking for student opinions can reveal knowledge level and takes very little time. In this final assessment chapter, the goal is to share several practical assessment tools and tips that you can use without taking much time away from physical activities.

Useful Tools for Assessing Fitness Knowledge

Cognitive assessment needs to be manageable and reflect what you have taught. Most experts recom-

mend that formal testing consume no more than 10 percent of total instructional time (Baumgartner and Jackson 1999; Lacy and Hastad 2003). Keep these parameters in mind as you review the assessment tools that can be applied to the cognitive domain, and remember that informal testing can be an effective substitute for formal assessment (see chapter 12).

Discussions, Polls, and Role Plays

Discussions that include questions centered on important fitness concepts, polls asking students which technique is correct (A or B?), and role plays are viable methods for assessing general student knowledge. The limitations of these techniques are that they enable students who don't know or understand concepts to hide or follow the responses of other students.

Written Tests

Written tests still have their place as a valid assessment tool. Be sure you do not overemphasize or overvalue them. Design written tests to parallel what you've taught and to cover important cognitive objectives, so that you can collect assessment data on what each individual knows and doesn't know. Carefully choose the format (e.g., objective tests—multiple-choice, true-false; subjective tests—short-answer, essay) that best fits the content you're teaching and the ages and abilities of the students you're testing. Consider take-home tests and computer-formatted tests that are taken out of class. Although the potential for cheating exists, looking up correct answers is a proven method of exposing students to a thorough review of important concepts.

Logs and Journals

Journal and log entries allow students to track physical activity data and record physiological and psychological reactions to physical activity. But you can also have students record their personal responses to discussion questions in their journals, allowing you to assess the level of student understanding. Student reflections provide information on the breadth and depth of knowledge related to the importance of or reasons for participation in activities, and they provide opportunities for students to demonstrate what they've learned using their own words.

Reports and Research Assignments

Reports and research assignments can enhance a student's learning across the entire school curriculum. Most upper elementary through high school students are capable of learning to research a topic. The ability to research is a life skill that is in line with most schools' overall mission to prepare students to learn how to learn. Certainly, research has its place in health-related physical fitness education. Through research, students take what they already know about health-related fitness and teach themselves more. Then you assess the quality and value of each student's research in relation to how it might help him or her pursue an active lifestyle.

Mohnsen (1997) asserts the following: "Research is a viable option related to every standard that has a cognitive component. As a physical educator, however, you must be sure that students possess the necessary skills to conduct the research." Work with teachers in other subject areas, such as language arts, math, and science, to help students develop research skills and to coordinate the writing of health-related fitness reports. Encourage use of the Internet, library books, and CD-ROMs as research tools. Consider having students work with partners or in small groups to collect data but report on it individually. Try assigning topics such as the following:

- Select an athlete, movie star, singer, or some other celebrity and research what that person does (or doesn't do) to stay physically active and fit. Pretend you are this person's personal trainer, and write an analysis of this person's personal fitness plan, based on what you've learned about health-related fitness. What does this person do well and what does this person do less well regarding fitness? Then make suggestions on what this person could do to improve his or her plan. If you believe the plan is already excellent, show why you think this. Either way, be sure to address each component of health-related fitness.

- Select a specific health condition (for example, cancer, diabetes, asthma, heart disease), and research what benefits physical activity can have in helping a person with this condition improve his or her health.

- Find diet ideas and products advertised and analyze them for safety, effectiveness, and value to health.

Another option when working with elementary or less experienced students is to provide "raw" research information in lecture settings and have students briefly summarize it orally or in writing. Here is another example of a developmental approach to research:

Step 1: Provide a Web site for them to open and print out as a simple and less threatening beginning to using electronic resources. Have them bring in the printout, and the grade is based on task accomplishment.

Step 2: Provide one or two Web sites. Have the students read and explore linked sites and print out the pages explored.

Step 3: Progress to having students reflect on the Web readings in journals or through responses to specific questions aligned with critical concepts.

Although having students create reports is appropriate at times, beware of spending too much physical education time on having students research, write, or share them. As mentioned, work with teachers across other disciplines to save physical education class time. Use such assignments as homework. Post reports in the gymnasium or display them at health fairs, parent events, or in the library. If you want to have students report orally, only have a few do so each day, until all have had a turn.

Projects

Projects allow students to use avenues of communication other than the written word to create products from their research and what you've taught them. The following is a list of sample group or individual project ideas you might use or adapt to assess fitness knowledge:

- Students design a strength-training circuit.

- Students create an audiotape explaining how body composition stems from the other components of health-related fitness.

- Students make a "newscast" video (or untaped skit) to dispel the latest health-related fitness myths.

- Students act out a commercial to sell physical activity to a "couch potato."

- Students write questions and answers that the class could use in a TV game show format on a rainy day or other designated time.

- Students prepare a collage of healthy foods and post it in the school cafeteria.

- Students assess the nutritional qualities of the foods in school vending machines and make suggestions on how to change eating habits during school hours.

■ If students work in small groups, you should design a method for assessing individual learning to use in tandem with the group activity, such as a short written test or journal entry as a follow-up assignment.

Work to use cognitive assessment as a teaching tool—not just a check for current understanding. You can do this by discussing each item on a returned written test, by having students share their research or projects with classmates (perhaps at one station in a circuit), by asking students how they think you can help them learn more, and by helping students design cognitive self-assessments and learning activities that they feel will be helpful to them and their peers. You might also borrow a TV game show format, such as *Jeopardy*, to liven up review sessions.

Grading and Cognitive Assessment

Remember, assessing and grading are not quite the same. But, at a certain point, you may need to assign a grade. A grade in physical education should convey to students and parents how an individual is progressing toward important standards in each learning domain (see chapter 12). For example, a student who does not understand health-related fitness concepts should not receive a good grade in physical education for merely behaving in class and trying hard. Instead, giving separate grades for affective, physical, and cognitive performances conveys a more accurate picture of student achievement of standards and desired learning outcomes.

Today's health-related physical fitness education program values knowledge as an important aspect of reaching the ultimate goal of producing adults who value and can independently pursue physical activity. Thus, assessment of knowledge needs to be part of a student's physical education grade. Fitness knowledge is a vital component in a well-designed physical education program, making it well worth the time it takes to assess. The following list summarizes ways to make the assessment process more meaningful and efficient:

■ Use less formal (less paperwork) methods, such as role playing and discussions, to screen for basic understanding.

■ Only occasionally use more formal methods, such as written tests.

■ Limit formal nonactivity testing time to about 10 percent of total instructional time.

■ Make sure you assess what you have taught, not what you planned to teach but didn't quite cover.

■ Use a variety of assessment tools.

■ Use knowledge assessment results as only part of a grade, and communicate your exact intentions to parents and students.

■ Alter your plans once you know what your students know.

■ Assess your students' ability to apply their knowledge.

Assessing Personal Responsibility

When students leave a quality physical fitness education program, they should be prepared to apply their health-related fitness knowledge and skills. In this section, we focus primarily on how to answer the following question: Can and does each student actually apply the knowledge in meaningful ways? This is an essential process in producing students who are capable of engaging safely and profitably in physical activity after they leave your program. Indeed, students who have mastered fitness skills have moved closer to independence on Corbin and Lindsey's Stairway to Lifetime Fitness (figure 9.1) and closer to mature levels of personal responsibility for their own physical activity (Hellison 2003).

Useful Tools for Assessing Personal Responsibility

As discussed in chapters 12 and 13, students need to develop many skills to become **self-reliant** in health-related fitness activities. Of course, exactly what you target for assessment directly depends on your curriculum (that is, what you've taught) and on what is age appropriate. For example, it is appropriate to expect kindergartners to be able to place a hand over the heart to "check" heart rate and to understand that a faster heartbeat means the heart is working harder, but not to count the pulse or calculate target heart rate zone. This section explores the tools necessary for assessing whether a student can and does apply his or her fitness knowledge.

Teacher Observations

A quick, informal way to see if students know how to apply fitness information is simply to observe them performing fitness skills and see if they are working on assigned tasks or goals as you circulate around the activity area. To take a closer look, post yourself at a station on a circuit and target a specific skill to check for. Videotaping a skill, such as a student's running stride, can better allow both you and the student to determine if he or she uses pacing correctly. Before an observation, determine the critical elements you want to see. A short checklist or rubric works well to help you focus during the observation. Asking students what their fitness goal is for the day also checks to see if they are working with purpose and self-direction.

Rubrics

Add a rubric to an observation, recording critical or missing elements, and it becomes more formal. Students can use rubrics to assess themselves and peers. This teaches students to analyze themselves so that they can continue to do so after your program. Keep in mind, too, that rubrics provide structure and focus, helping keep students on task. Figure 14.1 shows a rubric to assess jogging stride. Teachers can use rubrics created by others but are encouraged to develop their own rubrics designed to incorporate the specific learning outcomes from a unit. A rubric will include technique or critical elements. Students should be able to observe a peer and determine if form is correct. If not correct, students should be able to identify the errors and provide corrective feedback.

To use rubrics effectively for this purpose, teachers should ensure that rubrics

- are provided to students before assessing them to help guide their practice and application attempts,
- include a space marked "don't know" (to assess the knowledge of the peer assessor),

---

Jogging Criteria

Doer 1 _____   Date _____

Doer 2 _____   Class _____

Level III

Observer: Give the doer some pointers about his or her jogging form. Use the tips below to help you. Try to be friendly.

Doer: Jog at a moderate pace. When the teacher signals, slow down—then change roles.

	DOER 1			DOER 2		
	Yes	No	Don't Know	Yes	No	Don't Know
1. Runs tall, leans slightly forward.						
2. Swings legs from hip, knees bent.						
3. Lands on heels with weight rolling along the outside portion of foot to toes.						
4. Points toes straight ahead, lands heel directly under knees.						
5. Swings arms straight forward and backward, hands relaxed.						
6. Breathes from stomach in an even rhythm.						

■ **Figure 14.1** A rubric for assessing running stride. A reproducible version of this rubric is available in appendix A.

Adapted, by permission, from S.J. Virgilio, 1997, *Fitness education for children: Team approach* (Champaign, IL: Human Kinetics), 20.

▨ accurately reflect and identify the components and critical elements that the teacher has taught, and that are important to performing the skill safely,

▨ include only the components that the teacher has told students they'll be assessed on,

▨ list standards to assess by, and

▨ state components and standards clearly.

Role Plays

As an extension of class discussions, role playing is an effective way to assess whether or not students can apply fitness knowledge. Set up role play situations that call for students to demonstrate fitness skills in a real-life context. The following are examples of role play challenges that help a teacher determine fitness skill competence.

▨ The student practices how to teach a younger student to run correctly as pace changes. The student should demonstrate knowledge of the components of a good running stride.

▨ The student demonstrates two ways to take a pulse.

▨ With students in small groups, one student in each group teaches three safe stretches to the rest of the group, and explains what makes them safe.

▨ The student pretends that a partner has sprained an ankle. The student demonstrates how to help the partner treat the injury safely following the RICES guidelines (rest, ice, compression, elevation, support).

▨ One student takes the role of a famous local athlete. Other students interview this person to find out what the person has done to improve his or her athletic achievement (adapted from NASPE 1995).

Be sure to provide any necessary equipment for students to practice using, such as a clock with a second hand for counting heart rate or an "ice pack" (e.g., beanbag) for a sprained ankle.

Role playing simulates real-life situations, giving students valuable practice even as you assess their competence. Remember, assessment that teaches is a more efficient and effective way to use precious class time.

Middle School Assessment Example

Effective assessment requires a plan. Here's one example of how to plan assessments for middle school students.

Establish Desired Course Outcome

A physically educated person assesses, achieves, and maintains physical fitness.

Define Domain Analysis (What Will Be Assessed)

▨ Creation of and participation in a personal plan of activities and exercises to achieve and maintain a level of physical fitness determined by the needs and goals of the student

▨ Application of principles of training and FITT Guidelines

▨ Management of personal lifestyle and responsibilities for inclusion of participation in regular physical activity

Select Dimension Components (Which Dimensions Are Most Important)

This assessment is intended to determine mastery of both the processes (principles of training and management of adult life roles) and the product (participation and goals). Assess and score each student on an individual basis with the results used for the purpose of prescribing further

☞

sequential instruction, including remediation and enrichment. Focus on achieving cumulative skills and knowledge, resulting from multiple units of study on fitness education, goal setting, and motivation. Achievement will occur through participation in and out of the gymnasium. All students in the system will be assessed as a requirement for promotion to the high school level work.

Identify Implementation Characteristics (What Other Issues Need to Be Considered)

The student will design a personal fitness profile to be used to plan a realistic personal program of regular physical activity. The profile will use the results of previous health-related fitness tests, recognized standards for fitness levels for good health, and personally set goals. Allow instructional time for students to master the skills of fitness testing, review the requirements of the assessment, and assist students in researching information needed for both the profile and the plan. In addition, conference time outside of class may be needed to provide feedback relative to accuracy and completeness in designing, implementing, and reporting progress toward achievement of the assessment. The focus of this assessment on life skills for adult roles requires that students be responsible for solving the same problems related to engaging in regular physical activity that adults do. Therefore, the teacher becomes an advisor who guides the search for information.

Establish Specifications (What the Student Will Do)

Each student will complete a personal fitness profile (test results, current status of health fitness levels, and personally established realistic goals), create a personal fitness plan, implement the personal fitness plan (including appropriate warm-up, workout, and cool-down activities and principles of training and conditioning), and report on the results of participation in the plan. (Sample forms are provided in appendix A.) Achievement will be determined based on the following criteria:

- Accurately assess and interpret personal fitness status
- Set appropriate and realistic goals to improve or maintain fitness status
- Apply principles of training and conditioning in designing the personal plan
- Document (accurately and neatly) implementation of the designed plan
- Achieve personal fitness goal
- Reflect on enjoyment, benefits, and risks of participation in physical activity

Administration

This assessment, including scoring, should be presented to the students at the beginning of the school year. You may spend several class periods reviewing the skills required for assessing fitness status, interpreting personal data, and determining research needs and procedures. Time lines for the completion of each component should be established to ensure completion by deadline dates. Students may work in pairs when fitness status, goals, interests, and accessibility for implementing personal plans are similar.

Adapted, by permission, from PSAHPERD, 1994, *Designing assessments: Applications for physical education*, 39-45.

Logs and Journals

Students can learn to log physical activity participation information in their journals. As discussed in chapter 12, being able to review this information over time is highly motivating. Activity charts and graphs help students see evidence of how far they've progressed. This process can help students stay motivated as adults, as well. The continued self-monitoring helps create greater awareness of the real-life applications of health-related training principles. In assessing whether or not students can apply knowledge and comply with self-improvement behaviors, journal reflections rather than activity logs are most critical for providing teachers with information about student levels of understanding.

An example related to aerobic training and the use of the PACER is a good illustration. The student records the number of laps completed in three trials over six weeks. The log is the record of the number of laps. The teacher remarks on the progress of the student—and then asks the student to write how he feels today at the end of the PACER, and to compare that to his feelings on the first attempt. The teacher also asks the student to reflect on or consider why it would feel easier now than before to complete laps, or what the student might want to do to increase the number of laps in the next three weeks.

Goals

Students who can write personal goals and plan a personalized fitness program based on log and journal data are demonstrating the ability to apply fitness knowledge in the most appropriate fashion. Teachers should make a point of checking student goals, as well as progress toward goals. Students who set goals that are too easily or quickly accomplished are not comprehending the knowledge base or skills necessary for lifetime health and fitness.

Projects

Well-designed group and individual projects provide the time and space for students to thoroughly demonstrate how to apply fitness knowledge. The following are some examples of effective project assignments:

- The student designs and makes a poster that outlines an interesting aerobic fitness workout.

- The student keeps a log of the physical activity done outside of physical education class.

- The student designs a calendar for the month. The student should consider the FITT guidelines as she fills in each day's strategies (e.g., doing strength exercises on alternate days) and should address each component of health-related fitness.

- The student makes a resource file (using three-by-five-inch cards) of physical activities to do with family, by himself, at school, in the neighborhood, and with a friend. Then the student demonstrates that he has used the file over a three-week period by recording his activities in his journal.

The *Physical Best Activity Guides* offer many additional project ideas.

Portfolios

As outlined in chapter 12, a portfolio provides a comprehensive way to look at an individual student. A well-designed portfolio can provide valuable insights into a student's overall participation in physical activity, both in and out of school. The portfolio gives the student a chance to showcase mementos—certificates, ribbons, and so forth—that demonstrate his or her lifetime activities:

- Ribbons earned for running in 10K races

- Certificates earned for supporting community fund-raisers through walking

- Certificates for completing "Hoops for Heart" or "Jump Rope for Heart" events

- Workout logs from weight rooms or health clubs

- Reflections of feelings regarding how his or her self-image has changed as a result of any of these activities

A portfolio that reflects an enthusiasm for physical activity through a variety of extracurricular events, interests, and lifestyle activities with friends and family members indicates a student who values physical activity.

Timing Is Everything

Perhaps the most significant change Marian Franck (retired from McCaskey High School, Lancaster, Pennsylvania) made to her assessment program was when she gave assessment forms to students. The first year she used the forms, she passed them out at the end of the fitness unit and expected students to follow the fitness plan on the forms outside of class, while the class moved on to another unit. At that time, her fitness unit consisted of four lessons on each component of health-related fitness over a nine-week unit. The unit's final exam was completing the written plan using this form. She was disappointed when only about a quarter of the class could complete it to a meaningful level—that is, prepare an appropriate plan based on their decisions about the health-related component on which they chose to focus.

The second year, Marian spent three lessons summarizing the health-related components, did an initial fitness test to give students benchmark information about their status in all components, and then asked the students to select one on which they would focus for the rest of the nine weeks. She believes that this is when she really began to teach in a meaningful way, and behavior changes and fitness test scores reflected this. While it did mean managing five different components being worked on in the class at the same time, providing resource materials for all components at the same time, and monitoring the written and physical activity work of five different groups of students, much better communication with each individual resulted. This led to far more "need-to-know" questions and the teaching opportunities these bring. At the same time, there was very little repetition, because only those students who did not know something had to be taught.

The results were stunning! Students brought informational resources from home, athletes passed on learning to teammates, and self-testing skills skyrocketed. Students needed much less teacher guidance because they were so enthusiastic about what they were working on—because they chose their focus and goals. For example, students adhered to test protocols with less teacher prompting. Most important, discipline problems were minimized, because students felt empowered and engaged. At the end of the unit, she asked students to rewrite their plans, focusing on the same or a different component, and to continue using the plan outside of class during the next quarter. This time, using the form and activity as a final exam was authentic. To keep tabs on the implementation of plans, she required weekly reports to indicate regular physical activity participation, which were counted as homework over the next nine weeks, while the class moved on to another unit.

Marian learned that teaching students to be responsible for their own learning is a whole set of skills to cover in themselves. Once the students learn these skills, the process goes more quickly and smoothly. Moreover, individualizing instruction to include personal choice and realistic personal goals provides the incentive to try learning new things, even if a student has already decided he or she is not interested.

Personal Responsibility and Grading

We do not advocate giving a single grade in physical education, nor on grading students on fitness scores. Yet, in real life, teachers may have no choice but to assign a single letter grade. With standards-based education, assessment and grading should directly measure and reflect the desired learning outcomes. But, where and how does taking personal responsibility for health and fitness fit neatly into the grading scheme?

Referencing back to the NASPE Standards provides some specific answers to this question. According to four of the six NASPE standards, the role of personal responsibility is viewed as central to a quality physical education program and physical activity behaviors relect the physically educated student. So, central to any authentic grading scheme is assessment of whether or not students:

- Participate regularly in physical activity (#3);
- achieve and maintain a health-enhancing level of physical fitness (#4);
- exhibit responsible personal and social behavior that respects self and others in physical activity settings (#5); and
- value physical activity provides opportunities for health, enjoyment, challenge, self-expression, and/or social interaction (#6).

Personal responsibility is reflected behaviorally by monitoring and identifying student compliance with positive physical activity behaviors, and by student application of knowledge about health-related fitness in their daily activity. Teachers who focus upon student behaviors and identify the behaviors that are tied into the grade will find their students to be less threatened by the grade, and more motivated to change.

The purpose of grading should be to monitor physical activity and to report students' progress toward maintaining daily physical activity behaviors to parents. Changes in student behavior in the direction of the desired outcomes reflects learning, and to quantify such changes, programs such as the *ACTIVITYGRAM* are useful tools. Grading on the completion of activity logs, journal entries, and regular *ACTIVITYGRAMs* are logical tools to use to determine the level of students' compliance with physical activity goals. Using a system whereby students enter data themselves, and grading them on whether or not they comply with and complete the self-assessment assignment is an authentic reflection of the assumption of personal responsibility.

Quantifying the days of compliance, or number of entries becomes an easy record-keeping task for teachers to score and include in a grade. It is also more accurate than teacher observation of participation level or of dressing for participation. Furthermore, the student reflection becomes the basis for personal goal setting that leads to increases in daily physical activity. A student should be asked to reflect on statements such as: "Can and do I actually apply fitness knowledge in meaningful ways?"

Keep in mind that knowledge without the ability to apply it will not lead to adults who are physically active for life. Each student who passes through your program, then, must become equipped and empowered to seek fitness independently. For the second grader, this may mean, for example, knowing that "huffing and puffing" is a signal that the exercise is beneficial to the heart. For the seventh grader, this may mean being able to keep accurate accounts of physical activities to quantify the personal benefit of his participation. For the high school senior, this may mean regular participation in physical activity in a self-designed fitness program, as evidenced by setting personal goals and quantifying activity levels through technology such as pedometers and heart rate monitors.

Learning Self-Responsibility

The addition of a student interactive component is a feature of *FITNESSGRAM/ ACTIVITYGRAM*, revision 6.0. Students can enter their own scores into the student version of the software. The interactive software allows students to learn more about fitness and the importance of physical activity. By entering their own scores, students will also learn that fitness is personal and that they can take responsibility for their own fitness and physical activity.

Assessing Attitudes and Values: The Affective Domain

As with the cognitive and physical domains of physical education, parents need to know how their child is doing in the affective domain. With the ultimate goal of having your students become adults who value and enjoy physical activity as an important lifestyle choice, being tuned in to each student's **attitude** and motivation level is vital. But how should you go about deciding if an individual's attitude is "good" or motivation is "high"? Then what do you do with this information? Certainly, if you want students to be honest, you should not penalize anyone for revealing a dislike of an activity or of physical activity in general.

Useful Tools for Assessing Attitude and Motivation

Assessing attitudes toward physical activity necessitates assessing the affective domain. Authentic assessment in health-related physical fitness education will examine each student's desire to be active in the real world—outside of class. Students who exhibit behaviors of avoidance of physical activity should be surveyed or interviewed about their beliefs and their feelings about activities and also about physical education class.

Research into the reasons some students dislike physical education class and physical activity ties directly into the social or environmental factors surrounding the activity settting. Teachers who respond to student needs and interests with age-appropriate programming, who offer choice activities, and who provide a psychologically safe and supportive learning environment can help change student attitudes toward activity. Students are motivated when they can identify with the social group (class) and feel accepted by class members, when they are provided choice and feel they have some control, when they see the relevance of activities (through personal goals), and when they feel competent and capable of succeeding (Carron, Hausenblas, and Estabrooks 2003).

Therefore, the primary way to initially motivate students is to conduct a fun program in a supportive, caring, and well-managed environment. Then, to assess attitude and motivation, you must find ways to monitor not only a student's in-class attitude and motivation level, but also the student's self-initiated participation in physical activity outside your program.

The difficult part can be determining whether students are participating to get a good grade or simply because they want to, or whether students are unhappy because of the activity, their friends, the environment, or the teacher. Teachers hope students participate for the joy they find in physical activity, not for stickers or points. But the fact is that younger students rely on rewards externally provided, and older ones rely on social support.

You can assess attitude and motivation in a variety of formal and informal ways, many of which are also used in assessing cognitive knowledge. The best use of motivation data is to use it to alter your teaching. You cannot mandate that students be happy when they are not. Be sure, therefore, that you let the students know that their honest responses will help you make the class fun AND helpful to them. Then, make it safe for students to respond honestly. Here, we look at several specific strategies for monitoring and assessing attitude and motivation.

Discussions

Discussions can encourage students to share how they feel about an activity at the end of a lesson and can help you assess attitude and motivation. Ask questions such as the following:

- How do you feel about running the mile?
- How do you feel about stretching at home while watching TV?
- How do you feel about continuing to design ball games that help increase aerobic fitness?
- How do you feel about today's activity?

Although class discussions can put you on the spot more than private responses can, encourage students to respond honestly by letting them know you accept their opinions. For example, if a student proclaims, "That was the stupidest activity ever!" refrain from taking offense. Instead, ask probing questions that may uncover more helpful information, such as, "You sound frustrated, Joe. Can you tell us one part of the activity you found especially frustrating?" Then put the responsibility back on students by asking questions such as, "Class, how can we make this activity more helpful to people who were as frustrated as Joe?" Through this process, you teach students to be physical activity problem solvers—a powerful life skill to possess.

Discussion can also begin from written questionnaires you assign as homework, such as the one shown in figure 14.2, which is appropriate for upper elementary students. Follow up by reviewing student answers and discussing results with students in a future lesson. Consider making such questionnaires anonymous to increase the likelihood that students will be completely honest.

Polls

Quick polls after class help when you don't have enough time for a full discussion but still want to get a general feel for what students think of an activity. In addition, some types of poll taking also allow for anonymity.

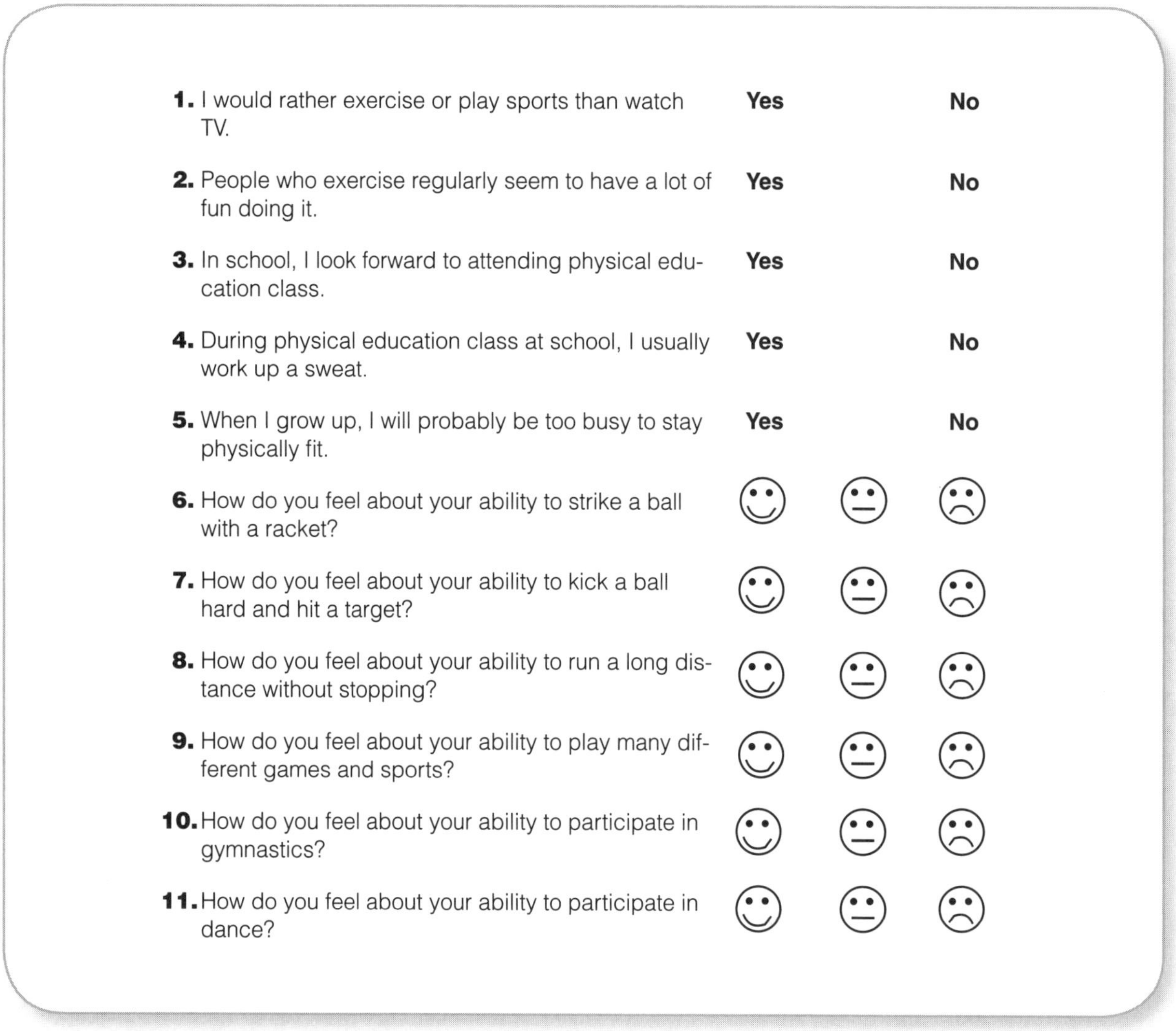

1. I would rather exercise or play sports than watch TV.   **Yes**   **No**

2. People who exercise regularly seem to have a lot of fun doing it.   **Yes**   **No**

3. In school, I look forward to attending physical education class.   **Yes**   **No**

4. During physical education class at school, I usually work up a sweat.   **Yes**   **No**

5. When I grow up, I will probably be too busy to stay physically fit.   **Yes**   **No**

6. How do you feel about your ability to strike a ball with a racket?   🙂 😐 🙁

7. How do you feel about your ability to kick a ball hard and hit a target?   🙂 😐 🙁

8. How do you feel about your ability to run a long distance without stopping?   🙂 😐 🙁

9. How do you feel about your ability to play many different games and sports?   🙂 😐 🙁

10. How do you feel about your ability to participate in gymnastics?   🙂 😐 🙁

11. How do you feel about your ability to participate in dance?   🙂 😐 🙁

Figure 14.2 Discussion can begin from written questions you assign as homework. A reproducible version of this figure is available in appendix A.

Reprinted, by permission, from G. Graham, 1992, *Teaching children physical education* (Champaign, IL: Human Kinetics), 159.

- For younger students, Graham (1992) suggests conducting a "smiley face exit poll." Students can deposit a smiley, neutral, or frowny face in a coffee can as they leave the lesson in answer to a question you have posed.

- Upper elementary and middle school students may respond with a thumbs-up or thumbs-down to indicate what they are thinking.

- High school students may prefer to mark a simple ballot or write "yes" or "no" on a slip of paper to turn in anonymously.

Hellison's *Teaching Responsibility Through Physical Activity* (2003) provides a variety of teacher strategies for student self-assessment with respect to their attitudes toward self and others during physical activity; this book is recommended reading for all teachers at the middle and high school levels. If responses are mostly negative, ask follow-up questions during the next lesson to help you plan how to better meet student needs and interests.

Role Plays

Role playing is a dynamic way to monitor attitude and motivation. Have groups of students act out how they feel about an activity or how they might change another person's opinion about physical activity. First, have groups brainstorm possible actions and statements among themselves. Next, have each group act out their ideas for the rest of the class. Then, discuss as a class which statements and actions are most likely to be helpful in a real-life situation. Ask students for suggestions of other issues they'd like to explore in this way.

Logs and Journals

Logs and journals provide a method for individual students to respond to your program privately. As a homework assignment, journaling offers the time to reflect and respond thoughtfully. Affective entries can simply be individual responses to discussion questions, or they can be more involved, such as logging feelings toward physical activity over several exercise sessions. Hichwa (1998) found it helpful to have his middle school students list the top 10 reasons why students enjoy physical education. He then found it personally and professionally helpful to list the 10 most important aspects of physical education (see figure 14.3).

Rubrics

Rubrics have been used successfully in many subject areas to assess affective performance. You can design rubrics that target, for example, such social behaviors as cooperating in a group (see figure 14.4) or atti-

tudes and levels of motivation (see figure 14.5). These examples are self-assessments, because this approach helps make students aware of important behaviors and attitudes. They also function as surveys of student attitudes and social behaviors, helping students reflect on their own affective development.

Portfolios

Portfolios can also provide invaluable insights into a student's overall attitude and motivation level. A portfolio that reflects the minimum of work in all areas may indicate the student is not very interested in physical activity. In contrast, a portfolio that reflects an enthusiasm for physical activity through up-to-date, detailed logs and thoughtful journal answers may indicate a student who values physical activity. Be careful, however, to confirm your hunches, because students with learning disabilities may have difficulty expressing their feelings in writing, and a student eager to please may mislead you. Of course, making such judgments can be a touchy issue. These extremes call for further investigation, perhaps in the form of private teacher–student conferences. You should also be sure to view the portfolio as a whole.

Students' Top 10 List	Teachers' Top 10 List
10. We get to grade ourselves.	**10.** Have enough equipment for each student.
9. We are taught to make goals for ourselves and to try our hardest to achieve them.	**9.** Chart each child's progress and motivate him/her to do his/her personal best.
8. We have plenty of supplies.	**8.** Play the game.
7. The activities are challenging.	**7.** Make lessons interesting, progressive, and challenging.
6. Physical education relieves stress from our day.	**6.** Keep the development of self-responsibility as a top priority.
5. We are always doing different things, so it's interesting, and you never get bored.	**5.** Develop individual and cooperative skills.
4. Teachers are supportive, understanding, and are easy to get along with.	**4.** Provide equipment that is developmentally appropriate.
3. We get a good workout.	**3.** Present a variety of offerings so that each child can experience success.
2. We are always active.	**2.** Keep students physically active as much as possible.
1. Teachers make physical education fun!	**1.** Treat each child fairly and with respect.

■ **Figure 14.3** John Hichwa had his students create a list of the top 10 reasons they enjoy physical education (on the left), and then he created his own list of what he felt were the 10 most important aspects of effectively teaching physical education (on the right).

Reprinted, by permission, from J. Hichwa, 1998, *Right fielders are people too* (Champaign, IL: Human Kinetics) 54-55.

What I think of my group . . .	Seldom	Sometimes	Always
I worked well with my group.			
I listened when others shared their ideas.			
I offered thoughtful comments to help others in my group improve.			
I followed the teacher's directions and used everyone's time wisely.			
I cheerfully tried others' suggestions.			
Share what you found the most difficult in working with this group: List at least two possible solutions to this problem:			

Name _____ Date _____

Figure 14.4 Sample rubric that targets social behaviors.

From *Physical Education for Lifelong Fitness: The Physical Best Teacher Guide*, 2nd edition. NASPE, 2004, Champaign, IL: Human Kinetics.

Name _____ Date _____

What I think of this activity...	Seldom	Sometimes	Always
I think the activities in this class can help me become more fit.			
I try class activities during my free time.			
I recommend class activities to friends.			
I like class activities.			
Write any other comments you would like to make:			

Figure 14.5 Sample rubric that targets motivation levels. A reproducible version of this rubric is available in appendix A.

Remember, it is a forum for viewing several different types of assessments collected over time to give you a more complete picture of a student's progress.

Grading and Affective Assessment

Affect or attitudes toward physical activity are also critical for ensuring students remain physically active for a lifetime. However, teachers should try to separate affective assessments from the knowledge and fitness assessments in the grading scheme, even if this means creating your own health-related physical fitness education report card. Assessing attitude and motivation, and then using that information wisely, are the keys to developing a health-related physical fitness education program that teaches students that physical activity is enjoyable and worthwhile.

Strive to get to know each student's likes, dislikes, and fears. Then help each student discover enjoyable physical activities to increase the likelihood that he or she will independently pursue physical activity. Include parents in this process by keeping them informed and asking them for suggestions. Finally, grade students on how thoughtful, timely, and thorough their responses are to affective assessment assignments—not on how much they say they liked an activity or not.

Make the care a student puts into completing affective assessment assignments the main focus—not a student's actual attitude toward physical activity. This encourages students to be honest.

Although the student who persistently poisons the class with unhelpful negative comments and refuses to join you in troubleshooting disliked areas needs feedback and correction, consider ways other than grades to attack the problem. At the opposite end, the student who never stops trying, despite poor physical abilities, probably deserves rewards and praise, but should not be graded solely on that effort. Both of these students especially need to know that their approach affects their relationships with others but is not tied to assessment of curriculum standards. The key is to be open and up front about what weight you plan to give a perceived attitude and motivation level in the final physical education grade (see "Weighty Matters" in chapter 12). From the beginning of the class, teachers should identify the content and behaviors to be assessed and must be able to tie these to important learning standards and outcomes—for example, level of out-of-class participation, expressiveness in written assignments, faithfulness and timeliness in completing affective assignments.

Summary

Accurate assessment of students' fitness knowledge, physical activity, and attitudes about fitness should be combined with fitness test assessments and assessment of activity level (FITT guidelines), which were described in chapter 13. By incorporating assessment of learning domains and providing feedback with suggestions for increasing knowledge and changing behaviors, teachers help students develop the tools necessary for continuing to be physically active in later years, long after they have passed through the teacher's classroom and gymnasium. As students learn to set appropriately challenging goals as an outcome of assessments and class activities, they will become self-directed learners. Motivation will be enhanced through education about ways to improve areas below healthy fitness zones and through recognition of individual strengths. Encourage students to recognize development in their peers and themselves. In this way, they will learn assessment skills that can be applied even as their interests and **aptitudes** change throughout their lives.

WORKSHEETS AND REPRODUCIBLES

Fitness Goals Contract

To improve my personal fitness level, I, with the help of my teacher, have set the following fitness goals. I will participate in the activities outlined in this plan to achieve improved physical fitness. Based on my current level of fitness, I believe that these goals are reasonable.

Fitness component test item	Score_____ Date: _____	My goal	Activities to improve physical fitness	Follow-up score_____ Date: _____
AEROBIC FITNESS				
One-mile walk/run				
PACER				
BODY COMPOSITION				
Percent body fat				
Body mass index				
MUSCULAR STRENGTH AND ENDURANCE				
Curl-up				
Trunk Lift				
Push-ups				
Modified pull-ups				
Pull-ups				
Flexed-arm hang				
FLEXIBILITY				
Back-saver sit-and-reach				
Shoulder stretch				

Student: _____ Date: _____ Teacher: _____

From *Physical education for lifelong fitness: The Physical Best teacher's guide*, 2nd edition. NASPE, 2004, Champaign, IL: Human Kinetics.

Activity Goals Contract

Week of _____   My plans are to do the following:

	Activity I plan to do	Time of day	Friends who will be active with me
Monday			
Tuesday			
Wednesday			
Thursday			
Friday			
Saturday			
Sunday			

Student: _____   Date: _____   Teacher: _____

From *Physical education for lifelong fitness: The Physical Best teacher's guide*, 2nd edition. NASPE, 2004, Champaign, IL: Human Kinetics.

Fitness Workout Plan

Name: _____ Date: _____

Week beginning:

Component	Activity	Mon	Tue	Wed	Thu	Fri	Weekend
	WARM-UP						
Aerobic fitness							
Muscular strength and endurance							
Flexibility							
Body composition							
	COOL-DOWN						

From *Physical education for lifelong fitness: The Physical Best teacher's guide*, 2nd edition. NASPE, 2004, Champaign, IL: Human Kinetics.

Muscular Strength and Endurance Training Log

Name						
Week						
Day						
	SET 1		SET 2		SET 3	
Exercise	Weight	Reps	Weight	Reps	Weight	Reps

Adapted, by permission, from W. Kraemer and S. Fleck, 1993, *Strength training for young athletes* (Champaign, IL: Human Kinetics), 23.

From *Physical education for lifelong fitness: The Physical Best teacher's guide*, 2nd edition. NASPE, 2004, Champaign, IL: Human Kinetics.

Goal-Setting Worksheet

Name:_____ Date:_____

M = Measure and monitor

In class, my *FITNESSGRAM* scores were as follows: _____

test _____ score _____

test _____ score _____

test _____ score _____

test _____ score _____

test _____ score _____

The scores below the healthy fitness zone were (list) _____ .

test _____ score _____

test _____ score _____

test _____ score _____

test _____ score _____

test _____ score _____

O = Outcomes defined that are optimally challenging

Based on my *FITNESSGRAM* scores, I wish to improve fitness in the following areas:
(Example: abdominal strength and endurance)

T = Time

I will accomplish my goal in _____ weeks.

I = Individualized

I will not compare my scores to my classmates' scores.
To reach the HFZ, I need to increase my score by _____ (the exercise).
(Example: 10 curl-ups)

V = Valuable

I have chosen a goal of _____ .
(Example: increasing abdominal strength)
This is important to me because . . .

A = Active

By completing this sheet, I am taking responsibility for increasing my health and fitness. _____
(initial)

T = Type

The following activities will help me to reach my goal: (list several activities)
(Example: curl-ups, pelvic thrusts, oblique curls)

I = Incremental

I will add _____ (a number of exercises) to my score or add _____ minutes

of _____ (activity) each week to achieve my goals.
(Example: 2 curl-ups each week or 5 minutes of jogging each week)

O = Overload

I will increase the weight or quantity of my activity each day by _____.
(Example: 10 curl-ups each day)

N = Necessary

The purpose of this activity is to help me . . .

A = Authentic assessment

Although I can perform the _____ test again to see my improvement, I can also know
I am achieving my goal by
(Examples: measuring waist circumference, seeing my clothes fit better)

L = Lifestyle

Unhealthy behaviors that I would like to change in the future include the following:
(Examples: Inactive television viewing, snacking on unhealthy foods)

P = Posted but private

I will post this sheet or keep it _____, where I can see it each day.

My goal partner is_____ .

E = Enjoyable

I know that work on this activity may not always be easy or fun, but I will be happier when I am healthy.
My reward to myself when I achieve this goal is _____.
(Example: I will go see a movie with my best friend)

My signature:_____

Teacher signature*: _____

(*Teacher has reviewed goal and believes it to be achievable for student.)

From *Physical education for lifelong fitness: The Physical Best teacher's guide*, 2nd edition. NASPE, 2004, Champaign, IL: Human Kinetics.

Bench Press Technique

Resistance used

40 to 50 percent of body weight

Starting position

Elbows are straight; feet are flat on the floor or flat on the end of bench or platform; buttocks and shoulders touch bench; back is not excessively arched; bar is over upper chest; bar is horizontal.

Points available: 0-6

Points earned: _____

Lowering (eccentric) phase

Descent of bar is controlled; elbows are out to side; forearms are perpendicular to the floor; bar touches chest at nipple level; there is no bounce on chest touch; bar is horizontal; feet stay flat on floor; back is not excessively arched; head stays still.

Points available: 0-7

Points earned: _____

Up (concentric) phase

Back is not excessively arched; elbows are out to sides; bar is horizontal; both arms straighten at same speed; motion is smooth and continuous; head stays still; feet stay flat on floor.

Points available: 0-9

Points earned: _____

Finishing position

Same position as starting position.

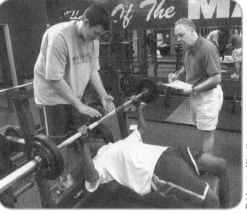

© Human Kinetics

Points available: 0-3

Points earned: _____

Total points available: 0-25

Total points earned: _____

Technique tips

- Inhale as you lower the weight and exhale as you lift it.
- A spotter should be behind the lifter's head and should assist the lifter with getting the barbell into the starting position and returning the barbell to the rack when finished. Impress on young weight trainers the importance of a spotter during the exercise because the bar is pressed over the lifter's face, neck, and chest.
- Learn this exercise with an unloaded barbell or long stick.
- Do not bounce the barbell off the chest, and do not lift your buttocks off the bench during this exercise.
- Avoid hitting the upright supports by positioning your body about three inches from the supports before you start.

Reprinted, by permission, from W. Kraemer and S. Fleck, 1993. Strength training for young athletes (Champaign, IL: Human Kinetics), 30.

From *Physical education for lifelong fitness: The Physical Best teacher's guide*, 2nd edition. NASPE, 2004, Champaign, IL: Human Kinetics.

Student Profile Sheet

Student: _____Date of birth:_____

Classroom teacher: _____ Physical education teacher: _____

Occupational therapist:_____ Physical therapist: _____

Speech and language therapist:_____

1. Medical information/precautions:

2. Speech/language programs used (devices):

3. Behavior program and/or protocol:

4. Positioning/adaptive equipment/braces:

5. Nursing plan:

6. Dressing:

From *Physical education for lifelong fitness: The Physical Best teacher's guide*, 2nd edition. NASPE, 2004, Champaign, IL: Human Kinetics.

Curl-Up Assessment

Name: _____ Date: _____

Directions:

Circle the level of assistance the individual requires in order to perform the task. Total each level of assistance column and place the subtotals in the sum of scores row. Total the sum of scores row and place the score in the individual's total score achieved row. Determine percent independence score based on the chart below. Place number of repetitions in the product score row.

Key to levels of assistance:

IND = Independent—the individual is able to perform the task without assistance

PPA = Partial Physical Assistance—the individual needs some assistance to perform the task

TPA = Total Physical Assistance—the individual needs assistance to perform the entire task

Curl-Up	IND	PPA	TPA
1. Lie on back with knees bent	3	2	1
2. Place feet flat on the floor with legs slightly apart	3	2	1
3. Place arms straight, parallel to the trunk	3	2	1
4. Rest palms of hands on the mat with fingers stretched out	3	2	1
5. Rest head on partner's hands	3	2	1
6. Curl body in a forward position	3	2	1
7. Curl back down until head touches partner's hand	3	2	1
Sum of scores:			
Total score achieved:			
Total possible points:	21		
% Independence score:			
Product score:			

Percentage of independence

7/21 = 33%	12/21 = 57%	17/21 = 80%
8/21 = 38%	13/21 = 61%	18/21 = 85%
9/21 = 42%	14/21 = 66%	19/21 = 90%
10/21 = 47%	15/21 = 71%	20/21 = 95%
11/21 = 52%	16/21 = 76%	21/21 = 100%

Reprinted, by permission, from AAHPERD, 1995, Physical best and individuals with disabilities: A handbook for inclusion in fitness programs (Champaign, IL: Human Kinetics), 100.

From *Physical education for lifelong fitness: The Physical Best teacher's guide*, 2nd edition. NASPE, 2004, Champaign, IL: Human Kinetics.

Assessing Knowledge of Calculating and Using Heart Rate Rubric

Student's name _____ Date _____ Score _____

Class _____

Target component	Score 1 point	Score 2 points
Can demonstrate sites at which to count the pulse	Knows one site	Knows two sites
Understands how heart rate information indicates intensity	Some understanding	Clearly understands
Can accurately count the pulse for a fraction of a minute, then accurately calculate heartbeats per minute with a calculator	Sometimes	Most of the time
Can describe ways and reasons to increase or decrease heart rate	Some understanding	Clearly understands

From *Physical education for lifelong fitness: The Physical Best teacher's guide*, 2nd edition. NASPE, 2004, Champaign, IL: Human Kinetics.

Family Steps

Name _____	Steps Day 1	Steps Day 2	Steps Day 3	Steps Day 4	Individual total
Parent/Guardian					
Parent/Guardian					
Daily total					
				Grand total	

Adapted, by permission, from R. Pangrazi, A. Beighle, and C. Sidman, 2003, *Pedometer power: 67 lessons for K-12* (Champaign, IL: Human Kinetics), 110.

From *Physical education for lifelong fitness: The Physical Best teacher's guide*, 2nd edition. NASPE, 2004, Champaign, IL: Human Kinetics.

Physical Education Progress Report: Grades 3-4

Student: _____ Date: _____

Teacher: _____

____ 1st qtr (Nov)   ____ 2nd qtr (Feb)   ____ 3rd qtr (Apr)   ____ 4th qtr (June)

	Working to achieve	Needs improvement	Achieved
Intellectual			
1. Knows rules and procedures governing movement activities and games	❐	❐	❐
2. Recognizes the effects of space, time, force, and flow on the quality of movement	❐	❐	❐
3. Applies basic mechanical principles that affect and control human movement	❐	❐	❐
Comments: _____			
Social			
1. Respects rights, opinions, and abilities of others	❐	❐	❐
2. Shares, takes turns, and provides mutual assistance	❐	❐	❐
3. Participates cooperatively in student-led activities	❐	❐	❐
Comments: _____			
Emotional			
1. Assumes responsibility for giving and following directions	❐	❐	❐
2. Makes decisions on an individual basis	❐	❐	❐
3. Responds freely and confidently through expressive bodily movement	❐	❐	❐
Comments: _____			
Values			
1. Carries out tasks to completion	❐	❐	❐
2. Displays preferences for various forms of movement	❐	❐	❐
3. Engages in movement activities voluntarily	❐	❐	❐
Comments: _____			
Physical			
1. Executes all locomotor movements in response to rhythmic accompaniments	❐	❐	❐
2. Controls body while balancing, rolling, climbing, and hanging	❐	❐	❐
3. Shows body control in manipulating playground ball, while stationary and moving	❐	❐	❐
Comments: _____			

Reprinted, by permission, from V.J. Melograno, 1998, *Professional and sport portfolios for physical education* (Champaign, IL: Human Kinetics), 109.

From *Physical education for lifelong fitness: The Physical Best teacher's guide*, 2nd edition. NASPE, 2004, Champaign, IL: Human Kinetics.

Running Stride Rubric

Jogging Criteria	
Doer 1 _____	Date _____
Doer 2 _____	Class _____

Level III

Observer: Give the doer some pointers about his or her jogging form. Use the tips below to help you. Try to be friendly.

Doer: Jog at a moderate pace. When the teacher signals, slow down—then change roles.

	DOER 1			DOER 2		
	Yes	No	Don't Know	Yes	No	Don't Know
1. Runs tall, leans slightly forward.						
2. Swings legs from hip, knees bent.						
3. Lands on heels with weight rolling along the outside portion of foot to toes.						
4. Points toes straight ahead, lands heel directly under knees.						
5. Swings arms straight forward and backward, hands relaxed.						
6. Breathes from stomach in an even rhythm.						

Adapted, by permission, from S.J. Virgilio, 1997, *Fitness education for children: Team approach* (Champaign, IL: Human Kinetics), 20.

From *Physical education for lifelong fitness: The Physical Best teacher's guide*, 2nd edition. NASPE, 2004, Champaign, IL: Human Kinetics.

Thinking About Physical Fitness and Activities

Name _____ Date _____ Class _____

1. I would rather exercise or play sports than watch TV. **Yes** **No**

2. People who exercise regularly seem to have a lot of fun doing it. **Yes** **No**

3. In school, I look forward to attending physical education class. **Yes** **No**

4. During physical education class at school, I usually work up a sweat. **Yes** **No**

5. When I grow up, I will probably be too busy to stay physically fit. **Yes** **No**

6. How do you feel about your ability to strike a ball with a racket? ☺ 😐 ☹

7. How do you feel about your ability to kick a ball hard and hit a target? ☺ 😐 ☹

8. How do you feel about your ability to run a long distance without stopping? ☺ 😐 ☹

9. How do you feel about your ability to play many different games and sports? ☺ 😐 ☹

10. How do you feel about your ability to participate in gymnastics? ☺ 😐 ☹

11. How do you feel about your ability to participate in dance? ☺ 😐 ☹

Reprinted, by permission, from G. Graham, 1992, *Teaching children physical education* (Champaign, IL: Human Kinetics), 159.

From *Physical education for lifelong fitness: The Physical Best teacher's guide*, 2nd edition. NASPE, 2004, Champaign, IL: Human Kinetics.

Thinking About Groups

Name _____ **Date** _____

What I think of my group . . .	Seldom	Sometimes	Always
I worked well with my group.			
I listened when others shared their ideas.			
I offered thoughtful comments to help others in my group improve.			
I followed the teacher's directions and used everyone's time wisely.			
I cheerfully tried others' suggestions.			
Share what you found the most difficult in working with this group: List at least two possible solutions to this problem:			

Thinking About Activities

Name _____ **Date** _____

What I think of this activity...	Seldom	Sometimes	Always
I think the activities in this class can help me become more fit.			
I try class activities during my free time.			
I recommend class activities to friends.			
I like class activities.			
Write any other comments you would like to make:			

NUTRIENT CONTENT CLAIMS

The regulations spell out what terms may be used to describe the level of a nutrient in a food and how those terms can be used. Alternative spelling of these descriptive terms and their synonyms is allowed—for example, *hi* and *lo*—as long as the alternatives are not misleading. These are the core terms:

■ Free. This term means that a product contains no amount of, or only trivial or "physiologically inconsequential" amounts of, one or more of these components: fat, saturated fat, cholesterol, sodium, sugars, and calories. For example, *calorie free* means fewer than 5 calories per serving, and *sugar free* and *fat free* both mean less than 0.5 grams per serving. Synonyms for *free* include *without*, *no*, and *zero*. A synonym for fat-free milk is *skim*.

■ Low. This term can be used on foods that can be eaten frequently without exceeding dietary guidelines for one or more of these components: fat, saturated fat, cholesterol, sodium, and calories. Synonyms for *low* include *little*, *few*, *low source of*, and *contains a small amount of*.

Thus, descriptors are defined as follows:

- Low fat: 3 grams or less per serving
- Low saturated fat: 1 gram or less per serving
- Low sodium: 140 milligrams or less per serving
- Very low sodium: 35 milligrams or less per serving
- Low cholesterol: 20 milligrams or less and 2 grams or less of saturated fat per serving
- Low calorie: 40 calories or less per serving

■ Lean and extra lean. These terms can be used to describe the fat content of meat, poultry, seafood, and game meats.

- Lean: less than 10 grams of fat, 4.5 grams or less of saturated fat, and less than 95 milligrams of cholesterol per serving and per 100 grams

- Extra lean: less than 5 grams of fat, less than 2 grams of saturated fat, and less than 95 milligrams of cholesterol per serving and per 100 grams

■ High. This term can be used if the food contains 20 percent or more of the daily value for a particular nutrient in a serving.

■ Good source. This term means that one serving of a food contains 10 to 19 percent of the daily value for a particular nutrient.

■ Reduced. This term means that a nutritionally altered product contains at least 25 percent less of a nutrient or of calories than the regular, or reference, product. However, a *reduced* claim can't be made on a product if its reference food already meets the requirement for a *low* claim.

■ Less. This term means that a food, whether altered or not, contains 25 percent less of a nutrient or of calories than the reference food. For example, pretzels that have 25 percent less fat than potato chips could carry a *less* claim. *Fewer* is an acceptable synonym.

■ Light. This descriptor can mean two things. First, it can mean that a nutritionally altered product contains one-third fewer calories or half the fat of the reference food. If the food derives 50 percent or more of its calories from fat, the reduction must be 50 percent of the fat. Second, it can mean that the sodium content of a low-calorie, low-fat food has been reduced by 50 percent. In addition, *light in sodium* may be used on food in which the sodium content has been reduced by at least 50 percent. The term *light* still can be used to describe such properties as texture and color, as long as the label explains the intent—for example, *light brown sugar* and *light and fluffy*.

■ More. This term means that a serving of food, whether altered or not, contains a nutrient that is at least 10 percent of the daily value more than the reference food. The 10 percent of daily value also applies to *fortified*, *enriched*, and *added*, *extra*, or *plus* claims, but in those cases, the food must be altered.

■ Healthy. A *healthy* food must be low in fat and saturated fat and contain limited amounts of cholesterol and sodium. In addition, if it's a single-item food, it must provide at least 10 percent of the recommended daily amount of one or more of the following: vitamins A or C, iron, calcium, protein, or fiber. Exempt from this "10 percent" rule are certain raw, canned, and frozen fruits and vegetables and certain cereal-grain products. These foods can be labeled *healthy* if they do not contain ingredients that change the nutritional profile, and, in the case of enriched grain products, conform to standards of identity, which call for certain required ingredients. If it's a meal-type product, such as frozen entrees and multicourse frozen dinners, it must provide 10 percent of two or three of these vitamins or minerals or of protein or fiber, in addition to meeting the other criteria. The sodium content cannot exceed 360 milligrams per serving for individual foods and 480 milligrams per serving for meal-type products.

Other Definitions

The regulations also address other claims. Among them are the following:

■ Percent fat free. A product bearing this claim must be a low-fat or a fat-free product. In addition, the claim must accurately reflect the amount of fat present in 100 grams of the food. Thus, if a food contains 2.5 grams of fat per 50 grams, the claim must be 95 *percent fat free*.

■ Implied. These types of claims are prohibited when they wrongfully imply that a food contains or does not contain a meaningful level of a nutrient. For example, a product claiming to be made with an ingredient known to be a source of fiber (such as *made with oat bran*) is not allowed unless the product contains enough of that ingredient (for example, oat bran) to meet the definition for *good source* of fiber. As another example, a claim that a product contains *no tropical oils* is allowed—but only on foods that are *low* in saturated fat because consumers have come to equate tropical oils with high saturated fat.

■ Meals and main dishes. Claims that a meal or main dish is *free* of a nutrient, such as sodium or cholesterol, must meet the same requirements as those for individual foods. Other claims can be used under special circumstances. For example, *low calorie* means the meal or main dish contains 120 calories or less per 100 grams. *Low sodium* means the food has 140 milligrams or less per 100 grams. *Low cholesterol* means the food contains 20 milligrams of cholesterol or less per 100 grams and no more than 2 grams of saturated fat. *Light* means the meal or main dish is *low fat* or *low calorie*.

■ Standardized foods. Any nutrient content claim, such as *reduced fat*, *low calorie*, and *light*, may be used in conjunction with a standardized term if the new product has been specifically formulated to meet the FDA's criteria for that claim, if the product is not nutritionally inferior to the traditional standardized food, and if the new product complies with certain compositional requirements set by the FDA. A new product bearing a claim also must have performance characteristics similar to the referenced traditional standardized food. If the product doesn't, and the differences materially limit the product's use, its label must state the differences (for example, not recommended for baking) to inform consumers.

Fresh

The FDA has issued a regulation for the term *fresh* although it is not mandated by NLEA. The agency took this step because of concern over the term's possible misuse on some food labels.

The regulation defines the term *fresh* when it is used to suggest that a food is raw or unprocessed. In this context, *fresh* can be used only on a food that is raw, has never been frozen or heated, and contains no preservatives. (Irradiation at low levels is allowed.) *Fresh frozen*, *frozen fresh*, and *freshly frozen* can be used for foods that are quickly frozen while still fresh. Blanching (brief scalding before freezing to prevent nutrient breakdown) is allowed.

Other uses of the term *fresh*, such as in *fresh milk* or *freshly baked bread*, are not affected.

Source: Food and Drug Administration, Center for Food Safety and Applied Nutrition, www.cfsan.fda.gov/~dms/hclaims.html.

EXERCISES FOR PREPUBERTY

From the multitude of exercises for strength training, the following exercises are guidelines only and not restrictions. You can use other exercises, depending on the environment and facilities.

Dumbbell Side Raise

Area worked: shoulders

1. The student stands with the feet apart and the arms at the side.
2. He or she lifts the dumbbells up above the head, and then returns to the starting position.

Dumbbell Curl

Area worked: biceps

1. The student stands with the arms extended down in front of the hips, and the palms facing upward.
2. He or she flexes the right elbow, lifting the dumbbell toward the right shoulder.
3. The student returns to the starting position, and then repeats with the left arm.

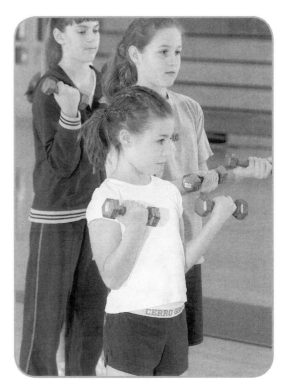

Adapted, by permission, from T.O. Bompa, 2000, *Total training for young champions* (Champaign, IL: Human Kinetics), 115-123.

Dumbbell Shoulder Press

Area worked: shoulders, especially trapezius

1. The student stands and holds the dumbbells at shoulder level.

2. He or she presses the dumbbells straight above the shoulders, and then returns them to the starting position.

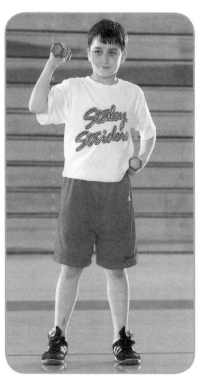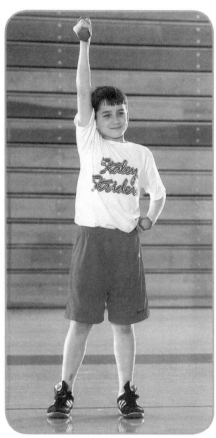

Dumbbell Overhead Raise

Area worked: shoulders

1. The student lies on back, with the arms along the body.

2. He or she raises both dumbbells up and over the head to the floor, and then returns them to the starting position.

Variation
The student repeats the same movement with each arm alternately.

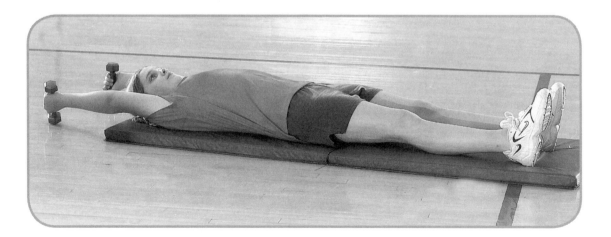

Adapted, by permission, from T.O. Bompa, 2000, *Total training for young champions* (Champaign, IL: Human Kinetics), 115-123.

Dumbbell Fly

Area worked: chest and shoulders

1. The student lies on back, with the arms extended to the sides.

2. He or she raises both arms to vertical (above the chest), and then returns to the starting position.

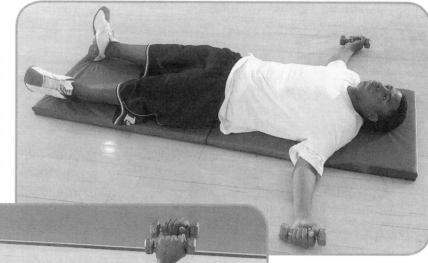

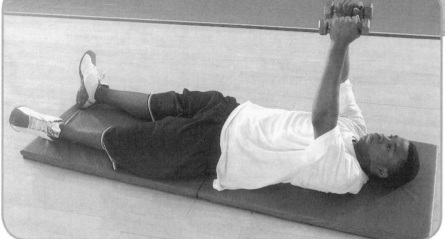

Medicine Ball Chest Throw

Area worked: shoulders and arm extensors (triceps)

1. Two partners face each other, standing 8 to 10 feet apart, with partner A holding a medicine ball in front of the chest.

2. Partner A extends the arms up and forward, throwing the ball toward the chest of partner B.

3. After catching the ball, partner B throws the ball back to partner A.

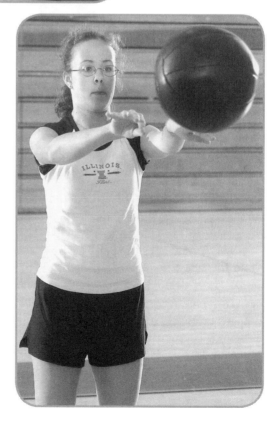

Adapted, by permission, from T.O. Bompa, 2000, *Total training for young champions* (Champaign, IL: Human Kinetics), 115-123.

Medicine Ball Zigzag Throw

Area worked: arms and shoulders

1. Two equal teams line up where they can throw a ball in zigzag: each team's players 10 feet aside and in front of each other. The first player on each team holds a medicine ball.

2. Players throw the ball with two hands, from player to player.

3. The first team that completes the course is the winner.

Variation

Players throw the ball with one hand, overhead with two hands, or from the side.

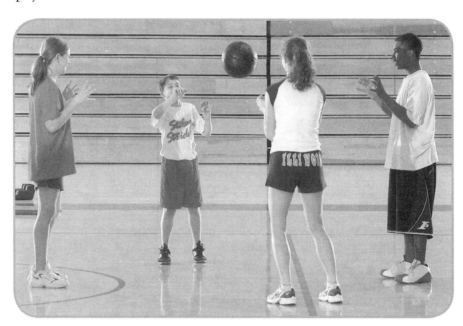

Medicine Ball Twist Throw

Area worked: arms, trunk, and oblique abdominal muscles

1. Partner A holds the ball at hip level, standing with his or her left side facing partner B.

2. Partner B faces partner A and anticipates the ball with arms extended forward.

3. Partner A turns the body to the left, extends the arms, and releases the ball to the side toward partner B.

4. After catching the ball, partner B takes the same starting position (side facing partner A), performs a rotation, and returns the ball to partner A in the same manner.

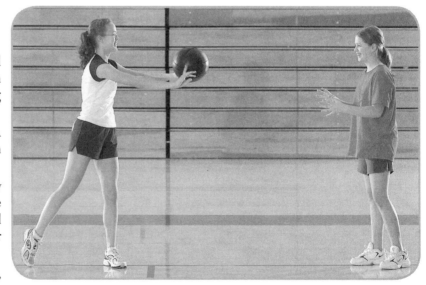

Adapted, by permission, from T.O. Bompa, 2000, *Total training for young champions* (Champaign, IL: Human Kinetics), 115-123.

Medicine Ball Forward Overhead Throw

Area worked: chest, shoulders, arms,
and abdominal muscles

1. Partners face each other, standing 8 to 10 feet apart, with partner A holding the ball above the head.

2. Partner A extends the arms backward, then immediately forward to release the ball toward the chest of partner B.

3. After catching the ball, partner B returns it to partner A with the same motion.

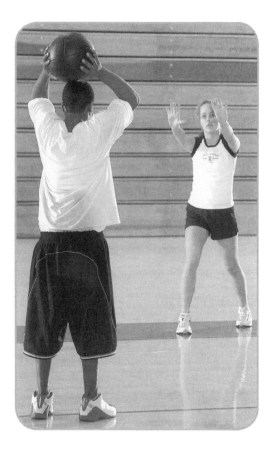

Medicine Ball Scoop Throw

Area worked: ankles; knees; hip extensors; and arm,
shoulder, and back muscles

1. The student stands with the feet apart and holds the ball between the legs.

2. He or she bends the knees, then immediately extends them, throwing the ball vertically with the arms.

3. The student extends the arms upward to catch the ball, and then returns to the starting position.

Variation
The student can perform the same exercise with a partner.

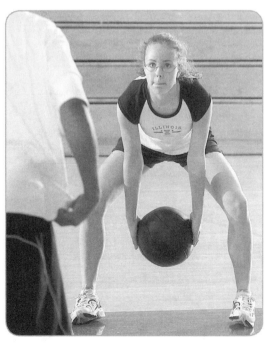

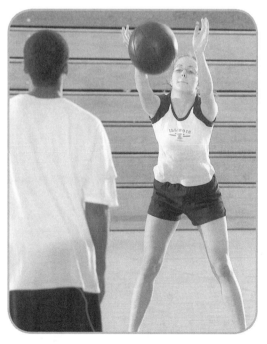

Adapted, by permission, from T.O. Bompa, 2000, *Total training for young champions* (Champaign, IL: Human Kinetics), 115-123.

Abdominal Crunch

Area worked: abdominal muscles

1. The student lies on the floor, with the arms along the body. The knees are slightly bent.

2. He or she raises the upper body up and forward, and then relaxes and brings the trunk slowly back to the starting position.

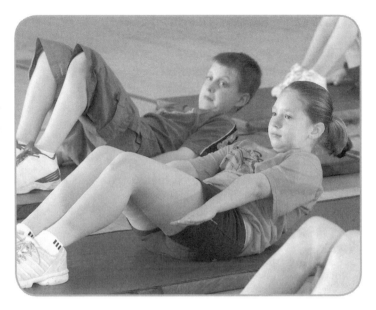

Medicine Ball Back Roll

Area worked: abdominals and hip flexors

1. The student lies on back, with the arms along the body, holding a medicine ball between the feet. The knees are slightly bent.

2. He or she raises the legs until the medicine ball is above the head, and then lowers the legs back to the starting position.

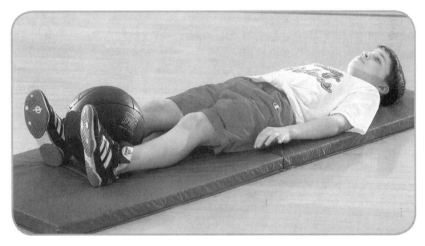

Variation

The student can perform the same exercise with a partner, throwing the ball backward overhead.

Safety note

When the ball is above the face, the student should place the palms over the face to catch the ball if it falls toward the face or head.

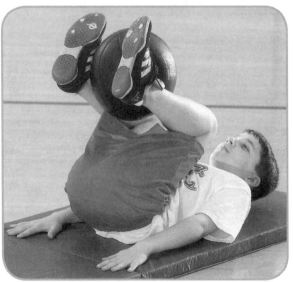

Adapted, by permission, from T.O. Bompa, 2000, *Total training for young champions* (Champaign, IL: Human Kinetics), 115-123.

Medicine Ball Side Pass Relay

Area worked: oblique abdominals and shoulders (deltoids)

1. Two equal teams sit with their feet apart. The players on each team are lined up in a straight line. (Calculate the distance between players so they can perform the pass comfortably.) The first player on each team holds a medicine ball.

2. The first player rotates to the right, passing the ball to the next player.

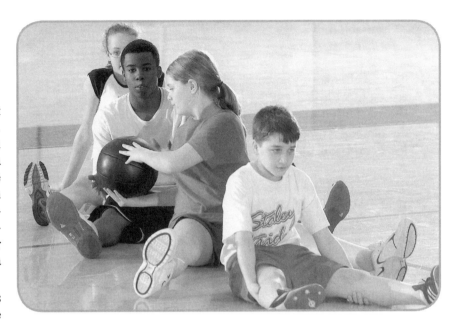

3. The players continue this as fast as possible to the end of the line.

4. After receiving the ball, the last player stands up, runs to the front as quickly as possible, sits down, and starts the series again.

5. The relay is over when the first player is at the end of the row. The winner is the team that finishes first.

Variations

■ Players pass the ball alternatively to each side.

■ Players pass the ball back over the head.

■ Players hold the ball between the feet, roll over, and pass the ball to the feet of the next player.

Trunk Twist

Area worked: oblique abdominals

1. The student sits with the feet resting under a heavy object or stall bars or with a partner holding the feet; the hands are behind the neck, and the knees slightly bent.

2. The student leans slightly back, with the trunk in an oblique position, and turns the trunk to the left as far as possible.

3. He or she returns to the starting position, and then turns the trunk to the right as far back as possible.

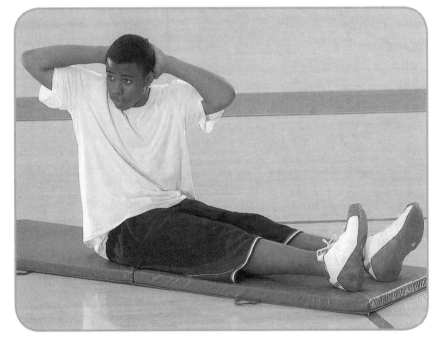

Adapted, by permission, from T.O. Bompa, 2000, *Total training for young champions* (Champaign, IL: Human Kinetics), 115-123.

Single-Leg Back Raise

Area worked: hip extensors and spine muscles

1. The student lies on the belly, with the arms extended forward.

2. He or she lifts the right leg upward as high as possible.

3. The student lowers the right leg to the floor and lifts the left leg.

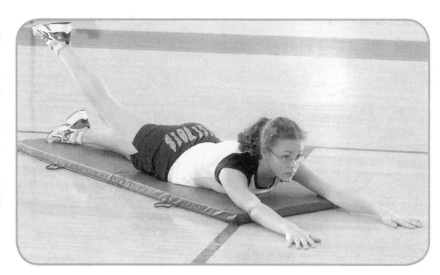

Chest Raise and Clap

Area worked: lower back muscles

1. The student lies on the belly, with the arms extended forward on the floor.

2. He or she raises the chest with the arms extended and performs two or three claps.

3. The student relaxes the trunk and lowers the arms to the floor.

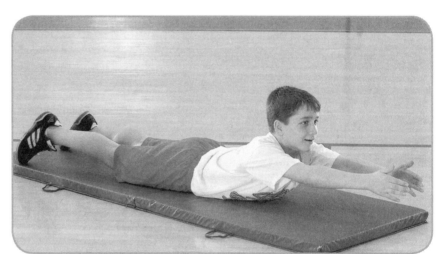

Seated Back Extension

Area worked: back and shoulder muscles

1. Two partners sit facing each other, with feet apart and arms extended in front of the shoulders. The partners grasp each other's hands firmly.

2. Partner B performs an upper body extension, and partner A resists it slightly so partner B can perform the motion slowly.

3. They repeat with the partners changing roles.

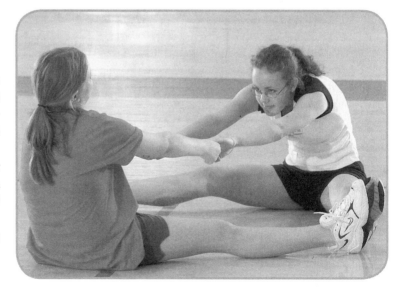

Adapted, by permission, from T.O. Bompa, 2000, *Total training for young champions* (Champaign, IL: Human Kinetics), 115-123.

Two-Leg Skip

Area worked: calf and knee extensor muscles

1. Two students hold the ends of a skipping rope, with a third student ready to skip the rope.

2. Rope holders rotate the rope, while the performer jumps up and down to avoid being hit by the rope.

3. They stop the action after 15 to 20 seconds, and change roles.

Variations

- One-leg skip on the spot.
- Two-leg forward skips.
- One-leg forward skips.
- Two-leg backward skips.
- One-leg backward skips.
- Alternate one- and two-leg skips forward and backward.

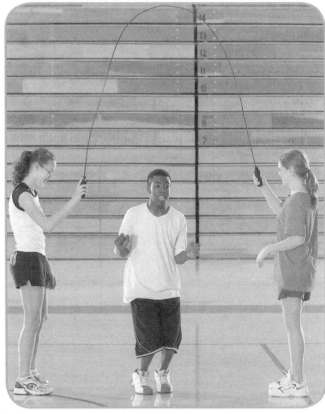

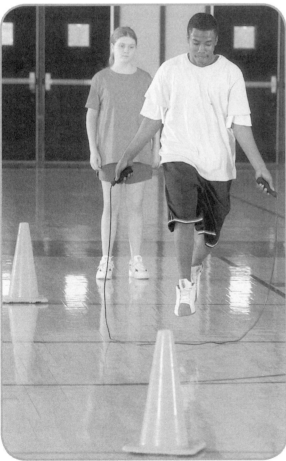

Loop Skip

Area worked: calf and knee extensors

1. Two teams are lined up behind a starting line. Each team has a cone 15 yards in front of them. The first player on each team has a skipping rope.

2. At the signal, the first player on each team skips the rope while moving forward, loops around the cone, and returns to the starting position.

3. The rope goes to the next player, and the first performer goes to the end of the line.

4. The players continue this, with each player skipping the rope as fast as possible.

5. The winning team is the one having all players skip over the course and finish line first.

Variation

Time individual performance (going over the course from start to finish).

Adapted, by permission, from T.O. Bompa, 2000, *Total training for young champions* (Champaign, IL: Human Kinetics), 115-123.

Dodge the Rope

Area worked: calf and knee extensors

1. A group of players form a circle. In the middle of the circle, there is a player holding the end of a skipping rope. The distance from the player in the middle to the circle is equal to the length of the rope.

2. The player in the middle swings the rope in a circle at ankle height. As the rope approaches each player, he or she jumps over it.

3. When the rope hits a player, he or she goes in the middle of the circle.

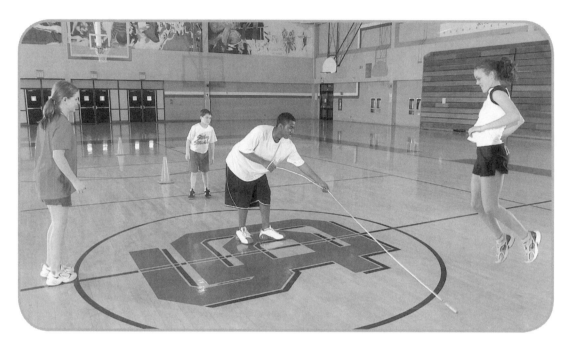

Adapted, by permission, from T.O. Bompa, 2000, *Total training for young champions* (Champaign, IL: Human Kinetics), 115-123.

ALTERNATIVES FOR QUESTIONABLE EXERCISES

Stretching can be harmful when the routine is too vigorous or too lengthy or when bouncing at the extreme ROM. The wrong choice of exercises also imposes serious risk of injury to joints. In fact, many popular stretching exercises used in the past are potentially harmful. Unfortunately, most people acquire their stretching knowledge by watching others. This informal, copycat approach has spawned a series of popular but dangerous exercises capable of damaging the knees, neck, spinal column, ankles, and lower back. The following material identifies a "hit list" of nine popular stretching exercises that should be avoided and offers safe substitutes that will effectively stretch the same muscle groups.

Questionable Exercises

Neck roll (circling)
Danger: Drawing the head backward could damage the disks in the neck area, and may even precipitate arthritis.

Safer Alternative Exercises

Forward neck roll
Description: Bend forward at the waist with the hands on the knees. Gently roll the head.

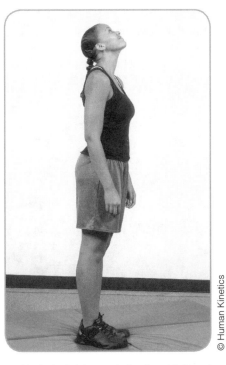

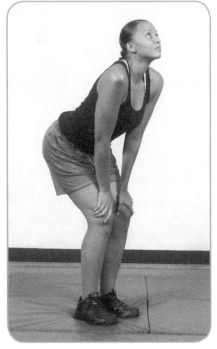

Figures and text adapted, by permission, from J.S. Greenberg, G.V. Dintiman, and B. Myers Oakes, 2004. *Physical fitness and wellness: Changing the way you look, feel, and perform,* 3rd edition (Champaign, IL: Human Kinetics), 151-153.

Questionable Exercises

Quadricep stretch

Danger: If the ankle is pulled too hard, muscle, ligament, and cartilage damage may occur.

Safer Alternative Exercises

Opposite leg pull

Description: Grasp one ankle with your opposite hand. Instead of pulling, attempt to straighten the leg you are stretching.

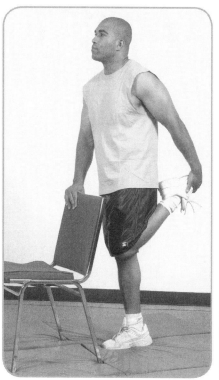

© Human Kinetics

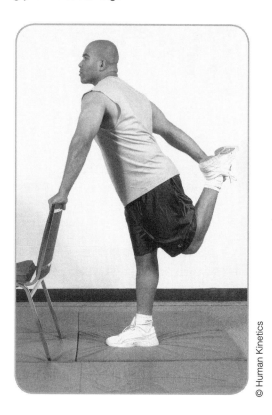

© Human Kinetics

Hurdler's stretch

Danger: Hip, knee, and ankle are subjected to abnormal stress.

Everted hurdler's stretch

Description: Bend the left leg at the knee and slide the foot next to the right knee. Pull yourself forward slowly by using a towel, or by grasping the toe.

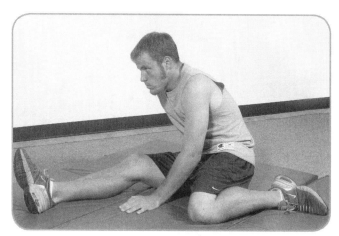

© Human Kinetics

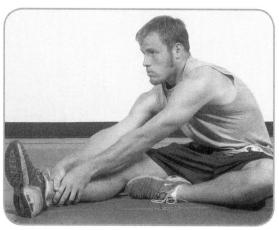

© Human Kinetics

Figures and text adapted, by permission, from J.S. Greenberg, G.V. Dintiman, and B. Myers Oakes, 2004. *Physical fitness and wellness: Changing the way you look, feel, and perform,* 3rd edition (Champaign, IL: Human Kinetics), 151-153.

Questionable Exercises

Deep knee bend (or any exercise that bends the knee beyond a right angle)

Danger: Excessive stress is placed on ligament, tendon, and cartilage tissue.

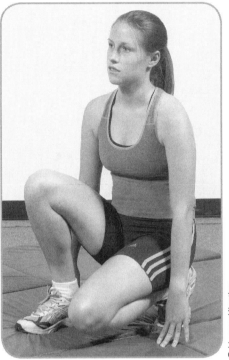

Safer Alternative Exercises

Single-knee lunge

Description: Place one leg in front of your body and extend the other behind. Bend forward at the trunk as you bend the lead leg to right angles.

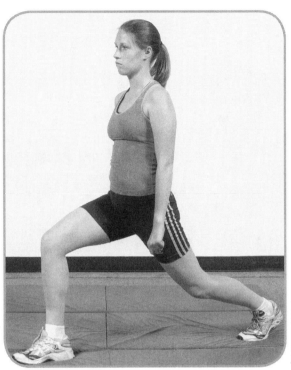

Yoga plow

Danger: This exercise could over-stretch muscles and ligaments, injure spinal disks, or cause fainting.

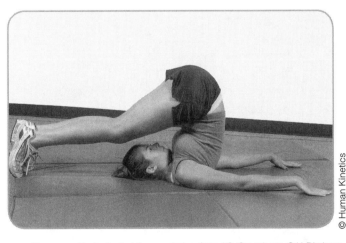

Extended one-leg stretch or Back-saver sit-and-reach

Description: Extend one leg and bend at the knee. With your foot on the floor, draw the knee of the other leg toward your chest. Bend forward at the trunk as far as possible.

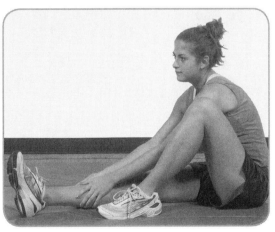

Figures and text adapted, by permission, from J.S. Greenberg, G.V. Dintiman, and B. Myers Oakes, 2004. *Physical fitness and wellness: Changing the way you look, feel, and perform,* 3rd edition (Champaign, IL: Human Kinetics), 151-153.

Questionable Exercises

Straight-leg curl-up

Danger: Produces back strain and sciatic nerve elongation. It also moves the hip flexor muscles and does not flatten the abdomen.

Safer Alternative Exercises

Bent-knee curl-up

Description: Cross both hands on your chest, with the knees slightly bent. Raise the upper body slightly to about 25° on each repetition. NOTE: *FIT-NESSGRAM* suggests that the arms remain straight along the body.

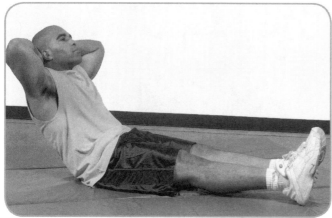

© Human Kinetics

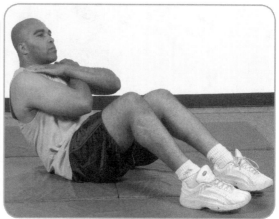

© Human Kinetics

Double leg raise

Danger: Stretches the sciatic nerve beyond its normal limits, and places too much stress on ligaments, muscles, and disks.

Knee-to-chest stretch

Description: Clasp both hands behind the neck. Draw the knee toward the chest, and hold that position of maximum stretch for 15-30 seconds.

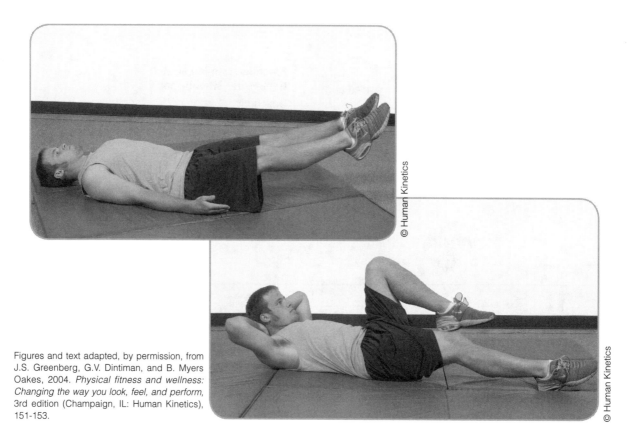

© Human Kinetics

© Human Kinetics

Figures and text adapted, by permission, from J.S. Greenberg, G.V. Dintiman, and B. Myers Oakes, 2004. *Physical fitness and wellness: Changing the way you look, feel, and perform*, 3rd edition (Champaign, IL: Human Kinetics), 151-153.

Questionable Exercises

Prone arch

Danger: Hyperextension of the lower back places extreme pressure on spinal disks.

Safer Alternative Exercises

Belly push-up

Description: Lie flat on your belly, resting on your elbows. Push with your arms slowly to raise the upper body as the lower torso remains pressured against the floor. Use caution in that you should not hyperextend your back.

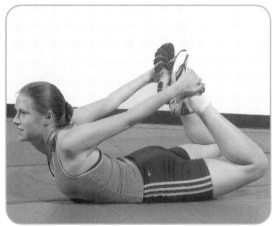

© Human Kinetics

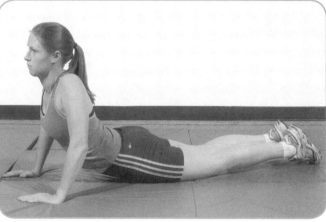

© Human Kinetics

Back bends

Danger: Spinal disks can easily be damaged.

No alternate exercise has been approved.

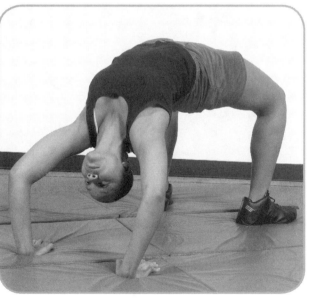

© Human Kinetics

Figures and text adapted, by permission, from J.S. Greenberg, G.V. Dintiman, and B. Myers Oakes, 2004. *Physical fitness and wellness: Changing the way you look, feel, and perform,* 3rd edition (Champaign, IL: Human Kinetics), 151-153.

BODY MASS AND COMPOSITION MEASURES

2 to 20 years: Boys
Body mass index-for-age percentiles

NAME _____

RECORD # _____

Date	Age	Weight	Stature	BMI*	Comments

*To Calculate BMI: Weight (kg) ÷ Stature (cm) ÷ Stature (cm) x 10,000
or Weight (lb) ÷ Stature (in) ÷ Stature (in) x 703

Published May 30, 2000 (modified 10/16/00).
SOURCE: Developed by the National Center for Health Statistics in collaboration with
the National Center for Chronic Disease Prevention and Health Promotion (2000).
http://www.cdc.gov/growthcharts

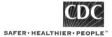

Figure E.1 BMI chart for males ages 2 to 20

http://www.cdc.gov/nchs/data/nhanes/growthcharts/set2clinical/cj411073.pdf

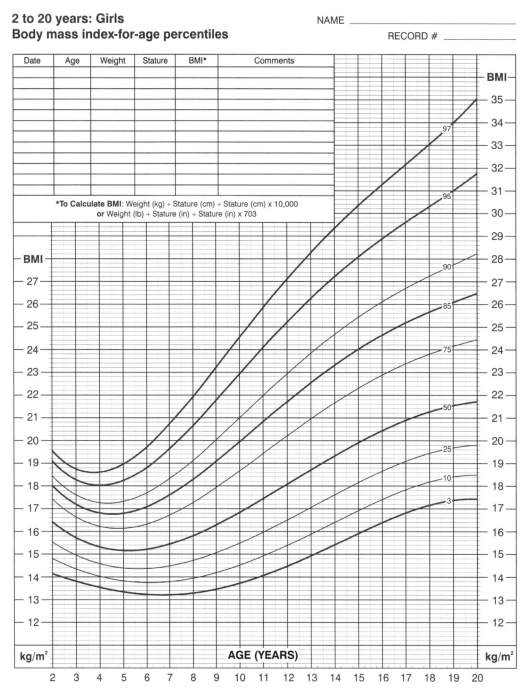

2 to 20 years: Girls
Body mass index-for-age percentiles

NAME _____

RECORD # _____

Date	Age	Weight	Stature	BMI*	Comments

*To Calculate BMI: Weight (kg) ÷ Stature (cm) ÷ Stature (cm) x 10,000
or Weight (lb) ÷ Stature (in) ÷ Stature (in) x 703

BMI

AGE (YEARS)

kg/m²

Published May 30, 2000 (modified 10/16/00).
SOURCE: Developed by the National Center for Health Statistics in collaboration with
the National Center for Chronic Disease Prevention and Health Promotion (2000).
http://www.cdc.gov/growthcharts

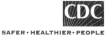

SAFER · HEALTHIER · PEOPLE™

■ **Figure E.2** BMI chart for females ages 2 to 20

http://www.cdc.gov/nchs/data/nhanes/growthcharts/set2clinical/cj411073.pdf

Skinfold Measurements

This section provides information on measuring skinfolds, including suggestions on how best to learn to do skinfold measurements.

Test Objective

To measure the triceps and calf (and abdominal for college students) skinfold thicknesses for calculating percent body fat.

Equipment and Facilities

A skinfold caliper is necessary to perform this measurement. The cost of calipers ranges from $5 to $200. Both the expensive and inexpensive calipers have been shown to be effective for use by teachers who have had sufficient training and practice.

Testing Procedures

The triceps and calf skinfolds have been chosen for *FITNESSGRAM* because they are easily measured and highly correlated with total body fatness. The caliper measures a double layer of subcutaneous fat and skin.

Measurement Location

The triceps skinfold is measured on the back of the right arm over the triceps muscle, midway between the elbow and the acromion process of the scapula. Using a piece of string to find the midpoint is a good suggestion. The skinfold site should be vertical. Pinching the fold slightly above the midpoint will ensure that the fold is measured right on the midpoint.

The calf skinfold is measured on the inside of the right leg at the level of maximal calf girth. The right foot is placed flat on an elevated surface with the knee flexed at a 90° angle. The vertical skinfold should be grasped just above the level of maximal girth and the measurement made below the grasp.

Measurement Technique

- Measure skinfolds on the person's right side.
- Instruct the student to relax the arm or leg being measured.
- Firmly grasp the skinfold between the thumb and forefinger and lift it away from the other body tissue. The grasp should not be so firm as to be painful.

- Place the caliper 1/2 inch below the pinch site.
- Be sure the caliper is in the middle of the fold.
- The recommended procedure is to do one measurement at each site before doing the second measurement at each site and finally the third set of measurements.

Scoring

The skinfold measure is registered on the caliper. Each measurement should be taken three times, with the recorded score being the median (middle) value of the three scores. To illustrate: If the readings were 7.0, 9.0, and 8.0, the score would be recorded as 8.0 millimeters. Each reading should be recorded to the nearest .5 millimeters. For teachers not using the computer software, a percent fatness look-up chart is provided in tables E.1 and E.2. *FITNESSGRAM* uses the formula developed by Slaughter and Lohman to calculate percent body fat (Slaughter et al., 1988).

Suggestions for Test Administration

- Skinfolds should be measured in a setting that provides the child with privacy.
- Interpretation of the measurements may be given in a group setting as long as individual results are not identified.
- Whenever possible, it is recommended that the same tester administer the skinfold measurement to the same students at subsequent testing periods.
- Practice measuring the sites with another tester and compare results on the same students. As you become familiar with the methods you can generally find agreement within 10% between testers.

Learning to Do Skinfold Measurements

Using video training tapes or participating in a workshop are excellent ways to begin to learn how to do skinfold measurements. The videotape *Practical Body Composition Video* (available from Human Kinetics) illustrates the procedures described in this manual.

TABLE E.1 *FITNESSGRAM* Body Composition Conversion Chart

BOYS									
Total MM	% Fat	Total MM	% Fat	Total MM	% Fat	Total MM	% Fat	Total MM	% Fat
1.0	1.7	16.0	12.8	31.0	23.8	46.0	34.8	61.0	45.8
1.5	2.1	16.5	13.1	31.5	24.2	46.5	35.2	61.5	46.2
2.0	2.5	17.0	13.5	32.0	24.5	47.0	35.5	62.0	46.6
2.5	2.8	17.5	13.9	32.5	24.9	47.5	35.9	62.5	46.9
3.0	3.2	18.0	14.2	33.0	25.3	48.0	36.3	63.0	47.3
3.5	3.6	18.5	14.6	33.5	25.6	48.5	36.6	63.5	47.7
4.0	3.9	19.0	15.0	34.0	26.0	49.0	37.0	64.0	48.0
4.5	4.3	19.5	15.3	34.5	26.4	49.5	37.4	64.5	48.4
5.0	4.7	20.0	15.7	35.0	26.7	50.0	37.8	65.0	48.8
5.5	5.0	20.5	16.1	35.5	27.1	50.5	38.1	65.5	49.1
6.0	5.4	21.0	16.4	36.0	27.5	51.0	38.5	66.0	49.5
6.5	5.8	21.5	16.8	36.5	27.8	51.5	38.9	66.5	49.9
7.0	6.1	22.0	17.2	37.0	28.2	52.0	39.2	67.0	50.2
7.5	6.5	22.5	17.5	37.5	28.6	52.5	39.6	67.5	50.6
8.0	6.9	23.0	17.9	38.0	28.9	53.0	40.0	68.0	51.0
8.5	7.2	23.5	18.3	38.5	29.3	53.5	40.3	68.5	51.3
9.0	7.6	24.0	18.6	39.0	29.7	54.0	40.7	69.0	51.7
9.5	8.0	24.5	19.0	39.5	30.0	54.5	41.1	69.5	52.1
10.0	8.4	25.0	19.4	40.0	30.4	55.0	41.4	70.0	52.5
10.5	8.7	25.5	19.7	40.5	30.8	55.5	41.8	70.5	52.8
11.0	9.1	26.0	20.1	41.0	31.1	56.0	42.2	71.0	53.2
11.5	9.5	26.5	20.5	41.5	31.5	56.5	42.5	71.5	53.6
12.0	9.8	27.0	20.8	42.0	31.9	57.0	42.9	72.0	53.9
12.5	10.2	27.5	21.2	42.5	32.2	57.5	43.3	72.5	54.3
13.0	10.6	28.0	21.6	43.0	32.6	58.0	43.6	73.0	54.7
13.5	10.9	28.5	21.9	43.5	33.0	58.5	44.0	73.5	55.0
14.0	11.3	29.0	22.3	44.0	33.3	59.0	44.4	74.0	55.4
14.5	11.7	29.5	22.7	44.5	33.7	59.5	44.7	74.5	55.8
15.0	12.0	30.0	23.1	45.0	34.1	60.0	45.1	75.0	56.1
15.5	12.4	30.5	23.4	45.5	34.4	60.5	45.5	75.5	56.5

TABLE E.2 FITNESSGRAM Body Composition Conversion Chart

GIRLS

Total MM	% Fat	Total MM	% Fat	Total MM	% Fat	Total MM	% Fat	Total MM	% Fat
1.0	5.7	16.0	14.9	31.0	24.0	46.0	33.2	61.0	42.3
1.5	6.0	16.5	15.2	31.5	24.3	46.5	33.5	61.5	42.6
2.0	6.3	17.0	15.5	32.0	24.6	47.0	33.8	62.0	42.9
2.5	6.6	17.5	15.8	32.5	24.9	47.5	34.1	62.5	43.2
3.0	6.9	18.0	16.1	33.0	25.2	48.0	34.4	63.0	43.5
3.5	7.2	18.5	16.4	33.5	25.5	48.5	34.7	63.5	43.8
4.0	7.5	19.0	16.7	34.0	25.8	49.0	35.0	64.0	44.1
4.5	7.8	19.5	17.0	34.5	26.1	49.5	35.3	64.5	44.4
5.0	8.2	20.0	17.3	35.0	26.5	50.0	35.6	65.0	44.8
5.5	8.5	20.5	17.6	35.5	26.8	50.5	35.9	65.5	45.1
6.0	8.8	21.0	17.9	36.0	27.1	51.0	36.2	66.0	45.4
6.5	9.1	21.5	18.2	36.5	27.4	51.5	36.5	66.5	45.7
7.0	9.4	22.0	18.5	37.0	27.7	52.0	36.8	67.0	46.0
7.5	9.7	22.5	18.8	37.5	28.0	52.5	37.1	67.5	46.3
8.0	10.0	23.0	19.1	38.0	28.3	53.0	37.4	68.0	46.6
8.5	10.3	23.5	19.4	38.5	28.6	53.5	37.7	68.5	46.9
9.0	10.6	24.0	19.7	39.0	28.9	54.0	38.0	69.0	47.2
9.5	10.9	24.5	20.0	39.5	29.2	54.5	38.3	69.5	47.5
10.0	11.2	25.0	20.4	40.0	29.5	55.0	38.7	70.0	47.8
10.5	11.5	25.5	20.7	40.5	29.8	55.5	39.0	70.5	48.1
11.0	11.8	26.0	21.0	41.0	30.1	56.0	39.3	71.0	48.4
11.5	12.1	26.5	21.3	41.5	30.4	56.5	39.6	71.5	48.7
12.0	12.4	27.0	21.6	42.0	30.7	57.0	39.9	72.0	49.0
12.5	12.7	27.5	21.9	42.5	31.0	57.5	40.2	72.5	49.3
13.0	13.0	28.0	22.2	43.0	31.3	58.0	40.5	73.0	49.6
13.5	13.3	28.5	22.5	43.5	31.6	58.5	40.8	73.5	49.9
14.0	13.6	29.0	22.8	44.0	31.9	59.0	41.1	74.0	50.2
14.5	13.9	29.5	23.1	44.5	32.2	59.5	41.4	74.5	50.5
15.0	14.3	30.0	23.4	45.0	32.6	60.0	41.7	75.0	50.9
15.5	14.6	30.5	23.7	45.5	32.9	60.5	42.0	75.5	51.2

Reprinted, by permission, from The Cooper Institute, 2004, *FITNESSGRAM/ACTIVITYGRAM Test Administration Manual,* (Champaign, IL: Human Kinetics), 96-97.

CDC'S GUIDELINES FOR SCHOOL AND COMMUNITY PROGRAMS TO PROMOTE LIFE-LONG PHYSICAL ACTIVITY AMONG YOUNG PEOPLE

1. Policy

Establish policies that promote enjoyable, lifelong physical activity among young people.

- Require comprehensive, daily physical education for students in kindergarten through grade 12.
- Require comprehensive health education for students in kindergarten through grade 12.
- Require that adequate resources, including budget and facilities, be committed for physical activity instruction and programs.
- Require the hiring of physical education specialists to teach physical education in kindergarten through grade 12, elementary school teachers trained to teach health education, health education specialists to teach health education in middle and senior high schools, and qualified people to direct school and community physical activity programs and to coach young people in sports and recreation programs.
- Require that physical education instruction and programs meet the needs and interests of all students.

2. Environment

Provide physical and social environments that encourage and enable safe and enjoyable physical activity.

- Provide access to safe spaces and facilities for physical activity in the school and the community.
- Establish and enforce measures to prevent injuries and illnesses related to physical activity.
- Provide time within the school day for unstructured physical activity.
- Discourage the use or withholding of physical activity as punishment.
- Provide health promotion programs for school faculty and staff.

3. Physical Education

Implement physical education curricula and instruction that emphasize enjoyable participation in physical activity and that help students develop the knowledge, attitudes, motor skills, behavioral skills, and confidence needed to adopt and maintain physically active lifestyles.

- Provide planned and sequential physical education curricula from kindergarten through grade 12 that promote enjoyable, lifelong physical activity.
- Use physical education curricula consistent with the national standards for physical education.
- Use active learning strategies and emphasize enjoyable participation in physical education class.

- Develop students' knowledge of and positive attitudes toward physical activity.
- Develop students' mastery of and confidence in motor and behavioral skills for participating in physical activity.
- Provide a substantial percentage of each student's recommended weekly amount of physical activity in physical education classes.
- Promote participation in enjoyable physical activity in the school, community, and home.

4. Health Education

Implement health education curricula and instruction that help students develop the knowledge, attitudes, behavioral skills, and confidence needed to adopt and maintain physically active lifestyles.

- Provide planned and sequential health education curricula from kindergarten through grade 12 that promote lifelong participation in physical activity.
- Use health education curricula consistent with the national standards for health education.
- Promote collaboration among physical education, health education, and classroom teachers, as well as teachers in related disciplines who plan and implement physical activity instruction.
- Use active learning strategies to emphasize enjoyable participation in physical activity in the school, community, and home.
- Develop students' knowledge of and positive attitudes toward healthy behaviors, particularly physical activity.
- Develop students' mastery of and confidence in the behavioral skills needed to adopt and maintain a healthy lifestyle that includes regular physical activity.

5. Extracurricular Activities

Provide extracurricular physical activity programs that meet the needs and interests of all students.

- Provide a diversity of developmentally appropriate competitive and noncompetitive physical activity programs for all students.
- Link students to community physical activity programs, and use community resources to support extracurricular physical activity programs.

6. Parental Involvement

Include parents and guardians in physical activity instruction and in extracurricular and community physical activity programs, and encourage them to support their children's participation in enjoyable physical activities.

- Encourage parents to advocate for quality physical activity instruction and programs for their children.
- Encourage parents to support their children's participation in appropriate, enjoyable physical activities.
- Encourage parents to be physically active role models and to plan and participate in family activities that include physical activity.

7. Personnel Training

Provide training for education, coaching, recreation, health care, and other school and community personnel that imparts the knowledge and skills needed to effectively promote enjoyable, lifelong physical activity among young people.

- Train teachers to deliver physical education that provides a substantial percentage of each student's recommended weekly amount of physical activity.
- Train teachers to use active learning strategies needed to develop students' knowledge about, attitudes toward, skills in, and confidence in engaging in physical activity.
- Train school and community personnel how to create psycho-social environments that enable young people to enjoy physical activity instruction and programs.
- Train school and community personnel how to involve parents and the community in physical activity instruction and programs.
- Train volunteers who coach sports and recreation programs for young people.

8. Health Services

Assess physical activity patterns among young people, counsel them about physical activity, refer them to appropriate programs, and advocate for physical activity instruction and programs for them.

- Regularly assess the physical activity patterns of young people, reinforce physical activity among active young people, counsel inactive young people about physical activity, and refer young people to appropriate physical activity programs.
- Advocate for school and community physical activity instruction and programs that meet the needs of young people.

9. Community Programs

Provide a range of developmentally appropriate community sports and recreation programs that are attractive to all young people.

- Provide a diversity of developmentally appropriate community sports and recreation programs for all young people.
- Provide access to community sports and recreation programs for young people.

10. Evaluation

Regularly evaluate school and community physical activity instruction, programs, and facilities.

- Evaluate the implementation and quality of physical activity policies, curricula, instruction, programs, and personnel training.
- Measure students' attainment of physical activity knowledge, achievement of motor and behavioral skills, and adoption of healthy behaviors.

Table F.1 Sample Progressive Scope and Sequence for Grades K-10

Essential learning goal: The student acquires the knowledge and skills necessary to maintain an active life: movement, physical fitness, and nutrition.				Essential learning goal: The student effectively analyzes health and safety information to develop health and fitness plans based on life goals.
Develops fundamental physical skills and progresses to complex movement activities as physically able	**Incorporates rules and safety procedures into physical activities**	**Understands the concepts of physical fitness, and plans and monitors personal fitness plans and goals**	**Understands nutrition and food nutrients and how they affect physical performance and the body**	**Develops a health and fitness plan and a monitoring system**
GRADE K LEARNING TARGETS				
• Demonstrates large muscle coordination in locomotor and nonlocomotor skills • Demonstrates an awareness of personal space • Demonstrates a feeling for beat and accent through rhythmic activities • Responds to visual and verbal signals • Performs various activities requiring body management	Demonstrates movement safety of self and others	• Meets age-appropriate health-related fitness criterion • Recognizes changes in heart rate during exercise and rest	• Explores the food pyramid and identifies food groups • Identifies healthy nutrition choices	Sets small group goals for specific activities
GRADE 1 LEARNING TARGETS				
• Demonstrates basic locomotor and nonlocomotor movement in combination • Demonstrates basic rhythm and dance movements • Manipulates simple apparatus with basic movement elements	Demonstrates movement safety of self and others using various movements and pathways	Meets age-appropriate health-related fitness criterion	• Identifies relationship of food to growth • Explains the concept of food as fuel	Identifies and establishes short-term class goals
GRADE 2 LEARNING TARGETS				
• Demonstrates basic movement and manipulative skills in combination in a variety of activities • Demonstrates mature movement patterns to teacher-selected rhythm, by using the body as a means of expression • Demonstrates balance skills using various apparatus	Participates safely during activities	• Meets age-appropriate health-related fitness criterion • Explains the relationship of fitness to health	• Demonstrates healthy nutritional choices • Explains the concept of variety and moderation in food selection • Explains the relationship of healthy food to healthy bodies	• Identifies goal-setting process and makes/monitors appropriate short-term goals • Assists in establishing class goals for health and fitness

GRADE 3 LEARNING TARGETS				
• Combines locomotor, nonlocomotor, and manipulative skills in game situations • Identifies and demonstrates appropriate movement to accents in music in a variety of ways	• Moves safely during activity • Demonstrates a basic knowledge of rules and specific safety procedures as related to physical activity	*• Meets age-appropriate health-related fitness criterion • Identifies the components of health-related fitness • Participates in activities that apply the concepts of duration and intensity as related to aerobic fitness	Identifies factors influencing nutritional choices within the family and nutritional sources for proteins and carbohydrates	Demonstrates the ability to develop health plans and predicts the benefits of healthy choices
GRADE 4 LEARNING TARGETS				
Combines locomotor, nonlocomotor, and manipulative skills in individual, dual, rhythmic, and team activities	Applies rules, safety procedures, and cooperation during active participation in a variety of activities	*• Meets age-appropriate health-related fitness criterion • Sets and monitors progress toward personal fitness goals • Identifies strength, flexibility, and aerobic fitness activities	Identifies nutrients provided by a variety of foods, and describes how the body and physical performance are affected	Establishes and monitors both short- and long-term personal health goals
GRADE 5 LEARNING TARGETS				
• Identifies, describes, and demonstrates increasingly complex movement combinations through previously learned progressions • Integrates multiple movement concepts and patterns in various rhythmic activities	Demonstrates knowledge of rules and safe participation in a variety of activities	*• Meets age-appropriate health-related fitness criterion *• Sets and monitors personal fitness goals • Analyzes health-related fitness components as they relate to personal lifestyles	Identifies the influence of advertising and food labeling on nutrition choices	Monitors progress toward personal health goals, and revises when appropriate
GRADE 6 LEARNING TARGETS				
• Performs multiple movement patterns in rhythmic activities • Demonstrates age and developmentally appropriate skills during participation in a variety of individual, dual, and team activities	Participates safely and cooperatively in physical activities	*• Meets age-appropriate health-related fitness criterion • Performs in personal, health-related fitness assessments, sets fitness goals, and creates/follows personal action plans to achieve fitness goals	Identifies components of the national dietary guidelines and sets/monitors personal nutrition patterns	Develops and implements a personal health and fitness action plan
GRADE 7 LEARNING TARGETS				
Performs age and developmentally appropriate physical skills and applies them in complex patterns, including leisure and rhythmic activities	Participates safely, follows rules, and acts cooperatively in a variety of physical activities	*• Meets age-appropriate health-related fitness criterion • Sets personal, health-related fitness goals and explores a variety of activities to maintain appropriate levels of health-related physical fitness	• Designs nutrition goals based on national dietary guidelines and individual activity needs • Understands the results of movement, fitness, and nutrition practices in relation to a healthy lifestyle	Develops a support system and record-keeping system to achieve health and fitness goals

(continued)

TABLE F.1 (continued)

Essential learning goal: The student acquires the knowledge and skills necessary to maintain an active life: movement, physical fitness, and nutrition.

Essential learning goal: The student effectively analyzes health and safety information to develop health and fitness plans based on life goals.

Develops fundamental physical skills and progresses to complex movement activities as physically able	Incorporates rules and safety procedures into physical activities	Understands the concepts of physical fitness, and plans and monitors personal fitness plans and goals	Understands nutrition and food nutrients and how they affect physical performance and the body	Develops a health and fitness plan and a monitoring system
GRADE 8 LEARNING TARGETS				
• Applies age and developmentally appropriate skills related to individual and leisure physical activities • Applies knowledge and skills to personal activity patterns outside of school setting	• Cooperatively and safely participates in a variety of physical activities • Analyzes the risks involved in participating in various physical activities	*• Meets age-appropriate health-related fitness criterion • Initiates a personal, health-related fitness plan that includes physical activity, nutrition, and reduction of risk-taking behaviors	• Identifies various noncommunicable diseases caused by or aggravated by poor nutritional choices and their specific effects on the body • Identifies how self-esteem, peer pressure, and the media influence nutritional practices	Modifies and continues to implement a personal fitness plan that includes physical activity, nutrition, and reduction of risk-taking
GRADE 9 LEARNING TARGETS				
Refines and applies age and developmentally appropriate skills in individual and leisure physical activities to participate at a recreational level	Applies rules and safety procedures	*• Meets age-appropriate health-related fitness criterion • Refines and monitors individual health-related fitness goals, based on a variety of physical activities, fitness profiles, and nutritional guidelines	Develops personal nutrition goals based on national dietary guidelines and individual needs	Refines personal health and fitness plans to include potential lifetime activities
GRADE 10 LEARNING TARGETS				
Applies knowledge and skills to personal activity patterns inside and outside of school setting	Applies rules and safety procedures, practices good sporting behavior, and participates in a variety of physical activities	*• Meets age-appropriate health-related fitness criterion • Monitors progress on individual health-related fitness goals, based on fitness profiles, individual physical capabilities, and national guidelines in relation to work and leisure goals	• Monitors personal nutrition goals based on national dietary guidelines and individual needs • Compares and contrasts the application of movement, fitness, and nutrition concepts to safe work practices and leisure activities	Implements and monitors a personal health and fitness plan, based on life goals for leisure and employment

*indicates taught in previous year

Reprinted, by permission, from A. Hass-Holcombe, 1997, *Fitness for a lifetime.* Courtesy of Corvallis School District 509J, Corvallis, Oregon.

302

STUDENT ASTHMA
ACTION CARD

 Asthma and Allergy Foundation of America

STUDENT ASTHMA ACTION CARD

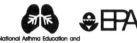

National Asthma Education and Prevention Program

Name:_____ Grade: _____ Age:_____

Homeroom Teacher:_____ Room: _____

Parent/Guardian Name: _____ Ph: (h): _____

 Address: _____ Ph: (w): _____

Parent/Guardian Name: _____ Ph: (h): _____

 Address: _____ Ph: (w): _____

ID Photo

Emergency Phone Contact #1_____
 Name Relationship Phone

Emergency Phone Contact #2_____
 Name Relationship Phone

Physician Treating Student for Asthma: _____ Ph: _____

Other Physician:_____ Ph: _____

EMERGENCY PLAN

Emergency action is necessary when the student has symptoms such as, _____ , _____ ,
_____ , _____ or has a peak flow reading of _____ .

• **Steps to take during an asthma episode**:
  1. Check peak flow.
  2. Give medications as listed below. Student should respond to treatment in 15-20 minutes.
  3. Contact parent/guardian if _____
  _____
  4. Re-check peak flow.
  5. Seek emergency medical care if the student has any of the following:
      ✔ Coughs constantly
      ✔ No improvement 15-20 minutes after initial treatment
        with medication and a relative cannot be reached.
      ✔ Peak flow of _____
      ✔ Hard time breathing with:
        • Chest and neck pulled in with breathing
        • Stooped body posture
        • Struggling or gasping
      ✔ Trouble walking or talking
      ✔ Stops playing and can't start activity again
      ✔ Lips or fingernails are grey or blue

}

IF THIS HAPPENS, GET EMERGENCY HELP NOW!

• **Emergency Asthma Medications**

Name	Amount	When to Use
1.		
2.		
3.		
4.		

See reverse for more instructions

www.aafa.org/public/pdfs/student.pdf

DAILY ASTHMA MANAGEMENT PLAN

• Identify the things which start an asthma episode (Check each that applies to the student.)

☐ Exercise   ☐ Strong odors or fumes   ☐ Other _____

☐ Respiratory infections   ☐ Chalk dust / dust   _____

☐ Change in temperature   ☐ Carpets in the room

☐ Animals   ☐ Pollens

☐ Food _____   ☐ Molds

Comments _____

• Control of School Environment

(List any environmental control measures, pre-medications, and/or dietary restrictions that the student needs to prevent an asthma episode.) _____

_____

_____

_____

• Peak Flow Monitoring

Personal Best Peak Flow number: _____

Monitoring Times: _____   _____   _____   _____

• Daily Medication Plan

	Name	Amount	When to Use
1.			
2.			
3.			
4.			

COMMENTS / SPECIAL INSTRUCTIONS

_____

_____

_____

FOR INHALED MEDICATIONS

☐ I have instructed _____ in the proper way to use his/her medications. It is my professional opinion that _____ should be allowed to carry and use that medication by him/herself.

☐ It is my professional opinion that _____ should not carry his/her inhaled medication by him/herself.

_____   _____
Physician Signature   Date

_____   _____
Parent/Guardian Signature   Date

AAFA • 1233 20th Street, N.W., Suite 402 , Washington, DC 20036 • www.aafa.org • 1-800-7-ASTHMA

02/00

GLOSSARY

active stretch—A stretch in which the person stretching provides the force of the stretch.

ACTIVITYGRAM—A feature of *FITNESSGRAM* that provides physical activity assessments. It includes detailed information about the student's activity habits and prescriptive feedback about how active he or she should be.

aerobic capacity—Another term for maximal oxygen consumption (see maximal oxygen consumption definition), which provides an indication of aerobic fitness.

aerobic fitness—The ability to perform large muscle, dynamic, moderate- to high-intensity exercise for prolonged periods. For a child, this definition may mean the ability to exercise or play for long periods of time without getting tired.

affective domain—The attitudes and values a student has toward and during physical activity. Although difficult to measure, affective behaviors can be assessed through journals, rubrics, questionnaires, and systematic observance of student behaviors, including effort and compliance with directions.

age or developmentally appropriate physical activity—Activity of a frequency, intensity, duration, and type that leads to optimal child growth and development and contributes to the development of future physically active lifestyles.

alternative assessment—Using tools other than traditional standardized testing—including tools such as portfolios, journals, and role playing—to collect evidence about student learning and achievement of program objectives.

anorexia nervosa—A serious and potentially fatal disease that is characterized by self-induced starvation and extreme weight loss. Symptoms include a refusal to maintain a normal body weight, an intense fear of weight and of getting "fat," feeling fat despite dramatic weight loss, an experience of loss of periods, and an extreme concern with body weight and appearance.

antagonist—Refers to muscles that have an opposite effect as the agonist or mover. The antagonist muscle opposes the contraction of the agonist or mover.

aptitudes—The potential for performance; learning potential.

assessment—Continuous collection and interpretation of information on student behaviors for the purpose of informing you and your students how they are improving in specific components.

attitudes—The feelings and values (affective domain) a student has toward and during physical activity.

authentic assessment—Observing students and collecting data in real-life activities and settings.

ballistic stretching—A type of stretching that involves moving quickly, bouncing, or using momentum to produce the stretch.

bingeing—The consumption of large amounts of food within a short period of time.

block scheduling—A type of scheduling that involves redesigning the school day to provide for greater learning time. This includes extending the length of class periods and reducing the number of courses a student takes in one day.

body building—A sport where competitors are judged on size, symmetry, and definition of muscle.

body composition—The amount of lean body mass compared to the amount of body fat. This is typically expressed in terms of percent body fat.

body mass index (BMI)—A ratio of height to weight that correlates with body fat in the general population. The health risk from weight greatly increases with BMIs of 30 and over.

bulimia—An eating disorder characterized by a destructive cycle of bingeing and purging of food. Most bulimics are of normal weight or are slightly overweight. Symptoms include bingeing, purging, and an extreme concern with body weight and shape.

carbohydrate—A category of nutrient that is the preferred source of energy for the body, particularly the brain. Carbohydrates are either simple or complex and contain carbon, hydrogen, and oxygen. All carbohydrates provide four kilocalories per gram.

circuit training—Training that involves several different exercises or activities. This type of training allows a physical educator to vary the intensity or type of activity as children move from station to station.

cognitive domain—Refers to knowledge about rules, procedures, safety, and critical elements, as well as fitness knowledge that will contribute to the ability to make healthy lifetime activity choices and to participate in a variety of physical activities throughout the lifetime.

communication systems—A means by which a student communicates through the use of assistive technology or systems such as sign language.

concentric contraction—A muscle contraction where the muscle shortens as it contracts.

continuous activity—Movement that lasts at least several minutes without rest periods.

cool-down—A period of light activity following exercise that allows the body to slow down and gradually return to near resting levels. The body needs this gradual recovery following exercise to ensure proper blood flow back to the heart, reduce muscle stiffness and soreness, remove lactic acid, and prevent light-headedness, dizziness, or even fainting.

cooperative learning—A teaching style that involves students working together to complete a specified task or assignment. It is an extremely flexible style that has the potential to incorporate all three learning domains, to use several intelligences, and to provide for a more positive learning environment.

criterion-referenced testing—A type of fitness testing in which student scores are compared to preset standard score ranges that indicate levels of health-related fitness necessary for good health and reduced risk of diseases associated with sedentary lifestyles. This method of scoring removes the competitive emphasis previously associated with fitness testing (norm-referenced tests) and puts the focus on the achievement of health-related fitness.

criterion score/zone—Preset standard scoring ranges used in criterion-referenced fitness testing to indicate levels of health-related fitness necessary for good health and reduced risk of diseases associated

with sedentary lifestyles. For example, in *FITNESS-GRAM*, the goal is to score in the healthy fitness zones (HFZs) in each component of health-related fitness.

cue words—Cue words or phrases that a student repeats while executing a skill so that he or she will learn the vocabulary that goes with the actions.

curriculum model—Examples of different physical education models include sport education, theme or skill based, movement education, activity based, wilderness or adventure education, concept or interdisciplinary based, fitness based, and student centered based. Many schools today use a more eclectic approach by combining models to meet the needs of their student population.

developmentally appropriate activities—Those activities that are appropriate based on a student's developmental level, age, ability level, interests, and previous experience and knowledge.

diet—The total intake of food and beverages consumed.

duration—How long the activity should be performed (time).

dynamic flexibility—The rate of increase in tension in relaxed muscle as it is stretched. Dynamic flexibility exercises are mostly utilized in sport-specific movements and physical therapy or rehabilitation settings.

eccentric contraction—A muscle contraction where the muscle lengthens as it contracts. Also known as negative exercise.

effort—Infers how hard a student tries.

elasticity—A muscle property that allows the tissue to stretch and return to its normal length following stretching.

energy balance—Calories injected must equal calories expended.

exercise—Physical activity that is planned, structured, and repetitive bodily movement done to improve or maintain one or more of the components of health-related fitness.

exercise-induced asthma—A narrowing of the airways that is brought on by exercise, making breathing difficult. For a person who has asthma, this may occur during or after exercise, and symptoms include wheezing, coughing, tightness of the chest, and breathlessness.

exercise prescription—The process of designing a routine of physical activity in a systematic and individualized manner (ACSM 2000).

exit outcomes—The ultimate desired achievements of students who graduate from a K-12 curriculum. The outcomes should specify what you expect students to know, understand, and be able to do by the time they complete high school.

extension—Increase in the angle of a joint.

external factors—Environmental (i.e., social and physical) influences on behavior.

extrinsic motivation—A person's desire to perform a particular task based on environmental or other personal influences. Occurs when a desired object or socially enhancing consequence is presented to increase the likelihood that a behavior will be repeated.

fartlek training—A modification of continuous training where periods of increased intensity are interspersed with continuous activity over varying and natural terrain.

fat—A category of nutrient that provides nine kilocalories per gram.

FITNESSGRAM—A health-related fitness assessment and computerized reporting system that has been endorsed as the assessment tool to be used in conjunction with the Physical Best program. It sets performance standards—called healthy fitness zones—that reflect the basic health-related fitness levels required for good health.

fitness knowledge—Knowledge that will contribute to the ability to make healthy lifetime activity choices and to participate in a variety of physical activities throughout the lifetime.

FITT guidelines—Describe how to safely apply the five principles of training (overload, progression, specificity, regularity, and individuality) by manipulating the frequency, intensity, time, and type of activity.

flexibility—The ability to move a joint through its complete ROM, or range of motion.

flexion—Decrease in the angle of a joint.

Food and Drug Administration (FDA)—The government agency that oversees food standards, food labeling, prescription drugs, and over-the-counter drug policies and standards in the United States.

frequency—How often a person performs the targeted health-related physical activity (e.g., three times a week).

Gardner's theory of multiple intelligences—A theory of learning that asserts that different individuals are strong in different "intelligences." The types of intelligence include bodily-kinesthetic intelligence, spatial intelligence, interpersonal intelligence, musical intelligence, logical-mathematical intelligence, intrapersonal intelligence, naturalistic intelligence, and linguistic intelligence.

grading—An attempt to communicate all that the individual has done in your physical education program. It involves assigning a summative score to student work—inferring value of student work.

health-related fitness—A measure of a person's ability to perform physical activities that require endurance, strength, or flexibility and are achieved through a combination of regular exercise and inherent ability. The components of health-related physical fitness are aerobic fitness (cardiorespiratory endurance), muscular strength, muscular endurance, flexibility, and body composition as they relate specifically to health enhancement.

health-related fitness domain—Refers to developing health-related fitness and most often is assessed through fitness testing.

heart rate monitor—A device that provides heart rate data. Students can use these data as an educational and self-assessment tool.

heart rate reserve—The difference between a person's maximal heart rate and resting heart rate.

hydrogenation—The process of adding hydrogen under pressure to unsaturated oils to produce a solid product such as shortening or margarine.

hyperextension—An exercise that takes a joint well beyond its normal range of motion (extension), which can cause an increased risk for the development of joint laxity and possible injury.

hyperflexion—An exercise that takes a joint well beyond its normal range of motion (flexion), which can cause an increased risk for the development of joint laxity and possible injury.

hypermobility—Excess ROM at a joint. This condition may predispose an individual to injury.

inclusion—The process of creating a learning environment that is open to and effective for all students whose needs and abilities fall outside of the general range of those for children of similar age or whose cultural or religious beliefs differ from that of the majority group. In short, inclusion means that *all* students are actively engaged in an appropriate manner, so that *all* students can reach their maximum potential.

inclusive—Although this term is generally used as a philosophical and programmatic descriptor relating to students with special needs or disabilities, the Physical Best program broadens this to mean creating physical activity opportunities that meet the needs of every student. This can be done by offering choices and modifying components of activities.

individuality principle—The principle of training that takes into account that each person begins at a different level of fitness, each person has personal goals and objectives for physical activity and fitness, and each person has different genetic potential for change.

intensity—How hard a person exercises during a physical activity period. Proper intensity should be determined based on the age, fitness level, and fitness goals of the participant.

internal factors—Personal (i.e., biological and psychological) influences on behavior.

interval training—Training that involves alternating short bursts of activity with rest periods.

intrinsic motivation—A person's internal desire to perform a particular task.

journal—A written account from the perspective of the individual. Often a reflection on daily events or logged activities.

kilocalorie—A measure of heat energy. Technically, it's the amount of energy required to raise the temperature of one kilogram of water one degree Celsius. Popular sources often shorten the term *kilocalories* to simply *calories*.

lanugo—A downy layer of hair growth that occurs as a side effect of anorexia nervosa.

laxity—The degree of abnormal motion of a given joint. Abnormal joint laxity means the ligaments connecting bone to bone can no longer provide stability to the joint.

lesson outcomes—What you expect students to know, understand, and be able to do as a result of a specific lesson. At this level, you are using lesson plans to help students work toward achieving the unit outcomes, thus leading to meeting the exit or program outcomes.

lipid—A technical term for fat. The term includes saturated as well as unsaturated fats.

log—A systematic record or accounting of behavior (usually without reflection) that is used mainly for recording performance and participation data. Logs provide a baseline record of behaviors and help form the basis to set personal goals related to exercise frequency, intensity, or duration.

maximal heart rate—Used when determining the appropriate exercise heart rate for monitoring training intensity. Maximal heart rate is calculated using this formula: $208 - (.7 \times \text{age})$.

maximal oxygen consumption—Considered to be the best measure of aerobic fitness. It is a laboratory test measuring the maximum amount of oxygen that an individual can consume despite an increase in the workload during a graded exercise test.

medicine ball—A heavy ball weighing 1 to 20 pounds and made of leather or rubber. Medicine balls can be employed in muscular fitness activities.

mineral—A nonorganic substance that is necessary for the normal functioning of the body, especially for growth and health maintenance. Minerals contain zero calories.

moderate physical activity—Activity of an intensity equal to brisk walking that can be performed for relatively long periods of time without fatigue.

motivational factors—Factors that push or pull to create behavior change. The behaviors of individuals are influenced by both internally and externally controlled factors.

muscle-tendon unit—The area of the muscle where the muscle and tendon connect to the bone. Stretching increases the length of the muscle-tendon unit.

muscular endurance—The ability of a muscle or muscle group to exert a submaximal force repeatedly over a period of time.

muscular fitness—In the Physical Best program, muscular fitness refers to the development of a combination of muscular strength and muscular endurance.

muscular power—The ability to exert a force rapidly. It can be calculated as force times distance divided by time.

muscular strength—The ability of a muscle or muscle group to exert a maximal force against a resistance one time through the full range of motion.

norm—The average score of all students who took a test.

norm-referenced scoring—A method of scoring in which an individual's score is compared to the average (norm) and standard deviation (average difference) of all the students who took a test or were measured on a factor.

nutrient density—The amount of a given nutrient per calorie in a food. For example, a vegetable has a higher nutrient density than a candy bar.

obesity—A condition of excess body fat, typically defined as 120 percent of ideal body weight or greater. Obesity increases a person's risk for weight-related complications as well as chronic diseases.

one-repetition maximum (1RM)—The amount of weight that can be lifted one time through the full range of motion. It is an assessment technique not recommended for children, but it can be determined by performing either a 10RM or 12RM and then using a table to estimate the 1RM.

overload principle—States that a body system (cardiorespiratory, muscular, or skeletal) must perform at a level beyond normal in order to adapt and improve physiological function and fitness.

overtraining—A condition caused by training too much or too intensely and not providing sufficient recovery time. Symptoms include lack of energy, decreased performance, fatigue, depression, aching muscles, loss of appetite, and proneness to injury.

PALA (Presidential Active Lifestyle Award)—An award offered through the Active Lifestyle program (part of the President's Challenge) to recognize youth and adults who participate regularly in physical activity. Students who are active for 60 minutes per day, five days a week, for six weeks are eligible to receive this award. The award can also be earned by keeping track of steps per day using a pedometer.

passive stretch—A stretch in which a partner provides the force of the stretch.

pedometer—A device that can be used to count the steps taken daily. Pedometers can be used as a motivational tool to provide feedback on the duration (distance) or intensity (distance over time) of physical activity.

peer assessment—An assessment method where students analyze the performance of other students. This method is useful to reduce student anxiety, to enhance student knowledge, and to empower students to take personal responsibility for assessment.

peer tutors—Students who work together to help each other learn. This teaching strategy also helps highly skilled students feel more challenged.

physical activity—Any bodily movement produced by skeletal muscles that results in an expenditure of energy.

plasticity—The property that establishes a new and greater resting length after passive stretching.

plyometrics—A muscular fitness training technique used to develop explosive power. It emphasizes pre-stretching (eccentric contraction) the muscle prior to engaging in concentric contractions, and it often involves hops, jumps, and throws.

PNF (proprioceptive neuromuscular facilitation)—A static stretch using combinations of the active and passive stretching techniques. Generally involves a precontraction of the muscle to be stretched and a contraction of the antagonist muscle during the stretch.

portfolio—A collection of a student's work—usually a combination of student-chosen and required material—demonstrating achievement of program goals.

power lifting—A competitive sport involving the dead lift, the squat, and the bench press.

process goals—Goals that are focused on the process, such as being active, rather than the product, such as achieving a fast time in the mile run.

progression—Refers to how an individual should increase the overload. Proper progression involves a gradual increase in the level of exercise that is manipulated by increasing either frequency, intensity, or time, or a combination of all three components.

protein—A category of nutrient that is primarily for cell growth and replacement. The body uses protein as a constituent of vital body parts. Protein contains carbon, hydrogen, oxygen, and nitrogen. Protein provides four kilocalories per gram.

psychomotor domain—Refers to skills and motor or movement patterns. It is commonly assessed during drills, skill tests, and gamelike activities.

purging—The use of laxatives, vomiting, or diuretics to prevent absorption of calories in the body and weight gain.

rating of perceived exertion (RPE)—A method of self-assessment of intensity of a person's workload on a scale of 6 to 20. (This is also known as the Borg Scale.)

regularity principle—States that physical activity must be performed on a regular basis to be effective, and that long periods of inactivity can lead to a loss of the benefits achieved during the training session.

repetition—The number of times an exercise is performed during one set.

resistance training or strength training—A systematic, preplanned program using a variety of methods (e.g., a person's own body weight or tension bands) or equipment (e.g., machines or free weights) that progressively stresses the musculoskeletal system to improve muscular strength, endurance, or power.

resting energy expenditure (REE)—The energy the body uses at rest.

rubric—A scoring tool that identifies the criteria used for judging student performance. Rubrics range in complexity from checklists to holistic in nature and can be used to assess skills, attitudes, and knowledge.

self-assessment—An assessment method where students use rubrics of critical elements, journals, or logs to monitor their own progress.

self-reliance—Having the skills and knowledge necessary to take control of your own health-related fitness (also referred to as self-responsibility). The goal of the Physical Best program is to help students become self-reliant so they can continue to pursue health-related fitness activities throughout their lifetime.

set—A group of repetitions followed by a rest period.

skill-related fitness—Skill-related fitness (sometimes referred to as sport-related fitness) components often go hand in hand with certain physical activities and are necessary for a person to accomplish or enhance a skill or task. The skill-related components include agility, coordination, reaction time, balance, speed, and power.

skinfold—A double layer of skin and subcutaneous fat.

skinfold caliper—Equipment used to measure a skinfold in body composition assessment.

specificity principle—States that explicit activities that target a particular body system must be performed to bring about fitness changes in that area.

The Spectrum Approach—An approach to teaching that involves using a "spectrum of teaching styles" that move along a continuum from direct instruction (teacher initiated) to independence (student-initiated instruction). The styles include command, practice, reciprocal, self-check, inclusion, guided discovery, convergent discovery, divergent production, learner-designed individual program, learner-initiated, and self-teaching.

spotting—A technique used in muscular fitness where a student or teacher helps ensure the safety of the student performing an exercise.

Stages of change (also transtheoretical model)—A model for behavioral change that focuses on motivation to change as it relates to stages of readiness and awareness. The model identifies typical behaviors of individuals at each stage and provides recommendations for moving through the stages of change.

Stairway to Lifetime Fitness—A health-related physical fitness education model that outlines the steps through which teachers must guide their students in order to have the students assume progressively more responsibility for their own health, fitness, and well-being.

static flexibility—The range of motion at a joint or group of joints. The limits of an individual's static flexibility are determined by his or her tolerance of the stretched position.

static stretch—A slow sustained stretch of the muscle that is held for 10 to 30 seconds. The person stretches the muscle-tendon unit to the point where mild discomfort is felt and then backs off slightly, holding the stretch at a point just prior to discomfort.

stiffness—Refers to the force needed to stretch and is related to the amount of elasticity in the muscle-tendon unit.

stride length—The distance between two heel strikes.

stride length calculation for steps—Some pedometers have the capacity to adjust the stride length. Teachers can instruct students on how to determine the number of steps per mile.

stroke volume—The amount of blood ejected in one heart beat.

task analysis—A process that involves breaking down a task into its component parts to help determine the level and type of support that you must provide for an individual with a disability. An individual may need a task to be broken down more or less, depending on his or her disability.

team teaching—A teaching strategy in which two or more teachers combine their students and provide instruction as a team. This strategy can help solve space, equipment, and scheduling issues, capitalize on each individual teacher's area of expertise, and allow one or more instructors greater interaction with individual students.

tidal volume—The volume of air either inhaled or exhaled in a normal resting breath.

time—How long the activity should be performed (duration).

traditional assessment—A process where results of tests are the main data used to measure or quantify student learning outcomes. In physical education, this has often taken the form of rules tests (e.g., for specific games and sports), skill test results, fitness tests, and teacher observation.

training adaptations—The basic physiological changes that occur over the course of a training period.

transfats—A type of unhealthy fat that is the result of the hydrogenation of vegetable oils.

type—Refers to mode or what kind of activity a person chooses to perform in each area of health-related fitness.

underweight—A low weight compared to a person's height. Typically defined as less than 90 percent of ideal body weight.

unit outcomes—What you expect students to know, understand, and be able to do at the completion of a specified set of lessons. Unit outcomes should be aligned with your exit or program outcomes.

ventilation—The volume of air moved (inspired or expired), generally expressed in liters per minute and calculated by multiplying respiratory rate times tidal volume.

vigorous physical activity—Movement that expends more energy or is performed at a higher intensity than brisk walking.

vitamin—An essential organic substance that contributes to the normal biological processes of the body. Vitamins contain zero calories.

volume—In muscular fitness, this is the number of sets and repetitions in a workout.

warm-up—A low-intensity activity done before a full-effort or main activity to prepare the body for upcoming more intense activity. A proper warm-up improves muscle function, maximizes blood flow to the muscles, and improves flexibility.

weightlifting—A competitive sport involving maximal lifts.

REFERENCES

Alter, M.J. 1998. *Sport Stretch*. 2nd ed. Champaign, IL: Human Kinetics.

American Academy of Pediatrics (AAP). 2000a. Intensive training and sports specialization in young athletes (RE9906). *Pediatrics* 106(1): 154-157.

American Academy of Pediatrics (AAP). 2000b. Physical fitness and activity in schools (RE9907). *Pediatrics* 105(5): 1156-1157.

American Academy of Pediatrics (AAP), Committee on Sports Medicine and Fitness. 2001. Policy statement: Strength training by children and adolescents. *Pediatrics* 107(6): 1470-1472.

American Association for Physical Education, Recreation and Dance (AAALF/AAHPERD). 1995. *Physical best and individuals with disabilities: A handbook for inclusion in fitness programs*. ed. J.A. Seaman, Champaign, IL: Human Kinetics.

American College of Sports Medicine (ACSM). 1998. ACSM Fitness Book. 2nd ed. Champaign, IL: Human Kinetics.

American College of Sports Medicine (ACSM). 2000. *ACSM's guidelines for exercise testing and prescription*. 6th ed. Philadelphia: Lippincott, Williams, and Wilkins.

American College of Sports Medicine (ACSM). 2001. *ACSM's resource manual for guidelines for exercise testing and prescription*. 4th ed. Philadelphia: Lippincott, Williams, and Wilkins.

Armstrong, N., J. Williams, J. Balding, P. Gentle, and B. Kirby. 1991. The peak oxygen uptake of British children with reference to age, sex, and sexual maturity. *European Journal of Applied Physiology* 62: 369-375.

Arthur, M., and B. Bailey. 1998. *Complete conditioning for football*. Champaign, IL: Human Kinetics.

Asthma and Allergy Foundation of America. 2000. Student asthma action card. www.aafa.org/public/pdfs/student.pdf.

Avela, J., H. Kyrolainen, and P.V. Komi. 1999. Altered reflex sensitivity after repeated and prolonged passive muscle stretching. *Journal of Applied Physiology* 86: 1283-1291.

Baechle, T.R., and R. Earle. 2000. *Essentials of strength training and conditioning*. 2nd ed. Champaign, IL: Human Kinetics.

Baechle, T.R., and B. Groves. 1998. *Weight training: Steps to success*. 2nd ed. Champaign, IL: Human Kinetics.

Bailey, D.A., W.D. Ross, R.L. Mirwald, and C. Weese. 1978. Size dissociation of maximal aerobic power during growth in boys. *Medicine and Science in Sport and Exercise* 11: 140-151.

Bailey, R.C., J. Olson, S.L. Pepper, J. Porszaz, T.J. Barstow, and D.M. Cooper. 1995. The level and tempo of children's physical activities: An observational study. *Medicine and science in sport and exercise* 27: 1033-1041.

Banks, J.A. 1988. *Multiethnic education: Theory and practice*. Needham Heights, MA: Allyn & Bacon.

Bar-Or, O. 1984. Children and physical performance in warm and cold environments. In *Advances in pediatric sport sciences*, Vol. 1, ed. R.F. Boileau, 117-130. Champaign, IL: Human Kinetics.

Bar-Or, O. 1993. Importance of differences between children and adults for exercise testing and exercise prescription. In *Exercise testing and exercise prescription for special cases*, 2nd ed., ed. J.S. Skinner, 57-74. Philadelphia: Lea and Febiger.

Bar-Or, O. 1994. Childhood and adolescent physical activity and fitness and adult risk profile. In *International proceedings and consensus statement*, ed. C. Bouchard, R.J. Shephard, and T. Stephens, 931-942. Champaign, IL: Human Kinetics.

Baumgartner, T., and A. Jackson. 1999. *Measurement for evaluation in physical education and exercise science*. 6th ed. Boston: WCB-McGraw-Hill.

Blair, S.N. 1995. Youth fitness: Directions for future research. In *Child health, nutrition, and physical activity*, ed. L.W.Y. Chueng and J.B. Richmond, 147-152. Champaign, IL: Human Kinetics.

Blair, S.N., H.W. Kohl, 3rd, C.E. Barlow, R.S. Paffenbarger Jr., L.W. Gibbons, and C.A. Macera. 1995. Changes in physical fitness and all-cause mortality: A prospective study of healthy and unhealthy men. *JAMA* 273: 1093-1098.

Blanchard, Y. 1999. Health-related fitness for children and adults with cerebral palsy. *American College of Sports Medicine current comment*, August.

Bompa, T.O. 2000. *Total training for young champions*. Champaign, IL: Human Kinetics.

Boreham, C.A., J. Twisk, L. Murray, M. Savage, J.J. Strain, and G.W. Cran. 2001. Fitness, fatness, and coronary heart disease risk in adolescents: The Northern Ireland Young Hearts Project. *Medicine and Science in Sport and Exercise* 33: 270-274.

Boreham, C.A., J. Twisk, M. Savage, G.W. Cran, and J.J. Strain. 1997. Physical activity, sports participation, and risk factors in adolescents. *Medicine and Science in Sport and Exercise* 29: 788-793.

Brown, J. 2002. *Nutrition now*. 3rd ed. Belmont, CA: Wadsworth Thomson Learning.

Bukowski, B.J., and D. Stinson. 2000. Physical educators' perceptions of block scheduling in secondary physical education. *JOPERD* 71(1): 53-57.

California Department of Education. 2002. *State study proves physically fit kids perform better academically*. www.cde.ca.gov/news/ releases2002/rel37.asp (accessed February 5, 2004).

Campbell, W., M. Crim, V. Young, and W. Evans. 1994. Increased energy requirements and changes in body composition with resistance training in older adults. *American Journal of Clinical Nutrition* 60: 167-175.

Cardinal, B.J. 2000. Are sedentary behaviors terminable? *Journal of Human Movement Studies* 38: 137-150.

Carron, A.V., H.A. Hausenblas, and P.A. Estabrooks. 2003. *The psychology of physical activity*. New York: McGraw-Hill.

Centers for Disease Control and Prevention (CDC). 1995.

Centers for Disease Control and Prevention (CDC). 2000b. CDC Growth Charts. www.cdc.gov/nchs/data/nhanes/growthcharts/set2clinical/cj411073.pdf (accessed February 5, 2004).

Centers for Disease Control and Prevention (CDC). 1997. Guidelines for school and community programs to promote lifelong physical activity among young people. *MMWR Morbidity and Mortality Weekly Report* 46(RR-6): 1-36.

Centers for Disease Control and Prevention (CDC). 1996. National Health and Nutrition Examination Survey III (1988-1994). Hyattsville, MD: National Center for Health Statistics.

Centers for Disease Control and Prevention (CDC). 2001a. *Profiles of the nation's health*.

Centers for Disease Control and Prevention, Department of Health and Human Services. 2001b. *CDC fact book 2000-2001*.

Centers for Disease Control and Prevention (CDC). 2002. Improving nutrition and increasing physical activity. www.cdc.gov.

Centers for Disease Control and Prevention (CDC). 2003. Summary of 2001 Youth Risk Behavior Survey Results. [Online]. Available: www.cdc.gov/nccdphp/dash/yrbs/2001/ summary_results/usa.htm [November 30, 2003].

Cohen, G. 1993. *Women in sport*. Newbury Park, CA: Sage.

The Cooper Institute. 2004. *FITNESSGRAM/ ACTIVITYGRAM Test Administration Manual*, 3rd. ed., ed. Gregory J. Welk and Marilu D. Meredith. Champaign, IL: Human Kinetics.

Corbin, C.B. 1994. The fitness curriculum: Climbing the stairway to lifetime fitness. In *Health and fitness through physical education*, ed. R.R. Pate and R.C. Hohn, 59-66. Champaign, IL: Human Kinetics.

Corbin, C.B., and R. Lindsey. 2002. *Fitness for life*. 4th ed. Champaign, IL: Human Kinetics.

Corbin, C.B., and R. Lindsey. 2004. *Fitness for life*. 5th ed. Champaign, IL: Human Kinetics.

Corbin, C.B., and L. Noble. 1980. Flexibility: A major component of physical fitness. *JOPERD* 51(6): 23-24, 57-60.

Corbin, C.B., and R.P. Pangrazi. 2002. Physical activity for children: How much is enough? In *FITNESSGRAM reference guide*, ed. G.J. Welk, R.J. Morrow, and H.B. Falls, 7. Dallas: The Cooper Institute.

Corbin, C.B., G.J. Welk, R. Lindsey, and W.R. Corbin. 2004. *Concepts of fitness and wellness*. 5th ed. New York: McGraw-Hill.

Council on Physical Education for Children (COPEC). 1992. *Developmentally appropriate physical education practices for children.* Reston, VA: NASPE.

Council on Physical Education for Children (COPEC). 1995. *Appropriate practices for middle school physical education.* Reston, VA: NASPE.

Coyle, E.F. 1990. Detraining and retention of training-induced adaptations. *Sports Science Exchange* 2(23). Chicago: Gatorade Sports Science Institute.

Coyle, E.F., W.H. Martin, D.R. Sinacore, M.J. Joyner, J.M. Hagberg, and J.O. Hollozy. 1984. Time course of loss of adaptations after stopping prolonged intense endurance training. *Journal of Applied Physiology* 57: 1857-1864.

Craft, D. 1994. Strategies for teaching inclusively. *Teaching Elementary Physical Education* 5(5): 8-9.

Craib, M.W., and V.A. Mitchell. 1996. The association between flexibility and running economy in sub-elite male distance runners. *Medicine and Science in Sports and Exercise* 28: 737-743.

Cumming, G.R., D. Everatt, and L. Hastman. 1978. Bruce treadmill test in children: Normal values in a clinic population. *American Journal of Cardiology* 59: 60-75.

Cumming, G.R., and S. Langford. 1985. Comparison of nine exercise tests used in pediatric cardiology. In *Children and exercise XI,* ed. R.A. Binkhorst, H.C.G. Kemper, and W.H.M. Saris, 58-68. Champaign, IL: Human Kinetics.

Darst, P., and R. Pangrazi. 2002. Dynamic physical education for secondary school students, 4th ed. San Francisco, CA: Benjamin Cummings.

Davison, B. 1998. *Creative physical activities & equipment: Building a quality program on a shoestring budget.* Champaign, IL: Human Kinetics.

DePauw, K. 1996. Students with disabilities in physical education. In *Student learning in physical education: Applying research to enhance instruction,* ed. S. Silverman and C. Ennis, 101-124. Champaign, IL: Human Kinetics.

Deurenberg, P., K. Van der kooy, R. Leenan, J.A. Westrate, and J.C. Seidell. 1991. Sex and age specific population prediction formulas for estimating body composition from bioelectrical impedance: A cross validation study. *International Journal of Obesity* 15: 17-25.

Dishman, R.K., and J.F. Sallis. 1994. Determinants and interventions for physical activity and exercise. In *Physical activity, fitness, and health: International proceedings and consensus statement,* ed. C. Bouchard, R.J. Shepard, and T. Stephens, 214-238. Champaign, IL: Human Kinetics.

Ennis, C.D. 1996. Designing curriculum for quality physical education programs. In *Physical education sourcebook,* ed. B.F. Hennessy, 13-37. Champaign, IL: Human Kinetics.

Epstein, L.H., A. Valoski, R.R. Wing, K.A. Perkins, M. Fernstrom, B. Marks, and J. McCurley. 1989. Perception of eating and exercise in children as a function of child and parent weight status. *Appetite* 12: 105-118.

Faigenbaum, A.D. 2001. Physical activity for youth: Tips for keeping kids healthy and fit. *ACSM Fit Society Page* (April-June): 3-4.

Faigenbaum, A.D. 2003. Youth resistance training. *PCPFS Research Digest* 4(3): 1-8.

Faigenbaum, A.D., W.J. Kraemer, B. Cahill, J. Chandler, J. Dziados, L.D. Elfink, E. Forman, et al. 1996. Youth resistance training: Position statement paper and literature review. *Strength and Conditioning* 18(6): 62-75.

Faigenbaum, A.D., and W.L. Westcott. 2000. *Strength and power for young athletes.* Champaign, IL: Human Kinetics.

Faigenbaum, A.D., W.L. Westcott, R. Loud, and C. Long. 1999. The effects of different resistance training protocols on muscular strength and endurance development in children. *Pediatrics* 104(1): e5.

Faigenbaum, A.D., L.D. Zaichkowsky, W.L. Westcott, L.J. Micheli, and A.F. Fehlandt. 1993. The effects of a twice-a-week strength training program on children. *Pediatric Exercise Science* 5: 339-346.

Faigenbaum, A. and D. Chu. 2001. Plyometric training for children and adolescents. *American College of Sports Medicine Current Comment,* December.

Falk, B., and G. Tenenbaum. 1996. The effectiveness of resistance training in children: A meta-analysis. *Sports Medicine* 3: 176-186.

Fleck, S.J. 1988. Cardiovascular adaptations to resistance training. *Medicine and Science in Sport and Exercise* 22: 265-274.

Food and Drug Administration. 1999. The Food Label. www.fda.gov/opacom/backgrounders/foodlabel/newlabel/html [May 1999].

Food and Drug Administration, Center for Food Safety and Applied Nutrition. 2003. Claims that can be made for conventional foods and dietary supplements. www.cfsan.fda.gov/~dms/hclaims.html (accessed February 6, 2004).

Food and Drug Administration, Office of Food Labeling. 2003. FDA's food label information on the Web. www.cfscan.fda.gov.label.html.

Food and Nutrition Board, Institute of Medicine. 2002. *Dietary reference intakes for energy, carbohydrates, fiber, fat, protein, and amino acid (micronutrients)*. Washington, DC: National Academics Press.

Foster, E.R., K. Hartinger, and K.A. Smith. 1992. *Fitness fun*. Champaign, IL: Human Kinetics.

Franks, B.D., and E.T. Howley. 1998. *Fitness leader's handbook*. 2nd ed. Champaign, IL: Human Kinetics.

Fredette, D.M. 2001. Exercise recommendations for flexibility and range of motion. In *ACSM's resource manual for guidelines for exercise testing and prescription*, 4th ed., 468-477. Philadelphia: Lippincott, Williams, and Wilkins.

Freedman, D.S., L.K. Khan, W.H. Dietz, S.R. Srinivasan, and G.S. Berenson. 2001. Relationship of childhood obesity to coronary heart disease risk factors in adulthood: The Bogalusa heart study. *Pediatrics* 108: 712-718.

Gardner, H. 1983. *Frames of mind: The theory of multiple intelligences*. New York: Basic Books.

Gardner, H. 1993. *Multiple intelligences: The theory in practice*. New York: Basic Books.

Gleim, G.W., and M.P. McHugh. 1997. Flexibility and its effects on sports injury and performance. *Sports Medicine* 24: 289-299.

Graham, G. 1992. *Teaching children physical education: Becoming a master teacher*. Champaign, IL: Human Kinetics.

Greenberg, J.S., Dintiman, G.V., and Myers Oakes, B. 2004. *Physical fitness and wellness: Changing the way you look, feel, and perform*. 3rd ed. Champaign, IL: Human Kinetics.

Greene, L. and R. Pate. 1997. *Training for Young Distance Runners*. Champaign, IL: Human Kinetics.

Griffin, J.C. 1998. *Client-centered exercise prescription*. Champaign, IL: Human Kinetics.

Grunbaum, J., L. Kann, S. Kinchen, B. Williams, J. Ross, R. Lowry, and L. Kolbe. 2002. Youth risk behavior surveillance—United States, 2001. June 28, 2002/51 (SS04); 1-64 www.cdc.gov/mmwr/preview/mmwrhtml/ss5104a1.htm (accessed February 5, 2004).

Guo, S.S., A.F. Roche, W.C. Chumlea, J.D. Gardner, and R. M. Siervogel. 1994. The predictive value of childhood BMI values for overweight at age 34 y. *American Journal of Clinical Nutrition*. 59: 1810-1819.

Halbertson, J.P.K., and L.N.H. Goeken. 1994. Stretching exercises: Effect on passive extensibility and stiffness in short hamstrings of healthy subjects. *Archives of Physical Medicine and Rehabilitation* 75: 976-981.

Harris, J., and J. Elbourn. 1997. *Teaching health-related exercise at key stages 1 and 2*. Champaign, IL: Human Kinetics.

Harrison, J.M., C.L. Blakemore, and M. Buck. 2001. *Instructional strategies for secondary school physical education*. 5th ed. New York: McGraw-Hill.

Harter, S. 1999. *The construction of the self: A developmental perspective*. New York: Guilford Press.

Harter, S., P.L. Waters, and N.R. Whitesell. 1998. Relational self-worth: Differences in perceived worth as a person across interpersonal contexts among adolescents. *Child Development* 69: 756-766.

Hass, C.J., M.S. Feigenbaum, and B.A. Franklin. 2001. Prescription of resistance training for healthy populations. *Sports Medicine* 31(14): 953-964.

Hastie, P. 2003. *Teaching for lifetime physical activity through quality high school physical education*. San Francisco: Benjamin Cummings.

Haynes-Dusel. 2001. Block scheduling: A catalyst for change in middle and high school physical education. *Research Quarterly for Exercise and Sport*, 72. A-67.

Hellison, D. 2003. *Teaching responsibility through physical activity*. 2nd ed. Champaign, IL: Human Kinetics.

Heyward, V.H. 2002. *Advanced fitness assessment and exercise prescription*. 4th ed. Champaign, IL: Human Kinetics.

Heyward, V.H., and L.M. Stolarczyk. 1996. *Applied body composition assessment*. Champaign, IL: Human Kinetics.

Hichwa, J. 1998. *Right fielders are people too: An inclusive approach to teaching middle school physical education*. Champaign, IL: Human Kinetics.

Himberg, C., G. Hutchinson, and J. Roussell. 2003. *Teaching secondary physical education:*

Preparing adolescents to be active for life. Champaign, IL: Human Kinetics.

Hopple, C., 2005. *Performance-based assessment in elementary education.* 2nd ed. Champaign, IL: Human Kinetics.

Horn, T.S., and C.A. Hasbrook. 1986. Informational components influencing children's perceptions of their physical competence. In *Sport for children and youth,* ed. M.R. Weiss and D. Gould, 81-88. Champaign, IL: Human Kinetics.

Horn, T.S., and C.A. Hasbrook. 1987. Psychological characteristics and the criteria children use for self-evaluation. *Journal of Sport Psychology* 9: 208-221.

Houston-Wilson, K. 1995. Alternate assessment procedures. In *Physical Best and individuals with disabilities: A handbook for inclusion in fitness programs,* ed. J.A. Seaman, 91-109. Reston, VA: AAHPERD.

Houtkeeper, L.B., S.B. Going, C.H. Westfall, A.F. Roche, and M. Van Loan. 1992. Bioelectrical impedance estimation of fat-free body mass in children and youth: A cross-validation study. *Journal of Applied Physiology* 72: 366-373.

Houtkeeper, L.B., T.G. Lohman, S.B. Going, and M.C. Hall. 1989. Validity of bioelectrical impedance for body composition assessment in children. *Journal of Applied Physiology* 66: 814-821.

Hutchinson, G.E. 1995. Gender-fair teaching in physical education. *Journal of Physical Education, Recreation and Dance* 60(2): 23-24.

Institute of Medicine of the National Academies. 2001. *Dietary reference intakes: Applications in dietary assessment.* Washington, DC: The National Academies Press.

International Life Sciences Institute (ILSI). 1997. Physical activity message for parents from new survey: No more excuses. Press release, July 1.

Jackson, A., J. Morrow, D. Hill, and R. Dishman. 2004. *Physical activity for health and fitness.* Champaign, IL: Human Kinetics.

Jacobs, J.E., and J.S. Eccles. 2000. Parents, task values, and real-life achievement related choices. In *Intrinsic motivation,* ed. C. Sansone and J.M. Harackiewicz, 405-439. San Diego: Academic Press.

Jacobs, J.E., S. Lanza, D.W. Osgood, J.S. Eccles, and A. Wigfield. 2002. Changes in children's self-competence and values: Gender and domain differences across grades one through twelve. *Child Development* 73(2): 509-527.

Janz, K.F., J.C. Golden, J.R. Hansen, and L.T. Mahoney. 1992. Heart rate monitoring of physical activity in children and adolescents: The Muscatine study. *Pediatrics* 89: 256-261.

Janz, K.F., S.M. Levy, T.L. Burns, J.C. Torner, M. C. Willing, and J.J. Warren. 2002. Fatness, physical activity and television viewing in children during the adiposity rebound period: The Iowa Bone Development Study. *Preventative Medicine* 35: 563-571.

Jobe, M. 1998. Disabilities awareness field days. *Teaching Elementary Physical Education* 9(1): 10-11.

Joint Committee on National Health Education Standards. *National health education standards: achieving health literacy.* (1995) American Cancer Society. Atlanta, GA.

Jones, B.H., and J.J. Knapik. 1999. Physical training and exercise-related injuries. *Sports Medicine* 27: 111-125.

Karlsson, M.K., H. Ahlborg, K.J. Obrant, F. Nyquist, H. Lindberg, and C. Karlsson. 2002. Exercise during growth and young adulthood is associated with reduced fracture risk in old ages. *Journal of Bone Mineral Research* 17(suppl. 1): S297.

Kim, H.K., K. Tanaka, F. Nakadomo, K. Watanabe, and Y. Marsuura. 1993. Fat-free mass in Japanese boys predicted from bioelectrical impedance and anthropometric variables. *Medicine and Science in Sport and Exercise* 25: S59. (Abstract).

Kirkpatrick, B., and B. Birnbaum. 1997. *Lessons from the heart: Individualizing physical education with heart rate monitors.* Champaign, IL: Human Kinetics.

Kleiner, S. 1999. Water: An essential but overlooked nutrient. *JADA* (Journal of the American Dietetic Association) v99: 200-206.

Knudson, D.V., P. Magnusson, and M. McHugh. 2000. Current issues in flexibility fitness. In C. Corbin and B. Pangrazi, eds., *The president's council on physical fitness and sports digest,* 3rd ser., no. 10, Washington, DC: Department of Health and Human Services.

Kokkonen, J., A.G. Nelson, and A. Cornwell. 1998. Acute muscle stretching inhibits maximal strength performance. *Research Quarterly for Exercise and Sport* 69: 411-415.

Kraemer, W.J., and S.J. Fleck. 1993. *Strength training for young adults.* Champaign, IL: Human Kinetics.

Kurtzweil, P. (2003). "Daily Values" encourage healthy diet. www.fda.gov/fdac/special/foodlabel/dvs.html.

Kushner, R.F., D.A. Schoeller, C.R. Field, and L. Danford. 1992. Is the impedance index (ht^2/R) significant in predicting total body water? *American Journal of Clinical Nutrition* 56: 835-839.

Lacy, A., and D. Hastad. 2003. *Measurement and evaluation in physical education and exercise science.* 4th ed. New York: Benjamin Cummings.

Lieberman, L., and C. Houston-Wilson. 2002. *Strategies for inclusion: A handbook for physical educators.* Champaign, IL: Human Kinetics.

Lindsey, E. 2003. *Strengthening your physical education program with innovative fitness strategies and activities (grades 6-12): Resource handbook.* Bellevue, WA: Bureau of Education and Research.

Lindsey, R., and C. Corbin. 1989. Questionable exercises—some safer alternatives. *Journal of Physical Education, Recreation and Dance* (October): 26-32.

Lohman, T.G. 1992. Advances in body composition assessment: Current issues in exercise science series. Monograph no. 3. Champaign, IL: Human Kinetics.

Lowry, S. 1995. A multicultural perspective on planning. *Teaching Elementary Physical Education* 6(3): 14-15.

Lukaski, H.C., P.E. Johnson, W.W. Bolonchuk, and G.I. Lykken. 1985. Assessment of fat-free mass using bioelectric impedance measurements of the human body. *American Journal of Clinical Nutrition* 41: 810-817.

Lund, J.L., and M.F. Kirk. 2002. *Performance-based assessment for middle and high school physical education.* Champaign, IL: Human Kinetics.

Malina, R.M. 1996. Tracking of physical activity and physical fitness across the life span. *Research Quarterly for Sport and Exercise* 67: 48-57.

Malina, R.M. 2001. Tracking of physical activity and physical fitness across the life span. *PCPFS Research Digest* 3(14): 1-8.

Martens, R. 2004. *Successful coaching.* Champaign, IL: Human Kinetics.

McCraken 2001. *It's not just gym anymore: Teaching secondary students how to be active for life.* Champaign, IL: Human Kinetics.

McDowell, M., R. Briefel, K. Alaimo, et. al. 1994. Energy and macronutrient intakes of persons ages 2 months and over in the United States: Third national health and nutrition examination survey, phase 1, 1988-1991. *Advance Data from Vital and Health Statistics,* no. 255. Hyattsville, MD: National Center for Health Statistics.

Melograno, V.J. 1998. *Professional and student portfolios for physical education.* Champaign, IL: Human Kinetics.

Middle and Secondary School Physical Education Council (MASSPEC). 1995. *Appropriate practices for middle school education.* Reston, VA: NASPE.

Mohnsen, B.J. 1997. *Teaching middle school physical education: A blueprint for developing an exemplary program.* Champaign, IL: Human Kinetics.

Mohnsen, B.J. 2003. *Teaching middle school physical education: A standards-based approach for grades 5-8.* Champaign, IL: Human Kinetics.

Morris, G.S.D., and J. Stiehl. 1998. *Changing kids' games.* 2nd ed. Champaign, IL: Human Kinetics.

Mosston, M., and S. Ashworth. 2002. *Teaching physical education.* 5th ed. San Francisco: Benjamin Cummings.

Mujika, I., and S. Padilla. 2001. Cardiorespiratory and metabolic characteristics of detraining in humans. *Medicine and Science in Sports and Exercise* 33(3): 413-421.

National Association for Sport and Physical Education (NASPE). 1995. *Moving into the future: National standards for physical education.* St. Louis: Mosby.

National Association for Sport and Physical Education (NASPE). 1998. *Physical activity for children: A statement of guidelines.* Reston, VA: NASPE.

National Association for Sport and Physical Education (NASPE). 1999. Healthy people 2010. *NASPE News,* no. 52 (winter): 1.

National Association for Sport and Physical Education (NASPE). 2004a. *Moving into the future:*

National standards for physical education. 2nd ed. Reston, VA: NASPE.

National Association for Sport and Physical Education (NASPE). 2004b. *Physical activity for children: A statement of guidelines for children ages 5-12.* 2nd ed. Reston, VA: Author.

National Association for Sport and Physical Education (NASPE). 2005a. *Physical best activity guide: Elementary level,* 2nd ed. Champaign, IL: Human Kinetics.

National Association for Sport and Physical Education (NASPE). 2005b. *Physical best activity guide: Middle and high school levels.* 2nd ed. Champaign, IL: Human Kinetics.

National Association for Sport and Physical Education (NASPE). 1993. *Shape of the nation 1993: A survey of state physical education requirements.* Reston, VA: NASPE.

National Center for Chronic Disease Prevention and Health Promotion (NCCDPHP), Centers for Disease Control and Prevention. 2003. *Physical activity and good nutrition: Essential elements to prevent chronic diseases and obesity.* www.cdc.gov/nccdphp/aag/.

National Cholesterol Education Program. 1991. *Report of the expert panel on population strategies for blood cholesterol reduction program.* Circulation 83: 2154-2232.

National Consortium for Physical Education and Recreation for Individuals With Disabilities. 1995. *Adapted physical education national standards.* Champaign, IL: Human Kinetics.

National Dance Association. National standards for dance education: What every young American should know and be able to do in dance. (1996). Reston, VA: Author.

National Eating Disorders Association. 2003. *Anorexia nervosa and bulimia nervosa.* www.nationaleatingdisorders.org.

National Strength and Conditioning Association (NSCA). 2000. *Essentials of strength training and conditioning.* Ed. T.R. Baechle and R.W. Earle. Champaign, IL: Human Kinetics.

Nilges, L. 1996. Ingredients for a gender equitable physical education program. *Teaching Elementary Physical Education* 7(5): 28-29.

Ormrod, J.E. 1995. *Educational psychology principles and applications.* Columbus, OH: Merrill.

Pangrazi, R.P., A. Beighle, and C.L. Sidman. 2003. *Pedometer power: 67 lessons for K-12.* Champaign, IL: Human Kinetics.

Pangrazi, R.P., and C. Corbin. 1994. *Teaching strategies for improving youth fitness.* 2nd ed. Reston, VA: AAHPERD.

Pate, R.R. 1995. Promoting activity and fitness. In *Child health, nutrition, and physical activity,* ed. L.W.Y. Cheung and J.B. Richmond, 139-145. Champaign, IL: Human Kinetics.

Payne, V.G., and J.R. Morrow Jr. 1993. Exercise and VO$_2$max in children: A meta-analysis. *Research Quarterly for Exercise and Sport* 64: 305-313.

Powers, S.K., and S.L. Dodd. 1997. *The essentials of total fitness: Exercise, nutrition, and wellness.* Boston: Allyn & Bacon.

President's Council on Fitness and Sports. 2003. The president's challenge: Physical activity and fitness awards program. www.presidentschallenge.org.

Prochaska, J.O., J.C. Norcross, and C.C. DiClemete. 1994. *Changing for good: The revolutionary program that explains the six stages of change and teaches you how to free yourself from bad habits.* New York: William Morrow.

PSA/HPERD. 1994. P.E.-L.I.F.E. Project, Designing Assessments: Applications for Physical Education.

Raffini, J.P. 1993. *Winners without losers: Structures and strategies for increasing student motivation to learn.* Needham Heights, MA: Allyn & Bacon.

Rink, J. 2002. *Teaching physical education for learning.* 4th ed. New York: McGraw-Hill.

Ross, R., J. Freeman, and P. Janssen. 2000. Exercise alone is an effective strategy for reducing obesity and related comorbidities. *Exercise and Sport Science Review* 28: 165-170.

Rowland, T.W. 1990. *Exercise and children's health.* Champaign, IL: Human Kinetics.

Rowland, T.W. 1996. *Developmental exercise physiology.* Champaign, IL: Human Kinetics.

Rowland, T.W. 2002. Telephone conversation and email with Jennie Gilbert, 3 December.

Sadker, M., and D. Sadker. 1995. *Failing at fairness: How our schools cheat girls.* New York: Simon & Schuster.

Sallis, J.F. 1994. Determinants of physical activity behavior in children. In *Health and fitness through physical education*, ed. R.R. Pate and R.C. Hohn, 31-43. Champaign, IL: Human Kinetics.

Sallis, J.F. 2000. Age-related decline in physical activity: A synthesis of human and animal studies. *Medicine and Science in Sports and Exercise* 32(9): 1598-1600.

Sallis, J.F., and K. Patrick. 1994. Physical activity guidelines for adolescents: Consensus statement. *Pediatric Exercise Science* 6: 302-314.

Sallis, J.F., J.J. Prochaska, W.C. Taylor, J.O. Hill, and J.C. Geraci. 1999. Correlates of physical activity in a national sample of girls and boys in grades 4 through 12. *Health Psychology* 18: 410-415.

Saltman, P., J. Gurin, and I. Mothner, 1993. *The University of California at San Diego nutrition book.* Boston: Little, Brown.

Schincariol, L. 1994. Including the physically awkward child. *Teaching Elementary Physical Education* 5(5): 10-11.

Schmidt, R.A., and C. Wrisberg. 2000. *Motor learning and performance.* 2nd ed. Champaign, IL: Human Kinetics.

Secretary of Health and Human Services and Secretary of Education. 2000. *Promoting better health for young people through physical activity and sports: A report to the president.*

Segal, K.R., B. Gutin, E. Presta, J. Wang, and T.B. Van Itallie. 1985. Estimation of human body composition by electrical impedance. *Federation Proceedings* 46: 1334. (Abstract).

Segal, K.R., M. Van Loan, P.I. Fitzgerald, J.A. Hodgdon, and T.B. Van Itallie. 1988. Lean body mass estimation by bioelectrical impedance analysis: A four-site cross-validation study. *American Journal of Clinical Nutrition* 47: 7-14.

Slaughter, M.H., Lohman, T.G., Boileau, R.A., Horswill, C.A., Stillman, R.J., Van Loan, M.D., and Benben, D.A. 1988. Skinfold equations for estimation of body fatness in children and youth. *Human Biology* 60: 709-723.

Sonstroem, R.J. 1984. Exercise and self-esteem. *Exercise and Sports Science Reviews* 12: 123-155.

Sportline, Inc. *Sportline's guide to walking* (brochure), Walk4Life. Campbell, CA: Sportline, Inc.

Tanaka, H., K.D. Monahan, and D.R. Seals. 2001. Age-predicted maximal heart rate revisited. *Journal of the American College of Cardiology* 37(1): 153-156.

Thomas, K., A. Lee, and J. Thomas. 2003. *Physical education methods for elementary teachers.* 2nd ed. Champaign, IL: Human Kinetics.

Tipton, J., and S. Tucker. 1998. Fund-raising can be fun! *Teaching Elementary Physical Education.* 9 (3): 14.

Turner, C.H., and A.G. Robling. 2003. Designing exercise regimens to increase bone strength. *Exercise and Sports Science Reviews* 31(1): 45-50.

Ulrich, D. 2000. *Test of gross motor development.* Austin, TX: Pro-Ed.

U.S. Department of Agriculture. 2002. Food guide pyramid. www.nal.usda.gov/fnic/Fpr/pyramid.html.

USDA Center for Nutrition Policy and Promotion, 2000. *Dietary guidelines for Americans.* 5th ed. Atlanta: U.S. Department of Health and Human Services, Government Printing Office.

U.S. Department of Education. 1994. *Prisoners of time: Report of the National Education Commission on time and learning.* Washington, DC: U.S. Department of Education.

U.S. Department of Health and Human Services (USDHHS), Centers for Disease Control and Prevention, National Center for Chronic Disease Prevention and Health Promotion. 1996. *Physical activity and health: A report of the Surgeon General.* Atlanta: U.S. Department of Health and Human Services, Government Printing Office.

U.S. Department of Health and Human Services (USDHHS). 1999. *Promoting physical activity.* Champaign, IL: Human Kinetics.

U.S. Department of Health and Human Services (USDHHS). 2000aa. *Healthy people 2010: Understanding and improving health.* Washington, DC: U.S. Department of Health and Human Services, Government Printing Office.

U.S. Department of Health and Human Services (USDHHS). 2000bb. *Promoting better health for young people through physical activity and sports.* Washington, DC: U.S. Department of Health and Human Services, Government Printing Office.

U.S. Department of Health and Human Services (USDHHS), Centers for Disease Control and Prevention. 2000a. *Physical activity and the health of young people: Fact sheet.* [Online]. Available: www.cdc.gov.

U.S. Department of Health and Human Services (USDHHS), Centers for Disease Control and Prevention. 2000b. *Fact sheet: Physical education and activity, school health policies and programs study.* [Online]. Available: www.cdc.gov.

U.S. Department of Health and Human Services (USDHHS), Centers for Disease Control and Prevention. 2000c. *Promoting lifelong physical activity, CDC guidelines for school and community programs.* [Online]. Available: www.cdc.gov.

Vallerand, R.J. 2001. A hierarchical model of intrinsic and extrinsic motivation in sport and exercise. In *Advances in motivation in sport and exercise,* ed. G.C. Roberts. Champaign, IL: Human Kinetics.

Vanden Auweele, Y., F. Bakker, S. Biddle, M. Durand, and R. Seiler. 1999. *Psychology for physical educators.* Champaign, IL: Human Kinetics.

Van Loan, M., and P.L. Mayclin. 1987. Bioelectrical impedance analysis: Is it a reliable estimator of lean body mass and total body water? *Human Biology* 59: 299-309.

Virgilio, S.J. 1997. *Fitness education for children: A team approach.* Champaign, IL: Human Kinetics.

Wall, A.E. 1982. Physically awkward children: A motor development perspective. In *Theory and research in learning disabilities,* ed. J.P. Das, R.F. Mulcahy, and A.E. Wall, 253-268. New York: Plenum Press.

Wardlaw, G. 1999. *Perspectives in nutrition.* 4th ed. Boston: WCB/McGraw-Hill.

Wardlaw, G. 2002. *Contemporary nutrition.* 5th ed. Boston: WCB/McGraw-Hill.

Watanabe, K., F. Nakadomo, K. Tanaka, K. Kim, and K. Maeda. 1993. Estimation of fat-free mass from bioelectrical impedance and anthropometric variables in Japanese girls. *Medicine and Science in Sports and Exercise* 25: S163. (Abstract).

Weiss, M.R., and T.S. Horn. 1990. The relation between children's accuracy of estimates of their physical competence and achievement-related characteristics. *Research Quarterly for Exercise and Sport* 61(3): 250-258.

Welk, G.J., and S.N. Blair. 2002. Health benefits of physical activity and fitness in children. In *FITNESSGRAM reference guide,* ed. G.J. Welk, J.R. Morrow, and H.B. Falls. Dallas: Cooper Institute.

Westcott, W.L. 1996. *Building strength and stamina.* Champaign, IL: Human Kinetics.

Weston, A.T., R. Petosa, and R.R. Pate, 1997. Validation of an instrument for measurement of physical activity in youth. *Medicine and Science in Sports and Exercise* 29 (1): 138-143.

Wickelgren, I. 1998. Obesity: How big a problem? *Science* 280 (May): 1364-1367.

Winnick, J.P. 1995. Personalizing measurement and evaluation for individuals with disabilities. In *Physical best and individuals with disabilities: A handbook for inclusion in fitness programs,* ed. J.A. Seaman, 21-31. Reston, VA: AAHPERD.

Winnick, J.P. 1999. Individualized education programs and the development of health-related physical fitness. In *The Brockport physical fitness training guide,* ed. J.P. Winnick and F.X. Short, 6. Champaign, IL: Human Kinetics.

Winnick, J.P. 2000. *Adapted physical education and sport.* 3rd ed. Champaign, IL: Human Kinetics.

Winnick, J.P., and F.X. Short. 1999a. *The Brockport Physical Fitness Test manual.* Champaign, IL: Human Kinetics.

Winnick, J.P., and F.X. Short, ed. 1999b. *The Brockport physical fitness training guide.* Champaign, IL: Human Kinetics.

Woods, A.M. 1997. Assessment of the cognitive domain. *Teaching Elementary Physical Education* 8(3): 28-29.

Zeigler, E., and L. Filer. 2000. *Present knowledge in nutrition.* 7th ed. Washington, DC: International Life Sciences Press.

Zwiren, L.D. 1988. Exercise prescription for children. In *Resource manual for guidelines for exercise testing and prescription,* ed. American College of Sports Medicine, 309-314. Philadelphia: Lea and Febiger.

INDEX

PLEASE NOTE: The italicized *f* or *t* following a page number represent a figure or table on the page indicated.

ABOUT PHYSICAL BEST

Physical Best is a comprehensive health-related fitness education program developed by physical educators for physical educators. Physical Best was designed to educate, challenge, and encourage all children in the knowledge, skills, and attitudes needed for a healthy and fit life. The goal of the program is to help students move from dependence to independence and responsibility for their own health and fitness by promoting regular, enjoyable physical activity. The purpose of Physical Best is to educate ALL children regardless of athletic talent, physical and mental abilities, or disabilities. This is implemented through quality resources and professional development workshops for physical educators.

Physical Best is a program of the National Association for Sport and Physical Education (NASPE). A nonprofit membership organization of over 18,000 professionals in the sport and physical education fields, NASPE is an association of the American Alliance for Health, Physical Education, Recreation and Dance dedicated to strengthening basic knowledge about healthy lifestyles among professionals and the general public. Putting that knowledge into action in schools and communities across the nation is critical to improved academic performance, social reform, and the health of individuals.

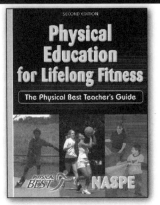
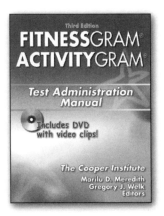
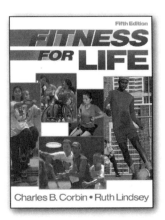
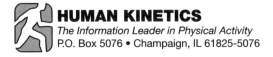